Vascular Disease in Older Adults

Rabih Chaer
Editor

Vascular Disease in Older Adults

A Comprehensive Clinical Guide

Springer

Editor
Rabih Chaer
Division of Vascular Surgery
University of Pittsburgh Medical Center
Pittsburgh, PA, USA

ISBN 978-3-319-29283-0 ISBN 978-3-319-29285-4 (eBook)
DOI 10.1007/978-3-319-29285-4

Library of Congress Control Number: 2017937369

Printed on acid-free paper

This Springer imprint is published by Springer Nature
The registered company is Springer International Publishing AG
The registered company address is: Gewerbestrasse 11, 6330 Cham, Switzerland

Dedication

To my children, the loves of my life, Maria the badass princess, Anthony my big boy with the biggest heart, and Michael the boss, without whom this book would have been completed a year earlier.

To all our frail elderly patients with vascular disease who inspired this book. You are the best! This one is for you.

Foreword

Vascular disease is one of the most challenging medical problems that we treat. It is not the interventions. The concepts behind these are quite simple. If a blockage is present, bypass around it or use a balloon to push it aside. Or if an artery is too large or aneurysmal, replace it or place a sleeve through its lumen. It is the judgments that make the specialty of vascular medicine and surgery challenging. And why are these judgments so difficult? For the most part, because vascular patients are elderly, frail, and plagued with comorbid conditions. I have often envied those who treat young and or middle-aged patients, for these individuals recover quickly, tolerate misadventure, and rarely have complications. Then, there is the elderly patient with vascular disease…

There have been very few attempts to create a compendium of knowledge regarding vascular disease in the elderly, and there is none that is contemporary. The need is great in that much has been learned in recent years, all essential knowledge for practitioners caring for these individuals. It is not surprising that Rabih Chaer would be the editor. Rabih is one of the nation's leading vascular surgeons with expertise and research penetration in almost every aspect of vascular disease. Rabih's work is characterized by an unparalleled level of comprehensiveness and accuracy. This is readily evident as one reads through *Vascular Disease in Older Adults*. Moreover, Rabih has recruited a superb lineup of experts; the chapters are written by individuals (with expertise in all aspects of vascular disease) who have published the definitive treatises on vascular disease in the elderly.

Over the past 20 years, treatments for vascular disease have evolved significantly. Options include no intervention, medical management, a minimally invasive alternative, or maximally invasive surgery. And not surprisingly, each of these choices is associated with advantages and disadvantages. Increasingly, we have learned that many patients with vascular disease benefit from either no intervention or medical treatment. Statins have stabilized carotid plaque, claudication will often improve on its own or the symptoms are overtaken by generalized arthritis, and small aneurysms rarely rupture. As minimally invasive interventions have evolved, this technology has become more refined, the results are improved, and they have greatly benefited our elderly patients. In terms of durability, traditional surgery for most vascular diseases remains the gold standard and in select patients it is the intervention of choice. The art of treating elderly patients with vascular disease is choosing which option should be used and when? The decisions are not easy, but when well made, the outcome can be extremely rewarding for the practitioner and the patient alike. These choices need to be individualized: each patient has their own story and particularly in the elderly, each story is different. The patient's social circumstances, morbidity, philosophy on life, and longevity are as important as their symptoms and anatomy. Although I have suggested that treating elderly patients with vascular disease is an art, there is also available a great deal of science accompanied by data, experience, and clinical studies. We now have access to a great deal of information about who to treat, how, and when. And of course all of this science can be found within the chapters of *Vascular Disease in Older Adults*.

If elderly vascular patients compose the majority of your practice, this book is a must read. For the occasional patient with a specific problem, the chapters are concise and advice can easily be found. Dr. Chaer is to be commended for his efforts to create a textbook that, if well used, has the potential to improve the lives and outcomes of thousands of elderly patients afflicted with this devastating disease. I hope you enjoy the read!

Ohio State University K. Craig Kent

Introduction

This textbook is intended to be a valuable resource to all medical and surgical specialties who manage elderly patients with vascular disease. Vascular surgery and vascular interventions have evolved tremendously over the last decade. The ongoing addition and refinement of surgical and minimally invasive endovascular techniques, as well as medical therapy, has made it safer for the elderly patients to get vascular care. As such, we believe it should be seldom the case nowadays to deny vascular care for the elderly patients based on chronological age. In addition, patient-centered interventions that can combine a hybrid approach of surgery, minimally invasive techniques, and medical therapy, can allow the geriatric patient to function and recover optimally even in the setting of multiple medical comorbidities.

Specific attention to the geriatric patients with vascular pathology is a must for multiple reasons. Not only can they present with more advanced vascular disease, but they can also be frail due to multiple other comorbidities. We recognize that optimization of their care starts preoperatively with coordination of care with their geriatrician, and possibly other specialties such as cardiology, pulmonary medicine, and endocrinology. In addition, obtaining a preoperative anesthesia consultation can allow the formulation of a proper anesthetic plan that can minimize side effects and complications. The perioperative care of the geriatric patients with vascular pathology can also be very intricate, as their recovery and quality of life will depend on their hospital stay, rehabilitation process, and eventual return to their social support system. To that effect, difficult ethical decisions have to be sometimes made, starting with the decision to offer care or deny it, and during recovery if the course does not go as planned.

This textbook provides a summary of different pathologies divided by vascular bed: aneurysm disease, cerebrovascular disease, peripheral vascular disease, renal failure, and venous disease. It aims at describing the pathophysiology of the disease process, as well as the decision making that goes into establishing a plan for vascular care, taking into account the extent of the pathology, the patient's frailty, and quality of life. The goals of care can therefore change and can be individualized based on the specific clinical presentation, as well as the patients' and their families' wishes.

We are proud to have rallied experts in the field to address the management of different vascular disease processes, including perioperative care, cutting-edge state-of-the-art vascular surgical and endovascular interventions, as well as ethical decision making. This book is a collaborative effort and does bring together multiple surgical and medical specialties, which is what is needed for the optimal care of the elderly patient with vascular disease.

Contents

Contributors

Huiting Chen, MD Section of Vascular Surgery, University of Michigan, Ann Arbor, MI, USA

Rafael S. Cires-Drouet, MD Vascular Medicine, University of Maryland Medical Center, Baltimore, MD, USA

Anthony J. Comerota, MD, FACS, FACC Jobst Vascular Institute, Toledo, OH, USA

University of Michigan, Ann Arbor, MI, USA

Michael S. Conte, MD Department of Surgery, University of California, San Francisco, San Francisco, CA, USA

Matthew J. Eagleton, MD Department of Vascular Surgery, Cleveland Clinic, Cleveland, OH, USA

Emily V. Finlayson, MD, MS UCSF Center for Surgery in Older Adults, Department of Surgery, University of California, San Francisco, San Francisco, CA, USA

Daniel E. Hall, MD, MDiv, MHSc Division of General Surgery, University of Pittsburgh, Pittsburgh, PA, USA

Jason M. Johanning, MD, MS Department of Surgery University of Nebraska Medical Center, Omaha VA Medical Center, The Nebraska Medical Center, Omaha, NE, USA

Jennifer Kaplan, MD Department of Surgery, University of California, San Francisco, San Francisco, CA, USA

Brajesh K. Lal, MD University of Maryland School of Medicine, University of Maryland Medical Center, Baltimore VA Medical Center, Baltimore, MD, USA

G. Matthew Longo, MD Department of Surgery University of Nebraska Medical Center, Omaha VA Medical Center, The Nebraska Medical Center, Omaha, NE, USA

Alyson Ashleigh Melin, DO Department of Surgery, University of Nebraska Medical Center, Omaha, NE, USA

Jon G. Quatromoni, MD Department of Vascular Surgery, Hospital of the University of Pennsylvania, Philadelphia, PA, USA

Bradley Reames, MD, MS Department of Surgery, University of Michigan, Ann Arbor, MI, USA

Shashank Saxena, MD Department of Anesthesiology, VA Pittsburgh Health Care Center, University of Pittsburgh School of Medicine, Pittsburgh, PA, USA

Mark L. Unruh, MD Chair and Professor of Medicine, Department of Internal Medicine, University of New Mexico School of Medicine, Albuquerque, NM, USA

Thomas W. Wakefield, MD Section of Vascular Surgery, Samuel and Jean Frankel Cardiovascular Center, University of Michigan, Ann Arbor, MI, USA

Grace J. Wang, MD Department of Vascular Surgery, Hospital of the University of Pennsylvania, Philadelphia, PA, USA

Max Wohlauer, MD Division of Vascular Surgery, Froedtert & the Medical College of Wisconsin, Milwaukee, WI, USA

Jun Xu, MD Division of Vascular Surgery, University of Pittsburgh Medical Center, Pittsburgh, PA, USA

Theodore H. Yuo, MD Assistant Professor of Surgery, Division of Vascular Surgery, Department of Surgery, University of Pittsburgh School of Medicine, Pittsburgh, PA, USA

Screening for Vascular Pathology: Current Guidelines and Recommendations

1

Jon G. Quatromoni and Grace J. Wang

1.1 Abdominal Aortic Aneurysm

Abdominal Aortic Aneurysms (AAAs) represent a significant vascular health problem. In the United States alone, an estimated 1.5 million people have AAAs, with 200,000 more diagnosed each year, and associated with at least 15,000 annual deaths [1, 2]. AAAs account for 4–5% of sudden deaths and represent the 13th most common cause of death overall [3]. An aneurysm is defined as an abnormal focal dilation of a blood vessel where the minimum diameter exceeds 3.0 cm in any perpendicular plane; this generally accepted threshold equates to 1.5 times the normal juxta-renal diameter [4]. As aneurysms grow, the vessel wall weakens, increasing the risk of rupture. AAA rupture is a life-threatening event with a high mortality rate due to the rapidity with which exsanguination occurs, often prior to the patient arriving at a medical facility for treatment. Thus, there is a rationale for screening to diagnose AAA and institute measures to reduce the growth of the aneurysm, as well as to stratify those who may need surgical treatment.

The benefit of treating AAAs electively is significant. An 80% improvement in mortality has been ascribed to elective AAA repair compared to emergent repair of a ruptured AAA (<5% vs. 80–90%, respectively) [5]; thus, the most effective method of reducing AAA-related mortality at the present time is early identification and elective repair. However, identifying only those patients who would most benefit from elective repair while at the same time limiting over-diagnosis and over-treatment is challenging, as any systematic program would uncover many previously undiagnosed AAAs that are unlikely to rupture. Thus, clear criteria for the population eligible for screening and the clinical handling of AAAs of all sizes need to be established and rigorously maintained. Unfortunately, there is no universal set of

J.G. Quatromoni • G.J. Wang (✉)
Department of Vascular Surgery, Hospital of the University of Pennsylvania, Philadelphia, PA, USA
e-mail: Grace.Wang@uphs.upenn.edu

R. Chaer (ed.), *Vascular Disease in Older Adults*,
DOI 10.1007/978-3-319-29285-4_1

guidelines set forth by which all practitioners abide; rather, multiple partially conflicting recommendations exist which confuse what should be a unified societal approach. This section of the chapter investigates the different published screening guidelines and the evidence upon which their recommendations are made.

1.1.1 Overview of Screening Guidelines

Multiple societies and governmental agencies have published AAA screening guidelines (Table 1.1). The major societies', and others', guidelines have been systematically reviewed elsewhere [6]. The most significant domestic sources include the United States Preventive Services Task Force (USPSTF), the American College of Cardiology/American Heart Association (ACC/AHA), the American College of Preventive Medicine (ACPM), and the Society for Vascular Surgery (SVS). Internationally, prominent groups include the Canadian and European Societies for Vascular Surgery (CSVS and ESVS, respectively) and the UK's National Health Service (NHS). While the NHS also serves as the main health insurance payer for eligible patients in the UK, Medicare covers most of the eligible patients in the United States under a recent piece of legislation entitled the Screening Abdominal Aortic Aneurysms Very Efficiently (SAAAVE) Act, reviewed later in the chapter.

Table 1.1 Summary of AAA screening recommendations by organization

	Men <65	Men 65–75		Women 65–75	
	Positive risk factors	Ever-smoker	Never-smoker	Ever-smoker	Never-smoker
USPSTF	Not addressed	Screen once	Selectively screen based on RFs	No recommendation	Do not screen
ACC/AHA	Screen once after *age 60* if (+) FHx in 1° relative	Screen once	Screen once if (+) FHx in 1° relative	Do not screen	Do not screen
SVS	Screen once after *age 55* if (+) FHx	Screen once	Screen once	Screen once	Screen once if (+) FHx
ACPM	Not addressed	Screen once	Not addressed	Do not screen	Do not screen
NHS	Not addressed	Screen once	Screen once	Do not screen	Do not screen
CSVS	Do not screen	Screen once	Screen once	Screen once	Screen once if (+) multiple RFs, i.e., CardioVascular Disease (CVD) or (+) FHx
ESVS	Consider screening if (+) RFs	Screen once	Screen once	No recommendation	Maybe screen with a (+) FHx

FHx family history, *N/A* not available, *RFs* risk factors

While differences in self-interests and audience exist between these bodies, the recommendations are generally concordant regarding populations for which strong supporting data exists [6]. The guidelines with the most influence in the United States are those of the USPSTF [7], which recommend one-time screening for AAA by ultrasonography in men aged 65–75 years who have ever smoked. It makes no definitive recommendation for or against screening in men aged 65–75 years who have never smoked, but endorses selective screening based on individual patient risk factors including their past medical and family history. It recommends against the routine screening for AAA in women who have never smoked and repeat screening in men who have had a negative ultrasound. Lastly, it makes no definitive statement regarding routine screening in women aged 65–75 years who have ever smoked because of “insufficient evidence” [7]. This current USPSTF recommendation on screening in the female population is an update from the 2005 guidelines, in which the USPSTF recommended against screening in all women regardless of smoking history [7]. The ACPM and the ACC/AHA agree with the USPSTF’s screening recommendation for men aged 65–75 who have ever smoked [4, 8]. However, the ACC/AHA deviate from the USPSTF guidelines by including a recommendation for screening in men over the age of 60 who have a family history of AAA in a first-degree relative [4]. Furthermore, neither group recommends screening in never-smoker men without a family history and in women altogether.

The original ACC/AHA guidelines were published in conjunction with the SVS; however, the SVS issued updated guidelines in 2009 that increased the pool of eligible recipients [9]. First, it recommended screening for all men older than 65, regardless of smoking history. Second, it recommended earlier screening at age 55 with a positive family history. Lastly, it definitively addressed the issue of screening in the female population with a recommendation in direct opposition to the USPSTF and ACC/AHA. While data from numerous sources suggests that the prevalence of AAAs in women is lower [10, 11], the SVS recommended screening for women older than 65 who have ever smoked or have a positive family history, with the rationale that women have both higher rates of rupture and longer expected lifespans [9, 11–15].

Internationally, the NHS recommends a screening ultrasound for all men at the age of 65, regardless of smoking history [16]. In fact, the NHS recently launched a screening program with the goal of reducing deaths from ruptured AAAs in men over 65 by 50%. It recommends against the screening of women, stating that “screening is inefficient” for this population. The CSVS and the ESVS largely agree with the SVS’s recommendations [17, 18]. Both these organizations support screening in all men aged 65–75, but they both have slightly different recommendations regarding women and men aged 55–65. The CSVS, in individualized cases, recommends screening for women over the age of 65 who have multiple risk factors; furthermore, it recommends against screening in men under the age of 65 regardless of risk factors. The ESVS agrees with the SVS on screening in the slightly younger male population with risk factors; however, it does not make a definitive statement about screening in women, stating that “screening in women who smoke may require further investigation” and screening of older women having a family history of AAA “might be recommended”.

1.1.2 Risk Factors for AAA

The most widely accepted risk factors that have been cited for AAA include male sex, older age, and smoking [19]. Population-based studies in adults older than 50 have consistently reported a higher prevalence of AAAs in men versus women. A recent study reported prevalence of 3.9–7.2% in men and 1.0–1.3% in women [19]. Most AAAs found in the population occurred in individuals over the age of 60, with a total prevalence of 4–9% [20, 21]. One cohort study demonstrated a 4.5-fold increase in the relative risk of AAA for males over 65 compared to those under 55 [22]. However, the majority of these aneurysms were small, with diameters less than 3.5 cm, and likely not clinically important during the patients' lifetime. More clinically important aneurysms over 4.0 cm exist in 1% of men between 55 and 64 years old, with incremental increases by 2–4% per decade thereafter [23]. Smoking is the most important risk factor , estimated to cause 75% of all AAAs over 4.0 cm and increasing risk of AAA by a factor of six [20, 24]. Other risk factors include positive family history, prior AAA, Caucasian or Native American ethnicity, cardiovascular disease, Hypertension (HTN), obesity, and aneurysms of the femoral or popliteal arteries [20, 22, 25, 26].

1.1.3 Natural History and Rationale for Screening for AAA

The natural history of AAAs is important to consider when establishing screening guidelines, as the risk for rupture and the expansion help determine surgical and surveillance planning. By projecting AAA growth curves, it is possible to estimate when the rupture risk is high and to intervene beforehand, as the case-fatality rate is 50% when surgery is performed emergently on the 40% of patients who even make it to the hospital [5, 27]. In contrast, the perioperative mortality from elective repair is reported to be 1–5%, and is largely dependent on patient comorbidities and the type of repair [3]. Fortunately, men without AAA by age 65 are unlikely (only about ~1%) to develop a new aneurysm over the course of the subsequent 5 years [28]. When aneurysms develop, however, larger aneurysms tend to grow faster than smaller aneurysms due to the increase in wall tension according to LaPlace's law. According to one systematic review, for each 0.5 cm increase in AAA diameter, growth rates increased on average by 0.59 mm per year and rupture rates by a factor of 1.91 [29]. Aneurysms less than 4.0 cm in transverse diameter have a very low (~0%) annual risk of rupture, with an exponential increase in risk thereafter: 4.0–4.9 cm (0.5–5%), 5–5.9 cm (3–15%), 6–6.9 cm (10–20%), 7–7.9 cm (20–40%), and greater than 8 cm (30–50%) [30]. Extending this risk out to 5 years, the overall cumulative rupture rate of incidentally diagnosed aneurysms in population-based samples is 25–40% for aneurysms larger than 5.0 cm compared to 1–7% for aneurysms 4–5 cm [31–33].

1.1.4 Screening Imaging Modalities

Before imaging tests were developed, AAA screening was based on physical exam. However, accuracy of physical exam is limited by patient factors such as obesity and smaller aneurysm size [34]. Clinical studies have confirmed the poor reproducibility of physical exam, with sensitivity and specificity estimated at 39–68% and 75–91% [7, 19]. Aside from exposing patients to ionizing radiation, computed tomography (CT) can over-estimate aneurysm size by 2 mm or more because the cross sectional diameter of the aorta obtained in axial CT imaging is often not in the transverse plane [9]. While CT is more reproducible and remains the primary modality for operative planning, ultrasound has become the primary method for AAA screening because of its high sensitivity and specificity, portability, ease-of-use, safety (i.e., lack of radiation), and relative low cost [7]. While somewhat user-dependent, the sensitivity and specificity of ultrasound both approach 100%. Thus, given these advantages, ultrasound remains the primary method for AAA screening.

1.1.5 Clinical Trials and Longitudinal Studies on Screening for AAA

Four large randomized controlled trials (RCTs) have been conducted to evaluate the effectiveness of population-based screening for AAAs using ultrasound: the Multicentre Aneurysm Screening Study (MASS), the Chichester, UK screening trial, the Viborg County, Denmark screening trial, and the Western Australia screening trial [35–38]. Multiple summative attempts have been made to combine these data sets, including a meta-analysis and two systematic reviews [19, 39, 40]. As these trials represent the highest-quality evidence in the literature, their cumulative data serves as the basis for all the major societal guidelines presented above. Overall, these trials showed that invitation to one-time screening for AAA is associated with a reduction in AAA-specific mortality in 65–75-year-old men. Follow-up reports for these trials have shown that this effect is both persistent, lasting up to 15 years [7, 41–44], and significant, with estimated relative reductions of 42% and 66% at 13 years in the two highest-quality trials [41, 44]. Other beneficial effects, including reductions in risk for AAA rupture and emergency surgery, persisted up to 13 years out from screening as well [7]. While these trials did not collect specific data about participants' smoking histories or other risk factors, given the increased AAA prevalence in men who have ever smoked (6–7% of this population [24, 45]), the presence of this risk factor increases the benefit of screening in this population. The data for screening in other populations, including women, is less definitive [7].

Together, the four large population-based screening RCTs accumulated 137,214 participants with mean (or median) ages ranging from 67.7 to 72.7 years [7]. In each trial, participants were selected from population registries or regional health directories and randomized to either invitation for one-time ultrasound screening or usual care. The MASS trial, the largest of the four, randomized 67,800 men aged 65–74.

This was the only trial that excluded participants based on health status; men that were too high risk to be screened by their primary care physicians, terminally ill, or had other serious health problems were excluded. Men with 3–4.4 cm aneurysms were followed with annual ultrasounds while those with 4.5–5.4 cm aneurysms were rescanned every 3 months. Surgery was offered to men with aneurysms greater than 5.5 cm, growth greater than 1 cm per year, or development of symptoms. Mean follow-up was 4.1 years in the original study but long-term data out to 13 years continues to be published [41, 42]. The Viborg trial included 12,658 men aged 65–73 years old. Participants with aneurysms above 3.0 cm were offered annual rescreening while those with aneurysms greater than 5.0 cm were offered surgery. While mean follow-up in the original study was 5.1 years, a subsequent report detailing results out to 10 years was published thereafter [44]. The Chichester trial was the only trial to include women, with a total of 15,775 randomized participants (6433 men, 9342 women), aged 65–80 years. Subjects with 3–4.4 cm aneurysms were followed with annual ultrasound, while those with 4.5–5.9 cm aneurysms were rescanned every 3 months. Surgery was offered to participants with aneurysms greater than 5.9 cm, growth greater than 1 cm per year, or development of symptoms. Lastly, the Western Australia trial involved 41,000 men aged 65–83 years. The structure of this study was unique in that it did not specify its post-screening ultrasound surveillance protocol. Men were provided with two copies of a letter detailing the outcome of their ultrasound: one for them and one for their primary care doctor. Follow-up care, whether rescreening or surgical referral, was left up to the discretion of the primary care doctor as they deemed appropriate. Median follow-up was 43 months.

In general, the statistical analysis plans and outcome variables among the trials were similar. All four trials were conducted via intention-to-treat analysis. Adherence to screening varied from 62.5% in the Western Australia trial, to 80.2% in the MASS trial. Less than 1% of the control groups crossed over in any trial to receive elective surgery, even at the longest follow-up of 13–15 years [19]. The primary outcome variable was AAA-specific mortality (all deaths related to AAAs and all deaths within 30 days of AAA surgical repair), but AAA rupture and all-cause mortality were also reported. In a recent systematic review that evaluated each trial according to USPSTF design-specific criteria [46], the MASS and Viborg trials were rated as "good-quality", while the Chichester and Western Australia studies were labeled as "fair-quality" [19].

The prevalence of AAAs across the four trials ranged from 4.0% to 7.6%, with the majority (70–82%) less than 4.0–4.5 cm, and only a small proportion (0.4–0.6%) greater than 5.5 cm. The two "good-quality" trials, MASS and Viborg, demonstrated statistically significant reductions in AAA-related mortality in the groups invited to screening compared with the control groups, up to 13 years after screening (13-year hazard ratio [HR], 0.58 [CI, 0.49–0.69] and 0.34 [CI, 0.20–0.57], respectively) [35, 36, 41, 42, 44, 47]. For the MASS trial, this was associated with an absolute risk reduction of 0.14%, or 1.4 fewer AAA-related deaths per 1000 men screened [7, 41]. Not surprisingly, these two trials also found that an invitation to screening was associated with both lower AAA rupture rates at the 13-year follow-up (MASS: HR, 0.57 [CI, 0.49–0.67] [41]; Viborg: HR 0.44, [CI, 0.24–0.79] [47]) and significantly fewer emergency surgeries (MASS: Relative Risk (RR), 0.48 [CI, 0.37–0.63] at mean follow-up of 13.1 years [41]; Viborg: RR, 0.25 [CI, 0.09–0.66] at mean follow-up of 10 years [36]). While the two "fair-quality" trials, Chichester and Western Australia, did not report statistically significant results, they both showed a trend toward reductions in AAA-related mortality (Chichester: HR, 0.88 [CI 0.6–1.30] at 15 years of follow-up; Western Australia: RR, 0.61 [CI, 0.33–1.11] at 3.6 years of follow-up) [37, 38]. Of note, on post hoc analysis in the Western Australia trial, an invitation to screening was associated with a significant reduction in AAA-related mortality for men 65–75 years (OR, 0.19 [CI, 0.04–0.89]) and a trend toward increased mortality in older men (more than 75 years). This suggests that with better participant selection (i.e., excluding men over 75 years, when their likelihood of dying from other causes increases, thus limiting the benefit from AAA screening/repair), the Western Australia results may have aligned with the MASS and Viborg studies. As expected, all trials that reported rates of elective procedures showed significant increases (by about twofold) in elective AAA operations in the groups invited for screening: RRs 2.17 (MASS), 2.01 (Viborg), and 2.19 (Chichester), respectively [41, 47, 48]. Pooled analyses of data from these four trials from three independent groups demonstrated a statistically significant reduction, by about 45–50%, in the odds of AAA-related mortality (OR, 0.55 [CI, 0.36–0.86], 0.60 [CI, 0.47–0.78], and 0.57 [CI, 0.45–0.74]) [39, 40, 49]. None of the four trials found that an invitation to AAA screening was associated with a statistically significant all-cause mortality benefit at any time point up to 15 years. Pooled analyses of the four trials using random effects analysis have all showed no effect on all-cause mortality (ORs, 0.98 [CI, 0.97–1.00], 0.98 [CI 0.95–1.02], 0.95, [CI 0.85–1.07], and 0.98, [CI 0.95–1.0]) [19, 39, 40, 49]. This was not entirely unexpected, as fewer than 3% of participant deaths were attributable to AAA across the trials [7].

Other longitudinal studies have been conducted that investigate the effectiveness of AAA screening programs. One such study, published in 2012, reported attendance rates, screening and surveillance outcomes, and intervention rates and outcomes resulting from an AAA screening program initiated in Gloucestershire, England 20 years after the program was initiated. Sixty-two thousand men were invited with an 85% participation rate. From this subpopulation, 148 men had an aortic diameter greater than 5.4 cm and were referred for treatment, and 4.6% had a diameter between 2.6 and 5.4 cm and entered an ultrasound surveillance program. Perioperative mortality for the 631 surgeries performed for screen-detected AAAs was 3.9%, in line with the expected percentages based on other trials. An additional 372 procedures were performed for aneurysms detected incidentally with a mortality of 6.7%. Most tellingly, the number of ruptured aneurysms treated annually fell significantly during the course of the program [50].

The clinical data supporting AAA screening in women lags behind that of men. As noted previously, only one of the four major ultrasound-based AAA-screening RCTs recruited women, who were aged 65–80 years [10]. This trial found that AAA prevalence in women was six times lower than men (1.3% vs. 7.6%), in agreement with screening reports from Sweden that found a prevalence of 0.8% and 2.0% in ever-smokers and current smokers, respectively [11]. While most (75%) screen-detected AAAs were small (<3.9 cm), meta-analysis has shown that women have a three- to fourfold higher risk for rupture than men at the same diameter [51]. Nonetheless, rupture rates (0.06% in both groups), AAA-specific mortality (<0.2% in both groups, no statistical analysis), or all-cause mortality (10.7% vs. 10.2%) did not significantly differ at 5 years in the invitation-to-screening and control groups [7, 10, 19, 37]. Unlike men from the same trial in which the majority of ruptures occurred prior to age 80, most (70%) of the AAA-related deaths in women occurred at age 80 or older (at a time of increased competing causes of death and a declining benefit-risk ratio for operative intervention) [10]. Ultimately, the low prevalence of AAA in women resulted in a trial that was underpowered to draw definitive conclusions regarding health outcomes in this population [7]. In combination with the paucity of available data from other trials, uncertainty remains regarding the benefit women receive from population-based AAA screening.

One topic currently under investigation is selective screening in high-risk populations. A history of smoking is the most important risk factor for developing an AAA and has been suggested as a possible criterion for selective AAA screening [52]. Even a relatively modest smoking history (i.e., half-pack or less per day for less than 10 years) increases the likelihood of developing a large AAA [52]; this effect has been estimated as a three- to fivefold increase in AAA prevalence across all age groups and an increase in AAA-related mortality [24, 49, 53]. Unfortunately, the population-based screening RCTs did not collect specific data about participants' smoking histories. As a result, modeling studies have been conducted to determine how the impact of screening would differ in those with a history of smoking as compared to those who had never smoked [49]. In one study of 100,000 hypothetical U.S. men aged 65–74 years, the invitation of only ever-smokers (69% of men in this population) to attend screening would account for 89% of the expected reduction in AAA-related mortality from population-based screening of all men 65–74 years of age [49]. In a simulation analysis based on participant data from the Viborg trial, selective screening in high-risk patients, defined as those having Chronic Obstructive Pulmonary Disease (COPD) or a cardiovascular condition, would have prevented half of all reported deaths at 5 years and required 72.9% fewer screening invitations compared to mass screening [54]. Other modeling studies have shown that screening strategies based on age, sex, and smoking history outperform strategies that use other risk factors, such as family history, coronary artery disease, or hypercholesterolemia [55, 56].

1.1.6 Cost-Effectiveness Analysis for Screening for AAA

A core requirement for policy-making regarding any potential AAA screening program is cost-effectiveness. The literature consists of data derived from the Viborg and MASS trials [42, 44, 57], as well as hypothetical data [58]. In the MASS trial, cost-effectiveness based on AAA mortality at 4, 7, and 10 years of follow-up was $44,900, $19,500, and $12,579, respectively, per life-year gained [42, 43, 59]. Likewise, the cost per life-year gained as determined in the Viborg trial also improved from $12,736 at 5 years to $2566 at 15 years [17, 44]. As expected, this incremental improvement in cost-effectiveness over time reflects the high initial cost of screening and elective surgery (for aneurysms >5.5 cm) followed by continued long-term benefit [42, 43, 57, 60]. As the survival advantage in terms of life-years gained continues to increase with time, predictive models based on MASS data estimate a cost of $3806 per life-year gained over the full lifetime of men aged 65, indicating an extremely cost-effective program [42, 57]. Other recent cost-effectiveness studies using MASS data have tried to account for recent changes in the management and epidemiology of AAAs (decreasing prevalence of AAA and new surgical approaches) and have still found that screening men was cost-effective and delivered significant clinical benefit [61]. Nevertheless, there are other reports that suggest AAA screening is not cost-effective [58]. This study utilized a hypothetical population in their prediction model and clinical cost profiles native to Denmark (i.e., for screening, elective surgery, emergency surgery) which differed significantly from the UK, which together are believed to explain the contrasting findings [62, 63].

1.1.7 Potential Harms Versus Benefits of Screening

As with any medical intervention, ultrasound screening represents a balance between benefits, i.e., identifying AAAs early on in the non-emergent setting when it is possible to undergo elective surgery, and risks. Unlike other forms of imaging, ultrasound has no known direct physical risks [64]; instead, its risk profile consists of two indirect effects: psychological distress in those who screen positive and adverse outcomes from operative management [65].

Anxiety/depression, decreased quality of life, and poor health perception comprise the most frequently investigated negative psychological outcomes from screening. Most of the data on these adverse effects was collected in the Viborg and MASS RCTs, in addition to five observational studies [35, 66–71]. Unfortunately, the aggregate results are conflicting, with four of the five observational studies showing no clinically significant decrease in quality-of-life measures in those who screened positive compared to unscreened control participants, the MASS trial demonstrating only a transient negative psychological effect that resolved after 6 weeks, and the Viborg trial finding a small, but significant, immediate negative change in the psychological profile of participants who screened positive after 1 month of conservative management. While it is difficult to generate definitive conclusions, these results suggest that a portion of the population who screen positive but do not require immediate intervention may develop mild, though likely transient, adverse psychological effects.

AAA repair, whether open or endovascular, remains associated with significant complications (surgical complication, hospitalization, or even death) [72]. The most feared complication of AAA repair, perioperative mortality, occurs in 2.7–5.8% of elective cases, depending on patient specific comorbidities, the type of procedures, and other operator-specific factors (surgeon experience, type of surgeon, hospital volume, etc.) [73–75]. A separate issue altogether is the relative mortality in patients undergoing elective open surgery compared to endovascular repair. One of the byproducts of screening programs is an increase in elective procedures, as borne out by data from the four population-based screening RCTs: the risk for any AAA-related operation in the invited group was approximately double that of the non-invited group at 3–5 years in all trials due to an uptick in elective procedures [35–38]. Concurrently, most screening trials reported associated decreases in emergency repairs (data presented above) in populations invited to screen [19]. While the complication rate may remain constant, estimated at 32% for elective AAA repairs [72], the total number of complications will inevitably rise. Thus, the increase in the overall rates of detection and surgery in the screening group potentially represents a harm, as a proportion of AAAs will never rupture due to cessation in growth or death from a competing cause. The extent of over-diagnosis and over-treatment is unfortunately difficult to estimate [7].

In conclusion, undetected AAAs represent a major public health concern because of the high rates of mortality with rupture. Ultrasound imaging has emerged as a viable screening modality because of its high sensitivity and specificity, reproducibility, portability, safety, and affordability. While separate guidelines have been published by multiple societies and governmental agencies, they share a consensus for those populations considered at high risk, i.e., men aged 65–75 with a history of smoking. Controversy still exists over other subpopulations for which the data is inconsistent or lacking altogether, i.e., women, younger non-smoking men, and those with risk factors other than smoking or a strong family history. Improved definition of those populations at high risk who will most benefit from screening is needed.

1.1.8 The SAAAVE Act: A Summary

Signed into law by President George W. Bush in 2007, the SAAAVE Act provides for a one-time AAA screening ultrasound as part of the "Welcome to Medicare Physical Exam" for patients with defined risk factors. More specifically, this population includes men aged 65–75 who have smoked at least 100 cigarettes and patients of either gender with a family history of AAA. Prior to 2007, screening for AAAs was not a covered Medicare benefit, requiring patients to pay out-of-pocket [76].

Although its intentions were supported by clinical evidence showing an AAA-related mortality benefit [35, 38, 39, 43, 49, 77], unfortunately the SAAAVE Act has been fraught with controversy since its inception. Opponents of the act point to a recent study from Stanford that found the act was associated with an increased number of abdominal ultrasounds, but without concurrent improvements in clinical outcomes [77]. The study, which compared a sample of Medicare enrollees eligible for screening to a control group that was not eligible for screening, found that while the use of abdominal ultrasound had increased 2.0% (7.6–9.6%) among SAAAVE-eligible men from 2004 to 2008, there were no apparent changes in the rates of AAA repair, AAA rupture, or all-cause mortality. Perhaps more concerning was that fewer than 10% of SAAAVE-eligible Medicare enrollees actually received the abdominal ultrasound. Proposed reasons for underutilization of abdominal aortic ultrasound screening include significant system factors, such as lack of awareness on the part of physicians and patients regarding the SAAAVE Act or the potential benefits of AAA screening, but also lack of in-depth history-taking to identify high-risk patients, and the misguided belief that AAAs can be easily palpated on physical examination [5, 77]. Other opponents contend that the modest impact of the SAAAVE Act on screening rates is based on a small absolute reduction in clinical events resulting from AAA screening, rather than a reduction in a significant percentage of those patients at risk [78]. They argue that the widespread adoption of AAA screening is not justifiable by medical practitioners because the population benefit is low relative to the time period upon which the USPSTF based their original screening recommendations. This conclusion is based on recent clinical evidence from Europe suggesting a decline in mortality from ruptured AAAs, and thus "clinically relevant aneurysms", over the past 10–15 years attributed to a decrease in the prevalence of smoking rather than the implementation of AAA screening or the rise of endovascular repair [79, 80].

Proponents of the SAAAVE Act are quick to point out that the 1-year follow-up in the study by Shreibati et al. might be too short to observe a reduction in all-cause mortality [77]. Randomized trials of AAA screening have shown that the reduction in AAA-related mortality is not apparent for at least 1 year after the initial AAA screening [35]. In addition, they argue that the requirements for patient eligibility and physician reimbursement prevent widespread adoption of AAA screening ultrasounds [76]. They point to the modest 2% increase in screening ultrasounds, still less than 10,000 total exams in 2007, after the implementation of the SAAAVE Act as evidence of the barriers for beneficiaries. Indeed, at-risk Medicare beneficiaries must obtain a referral for AAA screenings during their "Welcome to Medicare Physical Exam" and must be screened during their first 6 months of eligibility [81]. Furthermore, potential beneficiaries are required to pay a 20% co-payment out-of-pocket prior to screening [76]. Additionally, the millions of patients not newly enrolled in the Medicare program are not eligible.

A recent study conducted at the Geisinger Medical Center would suggest that more aggressive screening measures are in order [5]. The study investigated whether current screening guidelines under the SAAAVE Act, in conjunction with routine ambulatory medical care evaluation, were an effective way to identify and screen patients at risk for ruptured AAA. To do this, the authors retrospectively reviewed the pre-operative clinical data and outpatient office visit notes for all patients who presented with ruptured AAAs at their institution over a 6-year period. Notably, only 17% of patients who presented with a ruptured AAA would have been eligible for a screening ultrasound based upon the SAAAVE Act criteria at the time of rupture. The study also found significant gender disparities: while 30% (16 total women) of the study patients were women, only one would have been eligible for screening according to the SAAAVE Act. Further underscoring the importance of screening ultrasound was their finding that physical exam was inadequate to diagnose AAAs, as only 9.6% of patients had findings that the practitioner felt were suspicious for AAA. The authors rightfully concluded that current AAA screening guidelines, as currently constructed, are inadequate in reducing aneurysm-related mortality.

Another barrier to the provision of screening ultrasounds by a medical practitioner is the strict requirement for reimbursement. This suggestion was raised in response to one of the findings in the study by Shreibati et al. In the study, they found that the small increase in screening rates observed after the SAAAVE act was due to an increase in abdominal ultrasonography not reimbursed under the program (i.e., not an approved current procedural terminology [CPT] code under the act). While this may have purely been attributable to a lack of education regarding the proper CPT codes, one alternative explanation offered was that for some eligible patients, the screening ultrasound was billed under a different CPT code because it did not meet the complex criteria for reimbursement [77].

While the SAAAVE Act undoubtedly has its drawbacks, it nevertheless raised awareness of AAAs and lays the foundation for future progress toward the provision of potentially life-saving abdominal ultrasonography to all at-risk patients. Efforts by the SVS are already underway to introduce new legislation that would unlink AAA screening from the "Welcome to Medicare Physical Exam" as well as expand the one-time screening to 65–75-year-old at-risk Medicare beneficiaries. The largest hurdle may prove to be education of both primary care physicians and patients about AAAs. Indeed, multiple studies investigating patients presenting with ruptured AAAs have found that a high percentage (~30–40%) of them had a known AAA prior to rupture [5, 82]. In one of these studies, 40% of patients with radiographic evidence of AAA prior to rupture were never referred or evaluated in the vascular surgery clinic [5]. Akin to the disease processes of breast cancer and colorectal cancer, AAA screening reduces disease-specific mortality but not all-cause mortality [77]. However, awareness of AAA screening certainly lags behind the screening programs for these diseases, namely mammography and fecal occult blood testing, which receive ample attention in the press. This deficiency has not gone unnoticed, as companies such as Gore have created websites to raise awareness and provide patients with information on the SAAAVE Act [83].

Perhaps most important from a practical perspective, AAA screening has been shown to be cost-effective, with an estimated cost-effectiveness ratio of $19,500 per life-year gained [43]. Furthermore, evidence exists supporting the cost effectiveness and efficacy of a screening program. When a large-scale screening effort for identifying AAAs in patients in clinical practice was implemented, the prevalence of AAAs and aneurysm distribution reflected those reported in major clinical trials at a reasonable cost of $53 per ultrasound [81]. Given the marked improvement in mortality associated with elective AAA repair compared to emergent repair of a ruptured AAA [5] and the cost-effectiveness of AAA screening, the most effective method of reducing AAA-related mortality is early identification and elective repair. Within this context, the SAAAVE Act represents the foundation upon which future efforts will build a more thorough screening program that provides coverage to all at-risk beneficiaries.

1.2 Carotid Stenosis

1.2.1 Clinical Impact of Stroke and the Importance of Prevention

The American Stroke Association recently re-defined the term stroke as "acute cerebrovascular syndromes", to reflect the many pathological processes whose collective endpoint is neurologic tissue damage over a short period of time [84]. Stroke, as a clinical entity, is a major public health concern because it is one of the leading causes of death and disability. Not only is stroke the leading cause of death worldwide and the fourth leading cause of death in the United States, but it is associated with 20% mortality from the acute event and 40–50% survival at 5 years [85]. Of the people who survive a stroke, 18% are unable to return to work and one quarter of those over 65 require long-term institutional care [85, 86]. As the elderly population continues to grow, those at risk for stroke will increase; indeed, the prevalence of stroke has been rising in parallel with the expansion of this population [87]. Treatment options for patients who have had strokes are unfortunately limited. Only a small fraction of stroke patients are candidates for thrombolysis; for the remaining patients, treatment consists of damage control measures to limit the extent of brain injury. For this reason, stroke prevention represents the area with greatest potential impact on disease.

1.2.2 Carotid Stenosis as the Cause of Strokes

Ninety percent of strokes in the United States are ischemic strokes (thrombosis, embolism, or systemic hypoperfusion), and by far the predominant etiology [88]. Carotid artery stenosis (CAS), defined as atherosclerotic narrowing of the extracranial carotid arteries (either the internal or the common and internal carotid arteries), is thought to cause approximately 10% of ischemic strokes [89, 90], with a population-attributable risk of 1–7% [85, 91, 92]. CAS can be further subdivided based on the presence or absence of symptoms. Symptomatic CAS is defined by the presence of recent (i.e., within 6 months) transient or permanent focal neurologic symptoms related to high-grade stenosis of the affected artery [93]. Such symptoms include ipsilateral amaurosis fugax, contralateral weakness or numbness of an extremity or the face, dysarthria, or aphasia. This subset of patients, which will not be discussed in depth in this section, often benefit from early carotid revascularization [94]. The asymptomatic subtype, on the other hand, is defined by the degree of stenosis, with the cutoff ranging from 50% to 70%, depending on the study criteria [95–97].

Based on large US studies investigating the rate of progression of asymptomatic CAS, the 5-year risk for ipsilateral stroke is estimated at 5% for CAS greater than 70% [91]. In one of the largest trials in patients with asymptomatic CAS (defined in the trial as >60%), 11.8% of patients suffered from stroke or death at 5 years without surgical intervention [98]. Since this trial (in the 1990s), however, the annual risk of stroke in medically treated patients with asymptomatic CAS has decreased, mostly attributed to improved management of blood pressure, diabetes, and hypercholesterolemia. As shown by a meta-analysis in 2013 of 26 studies of patients with asymptomatic CAS, the rate of ipsilateral stroke was significantly lower for patients recruited between 2000 and 2010 than for those recruited earlier (11.3% vs. 2.4%) [99]. With current optimized medical therapy, it is estimated that the risk of stroke in these individuals may in fact be less than 1% per year and as low as 0.3% per year [100, 101].

Unfortunately, there are currently no validated, reliable methods to determine both who is at increased risk for CAS and who is at increased risk for stroke when CAS is present. The purpose of this section is to review the current evidence regarding the effectiveness of screening asymptomatic adults for CAS in reducing the risk of ipsilateral stroke.

1.2.3 Prevalence and Risk Factors for Carotid Stenosis

The overall prevalence of CAS varies depending on demographic factors, cut points for carotid stenosis, and methods of grading. For CAS greater than 70% in adults over 65 years, large US-based studies of the general population in the 1990s suggested a prevalence between 0.5% and 1% [90, 91]. Other more recent data from meta-analyses of 40 studies reported similar results, with an estimated prevalence of 1.7% in this population [102, 103]. Not surprisingly, older patients, men, smokers, and those with hypertension and heart disease were found to have a higher burden of disease. Indeed, age and sex were shown to significantly affect the prevalence of moderate stenosis in pooled results from 40 studies: CAS >50% for men and women under age 70 was 4.8% and 2.2%, respectively; this increased to 12.5% and 6.9%, respectively, for men and women over age 70 [102]. Other pertinent risk factors for CAS include diabetes and hyperlipidemia. While many of these risk factors are associated with CAS, some, such as hypertension, smoking, and hyperlipidemia, are directly associated with the development of strokes themselves. In fact, the population-attributable risk for stroke related to asymptomatic CAS (0.9%) is thought to pale in comparison to that of hypertension (>95%), smoking (12–14%), and hyperlipidemia (9%) [91, 92].

1.2.4 Screening Tests for Carotid Stenosis: Physical Exam and Non-invasive Imaging

Screening for CAS in the clinical setting has typically involved either auscultation of a carotid bruit during physical exam or non-invasive studies of the carotid artery, including duplex ultrasonography (DUS), CT angiogram (CTA), or magnetic resonance angiogram (MRA). While cerebral angiography is the gold standard for imaging, it is invasive, expensive, and associated with the risk of stroke and even death; for this reason, it is not frequently the first-line imaging modality.

Carotid bruits are often the initial finding in the primary care office that prompts further workup for CAS. Unfortunately, carotid bruits are fraught with multiple issues which make them a less-than-ideal screening test. Not only are bruits associated with a low degree of inter-observer reliability, estimated at 66% [104], but they are poor predictors of both underlying carotid stenosis and ipsilateral stroke risk in asymptomatic patients [105–107]. As a clinical tool for detecting underlying CAS, the estimated sensitivity and specificity for auscultation was only 46–77% and 71–98%, respectively, according to the USPSTF's review of four studies [105]. Similarly, the carotid bruit has failed to demonstrate utility as a predictor of ipsilateral stroke: in one study of nursing home residents, it was found that the 3-year cumulative incidence of cerebrovascular accidents was similar for patients with and without asymptomatic bruits [106]. Furthermore, 60% of bruits eventually disappeared without any correlation to the development of strokes. While bruits may not serve a useful purpose with regard to CAS screening, they in fact are thought to better predict general atherosclerotic disease rather than cerebrovascular disease [108]. In fact, patients with bruits are more likely to die from cardiovascular rather than cerebrovascular disease, and twice as likely to develop a myocardial infarction (MI) or die from cardiovascular disease than people without bruits [108, 109].

The three main non-invasive imaging techniques used for CAS screening are carotid DUS, MRA (contrast-enhanced MR angiography [CEMRA] if contrast-enhanced), and CTA. DUS has assumed the primary role as the screening method of choice due to its portability, inexpensiveness, lack of radiation, and accuracy. According to a meta-analysis of studies from 1996 to 2003 using angiography as a gold standard, DUS was associated with a sensitivity of 98% and specificity of 88% for CAS >50%; for CAS >70%, the accuracy was increased, with a sensitivity of 90% and specificity of 94% [110]. While this study also raised concerns regarding the reliability of DUS after finding variation between laboratories, other studies have shown that this is less of a concern for more pronounced CAS (>70%), in which 96% agreement has been reported between readers for this degree of disease [111].

Carotid DUS has performed well in comparative studies with other imaging techniques. In one meta-analysis, no significant difference was found in the ability of DUS or MRA to detect CAS >70% [112]. In another meta-analysis in 2006 of all four types of imaging, CEMRA was the most sensitive and specific compared to DUS, MRA, or CTA (sensitivity 94% vs. 89%, 88%, and 76%, respectively; specificity 93% vs. 84%, 84%, and 94%, respectively) [113]. In this study, DUS performed on par with MRA; CTA was less sensitive than both, but more specific [113]. Another more recent systematic review found similar results, with MRA having only a slightly higher sensitivity (95% vs. 86%) and specificity (90% vs. 87%) for detecting CAS of 70–99% than DUS [114].

1.2.5 Asymptomatic CAS: Effectiveness of Early Detection and Treatment

Unfortunately, no studies have been conducted that investigate the direct benefit of screening for asymptomatic CAS. However, three major randomized controlled trials (RCTs) have been published that examine the benefit of treating asymptomatic CAS with carotid endarterectomy (CEA): ACAS (Asymptomatic Carotid Atherosclerosis Study), VACS (Veterans Affairs Cooperative), and ACST (Asymptomatic Carotid Surgery Trial) [115–117]. The exact trial specifics are beyond the scope of this chapter. Nevertheless, it is important to briefly review the results because a discussion about the feasibility of a screening strategy without a subsequent intervention with proven benefit would be rendered moot.

In total, these three studies allocated 5226 subjects to medical therapy or CEA. The randomized patient sample lacked diversity: Caucasian men (no women were enrolled) in North America and Europe, aged 65–68 years old, with a life expectancy of at least 5 years. The criteria for inclusion was CAS >50% in the VACS and CAS >60% in the ACAS and ACTS studies. In general, pooled analysis of data from these three studies found that patients randomized to CEA experienced 2.0% fewer perioperative strokes or death or subsequent ipsilateral stroke than medical management. If the outcome measure under investigation was re-defined as all strokes or death, the benefit to patients undergoing CEA was even higher: 3.5% fewer patients experienced this outcome as opposed to those receiving medical therapy alone [105]. The absolute risk reduction was small, with an average of 1% per year [95]. Unfortunately, no studies exist that compare carotid angioplasty and stenting (CAAS) with medical therapy.

These RCTs had significant limitations that reduce the proposed benefit to patients undergoing CEA as compared to medical management. Most significantly, the medical arm was not standardized or defined in any of the trials (although ACAS and VACS patients received aspirin alone), no trials compared CEA to current best medical therapy (i.e., no statins or anti-hypertensive), patients with prior symptoms (>6 months prior to enrollment) suggesting ipsilateral symptomatic CAS were included along with asymptomatic patients (ACST), and only the most experienced surgeons were allowed to participate. These four factors, along with the inevitable decrease in effectiveness when implemented outside the strict confines of RCTs (i.e., in the more diverse general population), would likely limit the magnitude of benefit from surgical intervention in asymptomatic patients in the general population. As a result, conclusions regarding these trials are limited. At the most basic level, one may reasonably conclude that with patients and surgeons similar to those in the RCTs, treatment with CEA for asymptomatic CAS can result in a net absolute reduction in stroke rates in selected patients similar to those included in the trials (i.e., medically stable men with asymptomatic CAS of 60–99% who have a life expectancy of at least 5 years) with selected surgeons and must be weighed against the associated perioperative complications (discussed below) [95, 96].

1.2.6 Harms of Screening

As with any screening strategy, the benefits of identifying a disease process in the early stages must be weighed against the harms from both the screening technique and any subsequent intervention that occurs due to a positive screen. While carotid DUS has little, if any, direct harms, unnecessary CEA or CAAS in patients incorrectly diagnosed with CAS could lead to unnecessary interventions and result in significant harms.

Analysis of six trials with over 3000 patients comparing CEA to medical therapy under conditions similar to those in the three major RCTs determined that CEA was associated with a 30-day stroke or mortality rate of 2.4% in pooled analysis [90]. CAAS is also associated with significant risks, including stroke or death in 3.1% of patients, as shown in a meta-analysis of two trials with over 6000 patients [90]. These figures would likely increase in low-volume centers and with less experienced surgeons. Other post-operative complications post-CEA that should be considered include myocardial infarctions (0.8–2.2%), cranial nerve injury (3.8% patients), pulmonary embolism (1.4%), and local hematoma requiring reoperation (2.8%) [90, 105].

1.2.7 Screening of Asymptomatic Adults in the General Population for CAS

The purpose of a screening program is to identify people with an unrecognized condition (CAS) who would derive significant health benefits (prevention of stroke) from a treatment they would not have otherwise received [92]. Some argue that detecting asymptomatic CAS does not lead to an intervention, either medical or surgical, that benefits the patient. The reasons for this conclusion are multifold.

First, all risk factors for CAS should be medically managed aggressively regardless of the presence or absence of asymptomatic CAS. Not only are most of the risk factors for CAS associated with strokes themselves, but they are associated with strokes to a much more significant extent than CAS. Partly the result of the low prevalence of asymptomatic CAS in the general adult population (for these purposes, estimated at 0.90% in adults over 60), the population-attributable risk for stroke due to asymptomatic CAS (0.7%) is much smaller than that of hypertension (>95%), smoking (12–24%), and hyperlipidemia (9%) [88]. As a result, most of the population at risk for CAS are already medically optimized, such that the finding of asymptomatic CAS would only result in added benefit if an intervention or surgical procedure would reduce their risk of stroke [88]. Thus, evaluation of the efficacy of interventions after a positive screen should focus on surgical interventions (i.e., CEA or CAAS) and the risks and benefits of each.

Second, it has not been definitively shown that surgical intervention is superior to medical therapy in asymptomatic patients based on the available data. As discussed above, while the major RCTs found a statistically significant benefit of CEA as compared to medical therapy, the absolute risk reduction was small (average 1% per year) and the medical treatment arm was not representative of the current best practices [95]. Indeed, with recent advances in medical management (improved control of blood pressure, hyperlipidemia, and diabetes are thought to represent the most important factors, in decreasing order of importance [118]), observational studies now suggest that the rate of strokes with medical therapy may be at or below the 1% annual rates found in the trials' surgical groups [92]. If this is correct, complication rates associated with CEA or CAAS would need to be much lower than the previously recommended 3% to justify the intervention [88].

Lastly, as another consequence of low disease prevalence in the general population, the rate of false positives would be high. If a point prevalence of 0.9% asymptomatic CAS greater than 70% in adults over 60 is assumed, a sensitivity/specificity of 90%/94% would yield a positive predictive value of 12%. This would imply that 88% of subjects would undergo unnecessary further workup or interventions, which carry their own set of risks as outlined above [92].

1.2.8 Screening of High-Risk Asymptomatic Adults for CAS

Given the data presented above, it is not difficult to understand why all major medical societies, including the AHA, the SVS, and the USPSTF, recommend against the screening of asymptomatic CAS in the general adult population (see below). While not addressed by the USPSTF or the AHA directly, the SVS has endorsed the screening of asymptomatic patients at high risk for CAS (i.e., those with hypertension, smoking, diabetes). This approach is reasonable, as screening this subpopulation with presumably a higher prevalence would increase the positive predictive value of the carotid DUS. Unfortunately, no guaranteed method currently exists to identify groups of patients with this high a prevalence. In any case, probability models have been created to try and quantify the threshold prevalence in the high-risk population at which the benefit from CEA outweighs the risk of post-operative complications [119]. Results suggest that this prevalence estimate is 20%, but benefits would only be seen at centers where the duplex study has a demonstrated high sensitivity and specificity and where there was a low surgical risk.

1.3 The Major Societal Guidelines

1.3.1 USPSTF (2014) [105]

- Recommends against screening for asymptomatic CAS in the general adult population on the basis that the harms of screening outweigh the benefits.
- This is a grade D recommendation, meaning that the USPSTF discourages the use of this service.

1.3.2 Society for Vascular Surgery (2011) [120]

- Recommends against routine screening to detect clinically asymptomatic CAS in the general population. Screening is not recommended for the presence of a neck bruit alone without other risk factors. This is a Grade 1 recommendation based on level A evidence.
- Recommends that screening for asymptomatic CAS should be considered in individuals above the age of 65 with one of the following risk factors (hypercholesterolemia, smoking, coronary artery disease) or any individual with PAD as

long as the patient is a candidate for intervention or surgery and is willing to consider carotid intervention or surgery if a significant stenosis is discovered. The presence of a bruit in these patients increases the likelihood of a significant stenosis. This is a Grade 1 recommendation based on level B evidence.

- Screening may be reasonable in patients as part of the pre-operative evaluation prior to Coronary Artery Bypass Grafting (CABG). The presence of left main disease and PAD would increase the yield of the screening test in these individuals, based on level B evidence.
- Screening is not recommended in individuals with asymptomatic disease with prior history of head and neck radiation. They posit that the benefit of intervention in these patients has not been established, based on level B evidence.
- Screening is not recommended for individuals with AAA unless they fit one of the high-risk categories listed above, based on level B evidence.
- Recommends carotid DUS in an accredited vascular lab as the initial screening test of choice for asymptomatic CAS in high-risk patients. When non-diagnostic or stenosis of intermediate severity (50–69%) is found in an asymptomatic patient, follow-up imaging with MRA, CTA, or angiography is required prior to intervention. These are Grade 1 recommendations based on level B evidence.

1.3.3 American Heart Association (2011) [88, 121]

- Recommends against screening in low-risk populations for asymptomatic CAS. This is a class III recommendation based on level C evidence. This is made on the basis of concerns about lack of cost effectiveness, the potential adverse impact of false positives and false negatives in the general population, and the small absolute benefit of intervention.
- Recommends that it is reasonable to consider CEA in asymptomatic patients with >70% stenosis if the risk of perioperative stroke, MI, and death is low (<3%). However, effectiveness compared with contemporary best medical management is not well established. This is a class IIa recommendation based on level A evidence.

In conclusion, with the data available, the potential harms outweigh the benefits of population screening of adults, particularly elderly patients, for asymptomatic CAS. For this reason, this practice is discouraged by the major societal groups. Future work needs to be conducted with the goal of developing valid and reliable tools to determine which people are at high risk for CAS, as well as those who are at high risk for stroke once diagnosed with CAS. Once this population with a higher prevalence is identified, selective screening would prove more fruitful, as the positive predictive value of carotid DUS would increase and thus limit the false positives and unnecessary harms from further workup and interventions. While no current algorithm exists, it would be reasonable to adopt the approach of the SVS in terms of selective screening of asymptomatic patients with multiple risk factors for CAS at a point in which surgical intervention would be tolerated with minimal risk of perioperative stroke, MI, or death. Other areas of future work include comparing CEA and CAAS (carotid artery angioplasty and stenting) to current best medical practice to determine if there is truly a benefit from surgical intervention, which is being studied in CREST-2. These studies will also be more inclusive of a diverse patient sample, especially women and minorities, who were excluded from the three major RCTs of the 1990s.

1.4 Peripheral Artery Disease

The American Heart Association estimates that peripheral artery disease (PAD) afflicts eight million people over the age of 40 in the United States, and affects 12–20% of Americans above the age of 65 [122]. PAD, defined as atherosclerotic occlusion of the iliac, femoral-popliteal, and infrapopliteal arteries, causes impaired circulation to the lower extremities [123]. In addition to being a significant public health burden, PAD is a major source of morbidity and mortality resulting in functional impairment, limb loss, and death from cardiovascular causes. Timely diagnosis of PAD has allowed for primary and secondary prevention strategies aimed at reducing cardiovascular morbidity and mortality. Despite epidemiologic studies which have contributed to our understanding of PAD prevalence in defined populations and its association with traditional atherosclerotic risk factors, the recommendations for screening for PAD are somewhat inconsistent between governing bodies. We summarize the salient points of the American College of Cardiology/American Heart Association 2005 Practice Guidelines for the Management of Patients With Peripheral Arterial Disease [4], the 2011 ACCF/AHA Focused Update of the Guideline for the Management of Patients With Peripheral Artery Disease [124], and the U.S. Preventive Services Task Force Recommendation Statement [125].

1.4.1 ACC/AHA 2005 Practice Guidelines for the Management of Patients with Peripheral Arterial Disease

These practice guidelines represent a collaborative compilation effort between the ACC and AHA and have been officially endorsed by the Society for Cardiovascular Angiography and Interventions; Society for Vascular Medicine and Biology; Society for Vascular Surgery; and Society of Interventional Radiology; as well as by the American Association of Cardiovascular and Pulmonary Rehabilitation; National Heart, Lung, and Blood Institute; Society for Vascular Nursing; TransAtlantic Inter-Society Consensus; and Vascular Disease Foundation. For the purposes of this section of the chapter, we will focus on lower extremity PAD. With regard to the evaluation of a patient who is asymptomatic, these guidelines outline those populations who are at high risk and therefore most likely to benefit from further evaluation:

- Less than 50 years of age with diabetes and one other atherosclerotic risk factor such as smoking, dyslipidemia, hypertension, or hyperhomocysteinemia

- Age 50–69 years with history of diabetes or smoking
- Age >70 years
- Leg symptoms with exertion consistent with claudication or ischemic rest pain
- Abnormal lower extremity pulse exam
- Known disease in the coronary, carotid, or renal circulation

1.4.2 Detection of Symptomatic PAD

1.4.2.1 History and Physical Exam

In the high-risk populations as defined above, this document recommends that these patients should undergo a thorough history as well as vascular review of systems that evaluates for the presence of claudication symptoms, ischemic rest pain, or evidence of tissue loss. The review of systems should be thorough in its evaluation of possible organ systems affected. This assessment is not standardized, and the authors acknowledge that this may contribute at least partially to the underdetection of PAD. It also recommends that these individuals undergo a vascular-focused exam checking for pulses as well as evidence of tissue loss in the feet. The evidence for these recommendations was graded as level C in the 2005 guidelines, meaning that this recommendation was derived from case studies or a consensus of experts. In the evaluation of claudication symptoms, questionnaires have been derived for the detection of PAD, which can be added to the patient history, albeit each with its own limitations in terms of sensitivity. For reference, we have included a brief description of the questionnaires that have been utilized in the literature to define the prevalence of PAD (see below). They also recommend that these high-risk individuals undergo a through pulse exam as well as examination of their feet.

1.4.2.2 Claudication Questionnaires

The Rose/World Health Organization questionnaire was a field survey instrument designed to improve the definition of intermittent claudication for epidemiologic use [126]. The key characteristics of the survey include the presence of calf pain in one or both legs with walking that is not present with standing, exacerbation with exertion, and relief with rest. The San Diego Claudication Questionnaire [127] is a modified version of the Rose questionnaire which allows for the delineation of which leg is affected (right versus left), and also included thigh and buttock pain. The characterization of the pain also included atypical claudication pain, and incorporated pain, no pain, pain at rest, non-calf claudication, non-Rose calf claudication, and Rose claudication. These categories were further expounded by McDermott et al. [128], where those participants with pain at rest and exertion were further distinguished by their ability to walk through the discomfort. McDermott et al. also cautioned that one should distinguish between those who are asymptomatic because of physical inactivity versus a true lack of symptoms, since individuals with pain on exertion may limit their activity to avoid the discomfort, thus decreasing the detection of PAD. The Walking Impairment Questionnaire (WIQ) was designed to measure walking ability in patients with and without PAD. The questionnaire asks one to report on their walking endurance (WIQ distance score), walking speed (WIQ speed score), and ability to climb stairs (WIQ stair-climbing score) [129]. The study found that there was a correlation between the WIQ distance score and the six-min walk score and between the WIQ speed score and the four-m walking velocity, suggesting that these measures are more sensitive than prior questionnaires for the detection of PAD. Despite modifications of prior surveys, these epidemiologic surveys have been acknowledged in studies comparing them with non-invasive tests as limited by a lack of sensitivity and reproducibility [130].

1.4.2.3 Diagnostic Vascular Studies

The ankle brachial index (ABI) is an objective, standardized measurement which has been used in epidemiologic studies to define the presence of lower extremity PAD. It is calculated with the patient in the supine position, at rest. The systolic blood pressures at the ankle at the dorsalis pedis and posterior tibial arteries as well as brachial arteries are measured, and the higher of the two ankle pressures is divided by the higher brachial artery blood pressure. An ABI of <0.90 is considered diagnostic for PAD. The ACC/AHA guidelines make a class I recommendation that all individuals who have symptomatic PAD or are considered high risk (older than 50 years with a history of smoking or diabetes, or over 70 years of age) should undergo further testing with a bilateral ABI to confirm the diagnosis and to establish a baseline of degree of disease, based on level C evidence. Additionally, the toe-brachial index should be used to diagnose PAD in patients with non-compressible vessels, i.e., in diabetics and those with chronic renal insufficiency. Segmental pressure measurements are useful to diagnose PAD and in determining the level of disease when an intervention is contemplated, level of evidence B. The cuffs are placed at the high thigh, low thigh, calf, ankle, and metatarsal level and a gradient above 20 mmHg between levels is considered hemodynamically significant. Exercise testing in the form of toe-tip exercise testing or treadmill exercise testing can be used to unmask PAD in those individuals with a normal ABI at rest. Both the pre- and post-exercise ABIs should be compared to distinguish pseudoclaudication from claudication, level of evidence B. In the elderly who are not able to undergo exercise treadmill testing, a six-min walk test may be considered (Class IIb recommendation) to objectively assess the functional limitations due to PAD. Pulsed Volume Recordings can be useful to establish the diagnosis of PAD by measuring the amount of pulse blood volume passing through different levels of the leg (high thigh, low thigh, calf, ankle, metatarsal level), which correlates with blood flow, class IIa recommendation based on level B evidence. Duplex ultrasound can also be used to diagnose PAD as well as the location and severity of the lesions, class I recommendation and level A evidence. CTA or MRA might be considered to delineate the exact location of the lesions, as well as for the determination of access sites, and should only be performed if revascularization is contemplated, based on level B evidence. Arteriography is reserved for those instances where revascularization is being considered for treatment of PAD, or if the Glomerular Filtration Rate (GFR) is limited in that the contrast load from a CTA is prohibitive, and the risk of nephrogenic systemic fibrosis is too high to warrant MRA.

1.4.3 Management of Symptomatic PAD

Symptomatic patients should undergo a vascular physical exam including measurement of an ABI. If the resting ABI is normal in a symptomatic patient, then an exercise ABI should be performed, based on level B evidence. These guidelines state that revascularization should only be contemplated if the individual is significantly functionally impaired and there is an absence of other diseases such as angina, heart failure, orthopedic issues, or respiratory issues which might limit their exercise capacity, based on level C evidence. The document further outlines that individuals with symptomatic PAD being evaluated for revascularization therapy should be offered a supervised exercise regimen and pharmacotherapy, be given antiplatelet therapy and risk factor modification, have evidence of significant impairment because of PAD, and have an intervenable lesion with low risk and a high probability of success. They further state that an arteriogram is not necessary in patients with a normal post-exercise ABI, with the exception of unusual disease states such as entrapment syndrome or internal iliac artery disease, based on class C evidence.

1.4.4 Detection and Management of Asymptomatic PAD

There is a class I recommendation (Benefit>>>Risk) that the patient should undergo a thorough history and review of systems to elicit a history of walking impairment, claudication, rest pain, or tissue loss for those age 50 and older with atherosclerotic risk factors and all those age 70 and older, based on level C evidence. This may also be informed by questions derived from the claudication questionnaires referred to in the literature and described above. Asymptomatic patients who are at high risk for PAD as defined above should undergo a focused pulse exam as well as examination of the foot. They recommend further evaluation using the ABI in suspected individuals with PAD, based on level B evidence. Based on level C evidence, in those patients with a normal ABI (0.90–1.30) who are asymptomatic and do not have clinical evidence of atherosclerosis, an exercise ABI measurement is reasonable in order to detect PAD. A toe-brachial index in conjunction with pulsed volume recordings is also reasonable to detect PAD in those patients with non-compressible vessels such as those with diabetes or end stage renal disease who have an ABI greater than 1.3.

Once identified, individuals with asymptomatic PAD benefit from therapeutic interventions to decrease the risk of associated cardiovascular outcomes such as myocardial infarction, stroke, and death, based on level B evidence. These include treatment optimization for diabetes, hypertension, and hyperlipidemia, as well as smoking cessation. Antiplatelet therapy can be initiated to further decrease future cardiovascular events, based on level C evidence. Based on level C evidence, initiation of an Angiotensin Converting Enzyme inhibitor may be considered in those individuals with asymptomatic PAD to decrease cardiovascular morbidity.

1.4.5 2011 ACCF/AHA Focused Update of the Guideline for the Management of Patients with Peripheral Artery Disease (Updating the 2005 Guideline)

In this focused update, use of the resting ABI in individuals in those at high risk of having PAD or suspected of having PAD, such as those who are 50 years and older with diabetes or smoking, individuals above the age of 65, and those with exertional leg symptoms or tissue loss, was supported by level B evidence. The most notable change is that the age of screening was modified to all comers older than 65 [124].

1.4.5.1 Summary of ACCF/AHA Guidelines

The use of resting ABI for PAD screening is recommended in those individuals deemed at high risk, such as those with exertional leg symptoms or tissue loss, or those with diabetes or smoking above the age of 50, or all individuals older than 65.

1.4.6 US Preventive Services Task Force Recommendation

The US Preventative Services Task Force is an organization that evaluates the efficacy of preventative measures in the asymptomatic patient population, taking into account the potential harms and benefits of the test. The 2005 USPTF document recommended against screening for PAD, which was the same recommendation issued in 1996. The 2005 review, however, was limited to the symptoms and functional outcomes of PAD and did not evaluate the potential benefit of cardiovascular risk reduction. These weaknesses were addressed in an editorial which urged the USPSTF to reconsider their recommendations given the potential to reduce myocardial infarction, stroke, and death in patients who have been diagnosed with PAD [131]. The most recent USPSTF publication considered the potential effect of reducing future cardiovascular events, reviewed the evidence on the use of resting ABI alone for the diagnosis of PAD, and summarized its recommendations in a document published in 2013 [125]. It is important to note that they limited the population studied to asymptomatic adults seen in the primary care setting without PAD, cardiovascular disease, renal disease, or diabetes. They reasoned that patients with these disorders are already at high risk for cardiovascular events, and therefore should already be treated with antiplatelet and lipid-lowering therapies, with little additional benefit offered with screen-detected PAD. They felt that ABI was a reliable measure of PAD in symptomatic patients, but the benefit of screening and treatment of asymptomatic PAD in low-risk individuals was unclear. In a randomized trial of asymptomatic individuals with a low ABI, aspirin did not confer any added benefit with regard to cardiovascular morbidity [132]. They also point out that there is no data on the added benefit of lipid-lowering therapy in asymptomatic PAD patients without cardiovascular disease or diabetes. Thus, they concluded that there was no evidence that early treatment of screen-detected PAD improved outcomes.

1.4.7 Harms of Detection and Early Treatment

The USPSTF bases its recommendations on the potential harms and benefits of the screening tool. They did not find any studies which addressed the potential harms of screening for PAD with ABI. However, they acknowledge that the risks of the test itself are minimal. They list other potential harms such as false positive results, the need to undergo further testing via CTA or MRA for confirmation of the diagnosis, labeling, anxiety, and opportunity-related costs. The individual could undergo reclassification to a higher risk category, leading to additional therapies that may cause harm, or reclassification to a lower risk category, where discontinuation of therapies may be harmful. In addition, while earlier screening tests may allow for reduction of cardiovascular events, these identified individuals may never develop clinical signs of PAD, and yet may still be subjected to the harms of additional testing and treatments. Their overall assessment was that there was insufficient evidence to support screening via ABI for asymptomatic individuals without diabetes or cardiovascular disease, and therefore that the balance between risks and benefits could not be determined.

1.4.8 Cost

There is little cost associated with performance of an ABI. The main costs include the time to conduct the exam (15 min) and the staffing required to perform the test. Lost time on the part of the individual occurs as a result, potentially preventing them from undergoing other screening tests that may be beneficial for their health.

1.4.9 Summary of USPSTF Guidelines

The USPSTF current recommendation, aI statement, notes that there is insufficient evidence to evaluate the balance of harms and benefits in using ABI to screen for PAD in low-risk populations to prevent future cardiovascular morbidity.

Key Points

Abdominal aortic aneurysm

Undetected AAAs represent a major public health concern because of the high rates of mortality with rupture. Ultrasound imaging has emerged as a viable screening modality because of its high sensitivity and specificity, reproducibility, portability, safety, and affordability. While separate guidelines have been published by multiple societies and governmental agencies, they share a consensus for those populations considered at high risk, i.e., men aged 65–75 with a history of smoking. Controversy still exists over other subpopulations for which the data is inconsistent or lacking altogether, i.e., women, younger non-smoking men, and those with risk factors other than smoking or a strong family history. Improved definition of those populations at high risk who will most benefit from screening is needed.

Carotid Stenosis

With the data available, the potential harms outweigh the benefits of population screening of adults, particularly elderly patients, for asymptomatic CAS. For this reason, this practice is discouraged by the major societal groups. Future work needs to be conducted with the goal of developing valid and reliable tools to determine which people are at high risk for CAS, as well as those who are at high risk for stroke once diagnosed with CAS. Once this population with a higher prevalence is identified, selective screening would prove more fruitful, as the positive predictive value of carotid DUS would increase and thus limit the false positives and unnecessary harms from further workup and interventions. While no current algorithm exists, it would be reasonable to adopt the approach of the SVS in terms of selective screening of asymptomatic patients with multiple risk factors for CAS at a point at which surgical intervention would be tolerated with minimal risk of perioperative stroke, MI, or death. Other areas of future work include comparing CEA and CAAS (carotid artery angioplasty and stenting) to current best medical practice to determine if there is truly a benefit from surgical intervention, which is being studied in CREST-2. These studies will also be more inclusive of a diverse patient sample, especially women and minorities, who were excluded from the three major RCTs of the 1990s.

Peripheral Artery Disease

In select high-risk populations (age older than 50 with diabetes or smoking, age older than 65, those with exertional leg symptoms or tissue loss), using ABI as a screening tool can be effective for the diagnosis of PAD, as traditional questionnaires have limited sensitivity, and the prevalence of PAD in these patients is high. It remains to be determined if ABI should be used to screen the asymptomatic population without diabetes or cardiovascular or renal disease. Large population studies dedicated to better defining the prevalence and burden of asymptomatic, screen-detected PAD are needed. Large population intervention studies are also needed to better define the potential harms and benefits of this screening test.

References

1. Anderson RN. Deaths: leading causes for 2000. Natl Vital Stat Rep. 2002;50(16):1–85.
2. Bush RL, Lin PH, Lumsden AB. Endovascular management of abdominal aortic aneurysms. J Cardiovasc Surg (Torino). 2003;44(4):527–34.
3. Schermerhorn M. A 66-year-old man with an abdominal aortic aneurysm: review of screening and treatment. JAMA. 2009;302(18):2015–22.
4. Hirsch AT, Haskal ZJ, Hertzer NR, Bakal CW, Creager MA, Halperin JL, et al. ACC/AHA 2005 Practice Guidelines for the management of patients with peripheral arterial disease (lower extremity, renal, mesenteric, and abdominal aortic): a collaborative report from the American Association for Vascular Surgery/Society for Vascular Surgery, Society for Cardiovascular Angiography and Interventions, Society for Vascular Medicine and Biology, Society of Interventional Radiology, and the ACC/AHA Task Force on Practice Guidelines (Writing Committee to Develop Guidelines for the Management of Patients With Peripheral Arterial Disease): endorsed by the American Association of Cardiovascular and Pulmonary Rehabilitation; National Heart, Lung, and Blood Institute; Society for Vascular Nursing; TransAtlantic Inter-Society Consensus; and Vascular Disease Foundation. Circulation. 2006;113(11):e463–654.

5. Eckroth-Bernard K, Garvin RP, Ryer EJ, Elmore JR, Franklin DP. The SAAAVE act and routine ambulatory medical care fail to diagnose patients with abdominal aortic aneurysms prior to rupture: a single-institution experience. Int Scholarly Res Not. 2013;2013:134019.
6. Ferket BS, Grootenboer N, Colkesen EB, Visser JJ, van Sambeek MR, Spronk S, et al. Systematic review of guidelines on abdominal aortic aneurysm screening. J Vasc Surg. 2012;55(5):1296–304.
7. LeFevre ML, U.S. Preventive Services Task Force. Screening for abdominal aortic aneurysm: U.S. Preventive Services Task Force recommendation statement. Ann Intern Med. 2014;161(4):281–90.
8. Lim LS, Haq N, Mahmood S, Hoeksema L, ACPM Prevention Practice Committee, American College of Preventive Medicine. Atherosclerotic cardiovascular disease screening in adults: American College of Preventive Medicine position statement on preventive practice. Am J Prev Med. 2011;40(3):381.e1–10.
9. Chaikof EL, Brewster DC, Dalman RL, Makaroun MS, Illig KA, Sicard GA, et al. The care of patients with an abdominal aortic aneurysm: the Society for Vascular Surgery practice guidelines. J Vasc Surg. 2009;50(4 Suppl):S2–49.
10. Scott RA, Bridgewater SG, Ashton HA. Randomized clinical trial of screening for abdominal aortic aneurysm in women. Br J Surg. 2002;89(3):283–5.
11. Svensjo S, Bjorck M, Wanhainen A. Current prevalence of abdominal aortic aneurysm in 70-year-old women. Br J Surg. 2013;100(3):367–72.
12. Kent KC, Zwolak RM, Jaff MR, Hollenbeck ST, Thompson RW, Schermerhorn ML, et al. Screening for abdominal aortic aneurysm: a consensus statement. J Vasc Surg. 2004;39(1):267–9.
13. Mureebe L, Egorova N, Giacovelli JK, Gelijns A, Kent KC, McKinsey JF. National trends in the repair of ruptured abdominal aortic aneurysms. J Vasc Surg. 2008;48(5):1101–7.
14. Kung HC, Hoyert DL, Xu J, Murphy SL. Deaths: final data for 2005. Natl Vital Stat Rep. 2008;56(10):1–120.
15. Longo C, Upchurch Jr GR. Abdominal aortic aneurysm screening: recommendations and controversies. Vasc Endovascular Surg. 2005;39(3):213–9.
16. Davis M, Harris M, Earnshaw JJ. Implementation of the National Health Service Abdominal Aortic Aneurysm Screening Program in England. J Vasc Surg. 2013;57(5):1440–5.
17. Mastracci TM, Cina CS, Canadian Society for Vascular Surgery. Screening for abdominal aortic aneurysm in Canada: review and position statement of the Canadian Society for Vascular Surgery. J Vasc Surg. 2007;45(6):1268–76.
18. Moll FL, Powell JT, Fraedrich G, Verzini F, Haulon S, Waltham M, et al. Management of abdominal aortic aneurysms clinical practice guidelines of the European society for vascular surgery. Eur J Vasc Endovasc Surg. 2011;41(Suppl 1):S1–S58.
19. Guirguis-Blake JM, Beil TL, Senger CA, Whitlock EP. Ultrasonography screening for abdominal aortic aneurysms: a systematic evidence review for the U.S. Preventive Services Task Force. Ann Intern Med. 2014;160(5):321–9.
20. Lederle FA, Johnson GR, Wilson SE, Chute EP, Hye RJ, Makaroun MS, et al. The aneurysm detection and management study screening program: validation cohort and final results. Aneurysm detection and management veterans affairs cooperative study investigators. Arch Intern Med. 2000;160(10):1425–30.
21. Newman AB, Arnold AM, Burke GL, O'Leary DH, Manolio TA. Cardiovascular disease and mortality in older adults with small abdominal aortic aneurysms detected by ultrasonography: the cardiovascular health study. Ann Intern Med. 2001;134(3):182–90.
22. Tornwall ME, Virtamo J, Haukka JK, Albanes D, Huttunen JK. Life-style factors and risk for abdominal aortic aneurysm in a cohort of Finnish male smokers. Epidemiology. 2001;12(1):94–100.
23. Singh K, Bonaa KH, Jacobsen BK, Bjork L, Solberg S. Prevalence of and risk factors for abdominal aortic aneurysms in a population-based study: The Tromso Study. Am J Epidemiol. 2001;154(3):236–44.
24. Lederle FA, Johnson GR, Wilson SE, Chute EP, Littooy FN, Bandyk D, et al. Prevalence and associations of abdominal aortic aneurysm detected through screening. Aneurysm Detection

and Management (ADAM) Veterans Affairs Cooperative Study Group. Ann Intern Med. 1997;126(6):441–9.
25. Kent KC, Zwolak RM, Egorova NN, Riles TS, Manganaro A, Moskowitz AJ, et al. Analysis of risk factors for abdominal aortic aneurysm in a cohort of more than 3 million individuals. J Vasc Surg. 2010;52(3):539–48.
26. Salo JA, Soisalon-Soininen S, Bondestam S, Mattila PS. Familial occurrence of abdominal aortic aneurysm. Ann Intern Med. 1999;130(8):637–42.
27. Farooq MM, Freischlag JA, Seabrook GR, Moon MR, Aprahamian C, Towne JB. Effect of the duration of symptoms, transport time, and length of emergency room stay on morbidity and mortality in patients with ruptured abdominal aortic aneurysms. Surgery. 1996;119(1):9–14.
28. Emerton ME, Shaw E, Poskitt K, Heather BP. Screening for abdominal aortic aneurysm: a single scan is enough. Br J Surg. 1994;81(8):1112–3.
29. Collaborators RESCAN, Bown MJ, Sweeting MJ, Brown LC, Powell JT, Thompson SG. Surveillance intervals for small abdominal aortic aneurysms: a meta-analysis. JAMA. 2013;309(8):806–13.
30. Brewster DC, Cronenwett JL, Hallett Jr JW, Johnston KW, Krupski WC, Matsumura JS, et al. Guidelines for the treatment of abdominal aortic aneurysms. Report of a subcommittee of the Joint Council of the American Association for Vascular Surgery and Society for Vascular Surgery. J Vasc Surg. 2003;37(5):1106–17.
31. Lederle FA, Johnson GR, Wilson SE, Ballard DJ, Jordan Jr WD, Blebea J, et al. Rupture rate of large abdominal aortic aneurysms in patients refusing or unfit for elective repair. JAMA. 2002;287(22):2968–72.
32. Johansson G, Nydahl S, Olofsson P, Swedenborg J. Survival in patients with abdominal aortic aneurysms. Comparison between operative and nonoperative management. Eur J Vasc Surg. 1990;4(5):497–502.
33. Mortality results for randomised controlled trial of early elective surgery or ultrasonographic surveillance for small abdominal aortic aneurysms. The UK Small Aneurysm Trial Participants. Lancet. 1998;352(9141):1649–55.
34. Chervu A, Clagett GP, Valentine RJ, Myers SI, Rossi PJ. Role of physical examination in detection of abdominal aortic aneurysms. Surgery. 1995;117(4):454–7.
35. Ashton HA, Buxton MJ, Day NE, Kim LG, Marteau TM, Scott RA, et al. The Multicentre Aneurysm Screening Study (MASS) into the effect of abdominal aortic aneurysm screening on mortality in men: a randomised controlled trial. Lancet. 2002;360(9345):1531–9.
36. Lindholt JS, Juul S, Fasting H, Henneberg EW. Screening for abdominal aortic aneurysms: single centre randomised controlled trial. BMJ. 2005;330(7494):750.
37. Scott RA, Wilson NM, Ashton HA, Kay DN. Influence of screening on the incidence of ruptured abdominal aortic aneurysm: 5-year results of a randomized controlled study. Br J Surg. 1995;82(8):1066–70.
38. Norman PE, Jamrozik K, Lawrence-Brown MM, Le MT, Spencer CA, Tuohy RJ, et al. Population based randomised controlled trial on impact of screening on mortality from abdominal aortic aneurysm. BMJ. 2004;329(7477):1259.
39. Cosford PA, Leng GC. Screening for abdominal aortic aneurysm. Cochrane Database Syst Rev. 2007;(2):CD002945.
40. Takagi H, Goto SN, Matsui M, Manabe H, Umemoto T. A further meta-analysis of population-based screening for abdominal aortic aneurysm. J Vasc Surg. 2010;52(4):1103–8.
41. Thompson SG, Ashton HA, Gao L, Buxton MJ, Scott RA. Multicentre Aneurysm Screening Study (MASS) Group. Final follow-up of the Multicentre Aneurysm Screening Study (MASS) randomized trial of abdominal aortic aneurysm screening. Br J Surg. 2012;99(12):1649–56.
42. Thompson SG, Ashton HA, Gao L, Scott RA, Multicentre Aneurysm Screening Study Group. Screening men for abdominal aortic aneurysm: 10 year mortality and cost effectiveness results from the randomised Multicentre Aneurysm Screening Study. BMJ. 2009;338:b2307.
43. Kim LG, P Scott RA, Ashton HA, Thompson SG, Multicentre Aneurysm Screening Study Group. A sustained mortality benefit from screening for abdominal aortic aneurysm. Ann Intern Med. 2007;146(10):699–706.

44. Lindholt JS, Juul S, Fasting H, Henneberg EW. Preliminary ten year results from a randomised single centre mass screening trial for abdominal aortic aneurysm. Eur J Vasc Endovasc Surg. 2006;32(6):608–14.
45. Chun KC, Teng KY, Van Spyk EN, Carson JG, Lee ES. Outcomes of an abdominal aortic aneurysm screening program. J Vasc Surg. 2013;57(2):376–81.
46. U.S. Preventive Services Task Force. U.S. Preventive Services Task Force procedure manual. Rockville: Agency for Healthcare Research and Quality. 2008; Available at: www.uspreventiveservicestaskforce.org/uspstf08/methods/procmanual.htm. Accessed 05 Oct 2015.
47. Lindholt JS, Sorensen J, Sogaard R, Henneberg EW. Long-term benefit and cost-effectiveness analysis of screening for abdominal aortic aneurysms from a randomized controlled trial. Br J Surg. 2010;97(6):826–34.
48. Ashton HA, Gao L, Kim LG, Druce PS, Thompson SG, Scott RA. Fifteen-year follow-up of a randomized clinical trial of ultrasonographic screening for abdominal aortic aneurysms. Br J Surg. 2007;94(6):696–701.
49. Fleming C, Whitlock EP, Beil TL, Lederle FA. Screening for abdominal aortic aneurysm: a best-evidence systematic review for the U.S. Preventive Services Task Force. Ann Intern Med. 2005;142(3):203–11.
50. Darwood R, Earnshaw JJ, Turton G, Shaw E, Whyman M, Poskitt K, et al. Twenty-year review of abdominal aortic aneurysm screening in men in the county of Gloucestershire, United Kingdom. J Vasc Surg. 2012;56(1):8–13.
51. Sweeting MJ, Thompson SG, Brown LC, Powell JT, RESCAN Collaborators. Meta-analysis of individual patient data to examine factors affecting growth and rupture of small abdominal aortic aneurysms. Br J Surg. 2012;99(5):655–65.
52. Greco G, Egorova NN, Gelijns AC, Moskowitz AJ, Manganaro AJ, Zwolak RM, et al. Development of a novel scoring tool for the identification of large >/=5 cm abdominal aortic aneurysms. Ann Surg. 2010;252(4):675–82.
53. Lederle FA, Nelson DB, Joseph AM. Smokers' relative risk for aortic aneurysm compared with other smoking-related diseases: a systematic review. J Vasc Surg. 2003;38(2):329–34.
54. Lindholt JS, Juul S, Henneberg EW. High-risk and low-risk screening for abdominal aortic aneurysm both reduce aneurysm-related mortality. A stratified analysis from a single-centre randomised screening trial. Eur J Vasc Endovasc Surg. 2007;34(1):53–8.
55. Spencer CA, Jamrozik K, Norman PE, Lawrence-Brown MM. The potential for a selective screening strategy for abdominal aortic aneurysm. J Med Screen. 2000;7(4):209–11.
56. Lindholt JS, Henneberg EW, Fasting H, Juul S. Mass or high-risk screening for abdominal aortic aneurysm. Br J Surg. 1997;84(1):40–2.
57. Kim LG, Thompson SG, Briggs AH, Buxton MJ, Campbell HE. How cost-effective is screening for abdominal aortic aneurysms? J Med Screen. 2007;14(1):46–52.
58. Ehlers L, Overvad K, Sorensen J, Christensen S, Bech M, Kjolby M. Analysis of cost effectiveness of screening Danish men aged 65 for abdominal aortic aneurysm. BMJ. 2009;338:b2243.
59. Multicentre Aneurysm Screening Study Group. Multicentre aneurysm screening study (MASS): cost effectiveness analysis of screening for abdominal aortic aneurysms based on four year results from randomised controlled trial. BMJ. 2002;325(7373):1135.
60. Spronk S, van Kempen BJ, Boll AP, Jorgensen JJ, Hunink MG, Kristiansen IS. Cost-effectiveness of screening for abdominal aortic aneurysm in the Netherlands and Norway. Br J Surg. 2011;98(11):1546–55.
61. Svensjo S, Mani K, Bjorck M, Lundkvist J, Wanhainen A. Screening for abdominal aortic aneurysm in 65-year-old men remains cost-effective with contemporary epidemiology and management. Eur J Vasc Endovasc Surg. 2014;47(4):357–65.
62. Thompson S, Kim L, Gao L. Abdominal aortic aneurysm. Comparing studies for cost effectiveness of screening. BMJ. 2009;339:b3044.
63. Buxton MJ. Screening for abdominal aortic aneurysm. BMJ. 2009;338:b2185.
64. Barnett SB, Ter Haar GR, Ziskin MC, Rott HD, Duck FA, Maeda K. International recommendations and guidelines for the safe use of diagnostic ultrasound in medicine. Ultrasound Med Biol. 2000;26(3):355–66.

65. Johansson M, Hansson A, Brodersen J. Estimating overdiagnosis in screening for abdominal aortic aneurysm: could a change in smoking habits and lowered aortic diameter tip the balance of screening towards harm? BMJ. 2015;350:h825.
66. Lindholt JS, Juul S, Fasting H, Henneberg EW. Hospital costs and benefits of screening for abdominal aortic aneurysms. Results from a randomised population screening trial. Eur J Vasc Endovasc Surg. 2002;23(1):55–60.
67. Lesjak M, Boreland F, Lyle D, Sidford J, Flecknoe-Brown S, Fletcher J. Screening for abdominal aortic aneurysm: does it affect men's quality of life? Aust J Prim Health. 2012;18(4):284–8.
68. Spencer CA, Norman PE, Jamrozik K, Tuohy R, Lawrence-Brown M. Is screening for abdominal aortic aneurysm bad for your health and well-being? ANZ J Surg. 2004;74(12):1069–75.
69. Wanhainen A, Rosen C, Rutegard J, Bergqvist D, Bjorck M. Low quality of life prior to screening for abdominal aortic aneurysm: a possible risk factor for negative mental effects. Ann Vasc Surg. 2004;18(3):287–93.
70. Lindholt JS, Vammen S, Fasting H, Henneberg EW. Psychological consequences of screening for abdominal aortic aneurysm and conservative treatment of small abdominal aortic aneurysms. Eur J Vasc Endovasc Surg. 2000;20(1):79–83.
71. Lucarotti ME, Heather BP, Shaw E, Poskitt KR. Psychological morbidity associated with abdominal aortic aneurysm screening. Eur J Vasc Endovasc Surg. 1997;14(6):499–501.
72. Huber TS, Wang JG, Derrow AE, Dame DA, Ozaki CK, Zelenock GB, et al. Experience in the United States with intact abdominal aortic aneurysm repair. J Vasc Surg. 2001;33(2):304–10; discussion 310–1.
73. Lederle FA, Freischlag JA, Kyriakides TC, Padberg Jr FT, Matsumura JS, Kohler TR, et al. Outcomes following endovascular vs open repair of abdominal aortic aneurysm: a randomized trial. JAMA. 2009;302(14):1535–42.
74. Lederle FA, Wilson SE, Johnson GR, Reinke DB, Littooy FN, Acher CW, et al. Immediate repair compared with surveillance of small abdominal aortic aneurysms. N Engl J Med. 2002;346(19):1437–44.
75. United Kingdom Small Aneurysm Trial Participants. Long-term outcomes of immediate repair compared with surveillance of small abdominal aortic aneurysms. N Engl J Med. 2002;346(19):1445–52.
76. Society for Vascular Surgery. SAAAVE Act Background. 2010; Available at: https://www.vascularweb.org/healthpolicyandgovernmentrelations/Pages/saaave-act-background.aspx.
77. Shreibati JB, Baker LC, Hlatky MA, Mell MW. Impact of the Screening Abdominal Aortic Aneurysms Very Efficiently (SAAAVE) Act on abdominal ultrasonography use among Medicare beneficiaries. Arch Intern Med. 2012;172(19):1456–62.
78. Harris R, Sheridan S, Kinsinger L. Time to rethink screening for abdominal aortic aneurysm? Arch Intern Med. 2012;172(19):1462–3.
79. Hadjibashi AA, Ng T, Mirocha J, Cossman D, Gewertz B. Reduction in ruptured aortic aneurysms is not due to increases in endovascular repairs. Am Surg. 2011;77(10):1395–8.
80. Anjum A, Powell JT. Is the incidence of abdominal aortic aneurysm declining in the 21st century? Mortality and hospital admissions for England & Wales and Scotland. Eur J Vasc Endovasc Surg. 2012;43(2):161–6.
81. Lee ES, Pickett E, Hedayati N, Dawson DL, Pevec WC. Implementation of an aortic screening program in clinical practice: implications for the Screen For Abdominal Aortic Aneurysms Very Efficiently (SAAAVE) Act. J Vasc Surg. 2009;49(5):1107–11.
82. Macdonald AJ, Faleh O, Welch G, Kettlewell S. Missed opportunities for the detection of abdominal aortic aneurysms. Eur J Vasc Endovasc Surg. 2008;35(6):698–700.
83. Gore. The Ultimate SAAAVE. 2010; Available at: http://ultimatesaaave.com/.
84. Sacco RL, Kasner SE, Broderick JP, Caplan LR, Connors JJ, Culebras A, et al. An updated definition of stroke for the 21st century: a statement for healthcare professionals from the American Heart Association/American Stroke Association. Stroke. 2013;44(7):2064–89.
85. Roger VL, Go AS, Lloyd-Jones DM, Benjamin EJ, Berry JD, Borden WB, et al. Executive summary: heart disease and stroke statistics – 2012 update: a report from the American Heart Association. Circulation. 2012;125(1):188–97.

86. Gresham GE, Fitzpatrick TE, Wolf PA, McNamara PM, Kannel WB, Dawber TR. Residual disability in survivors of stroke – the Framingham study. N Engl J Med. 1975;293(19):954–6.
87. Rothwell PM, Coull AJ, Giles MF, Howard SC, Silver LE, Bull LM, et al. Change in stroke incidence, mortality, case-fatality, severity, and risk factors in Oxfordshire, UK from 1981 to 2004 (Oxford Vascular Study). Lancet. 2004;363(9425):1925–33.
88. Goldstein LB, Bushnell CD, Adams RJ, Appel LJ, Braun LT, Chaturvedi S, et al. Guidelines for the primary prevention of stroke: a guideline for healthcare professionals from the American Heart Association/American Stroke Association. Stroke. 2011;42(2):517–84.
89. Kistler JP, Furie KL. Carotid endarterectomy revisited. N Engl J Med. 2000;342(23):1743–5.
90. Jonas DE, Feltner C, Amick HR, Sheridan S, Zheng ZJ, Watford DJ, et al. Screening for asymptomatic carotid artery stenosis: a systematic review and meta-analysis for the U.S. Preventive Services Task Force. Ann Intern Med. 2014;161(5):336–46.
91. Longstreth Jr WT, Shemanski L, Lefkowitz D, O'Leary DH, Polak JF, Wolfson Jr SK. Asymptomatic internal carotid artery stenosis defined by ultrasound and the risk of subsequent stroke in the elderly. The Cardiovascular Health Study. Stroke. 1998;29(11):2371–6.
92. Goldstein LB. Screening for asymptomatic carotid artery stenosis: caveat emptor. Ann Intern Med. 2014;161(5):370–1.
93. Lanzino G, Rabinstein AA, Brown RD Jr. Treatment of carotid artery stenosis: medical therapy, surgery, or stenting? Mayo Clin Proc. 2009;84(4):362–87; quiz 367–8.
94. Rothwell PM, Eliasziw M, Gutnikov SA, Warlow CP, Barnett HJ, Carotid Endarterectomy Trialists Collaboration. Endarterectomy for symptomatic carotid stenosis in relation to clinical subgroups and timing of surgery. Lancet. 2004;363(9413):915–24.
95. Chambers BR, Donnan GA. Carotid endarterectomy for asymptomatic carotid stenosis. Cochrane Database Syst Rev. 2005;(4):CD001923.
96. Endarterectomy for asymptomatic carotid artery stenosis. Executive Committee for the Asymptomatic Carotid Atherosclerosis Study. JAMA. 1995;273(18):1421–8.
97. Fine-Edelstein JS, Wolf PA, O'Leary DH, Poehlman H, Belanger AJ, Kase CS, et al. Precursors of extracranial carotid atherosclerosis in the Framingham Study. Neurology. 1994;44(6):1046–50.
98. Halliday A, Mansfield A, Marro J, Peto C, Peto R, Potter J, et al. Prevention of disabling and fatal strokes by successful carotid endarterectomy in patients without recent neurological symptoms: randomised controlled trial. Lancet. 2004;363(9420):1491–502.
99. Raman G, Moorthy D, Hadar N, Dahabreh IJ, O'Donnell TF, Thaler DE, et al. Management strategies for asymptomatic carotid stenosis: a systematic review and meta-analysis. Ann Intern Med. 2013;158(9):676–85.
100. Abbott AL. Medical (nonsurgical) intervention alone is now best for prevention of stroke associated with asymptomatic severe carotid stenosis: results of a systematic review and analysis. Stroke. 2009;40(10):e573–83.
101. Marquardt L, Geraghty OC, Mehta Z, Rothwell PM. Low risk of ipsilateral stroke in patients with asymptomatic carotid stenosis on best medical treatment: a prospective, population-based study. Stroke. 2010;41(1):e11–7.
102. de Weerd M, Greving JP, de Jong AW, Buskens E, Bots ML. Prevalence of asymptomatic carotid artery stenosis according to age and sex: systematic review and metaregression analysis. Stroke. 2009;40(4):1105–13.
103. de Weerd M, Greving JP, Hedblad B, Lorenz MW, Mathiesen EB, O'Leary DH, et al. Prevalence of asymptomatic carotid artery stenosis in the general population: an individual participant data meta-analysis. Stroke. 2010;41(6):1294–7.
104. Chambers BR, Norris JW. Clinical significance of asymptomatic neck bruits. Neurology. 1985;35(5):742–5.
105. LeFevre ML, U.S. Preventive Services Task Force. Screening for asymptomatic carotid artery stenosis: U.S. Preventive Services Task Force recommendation statement. Ann Intern Med. 2014;161(5):356–62.

106. Van Ruiswyk J, Noble H, Sigmann P. The natural history of carotid bruits in elderly persons. Ann Intern Med. 1990;112(5):340–3.
107. McColgan P, Bentley P, McCarron M, Sharma P. Evaluation of the clinical utility of a carotid bruit. QJM. 2012;105(12):1171–7.
108. Pickett CA, Jackson JL, Hemann BA, Atwood JE. Carotid bruits as a prognostic indicator of cardiovascular death and myocardial infarction: a meta-analysis. Lancet. 2008;371(9624): 1587–94.
109. Chambers BR, Norris JW. Outcome in patients with asymptomatic neck bruits. N Engl J Med. 1986;315(14):860–5.
110. Jahromi AS, Cina CS, Liu Y, Clase CM. Sensitivity and specificity of color duplex ultrasound measurement in the estimation of internal carotid artery stenosis: a systematic review and meta-analysis. J Vasc Surg. 2005;41(6):962–72.
111. Sabeti S, Schillinger M, Mlekusch W, Willfort A, Haumer M, Nachtmann T, et al. Quantification of internal carotid artery stenosis with duplex US: comparative analysis of different flow velocity criteria. Radiology. 2004;232(2):431–9.
112. Blakeley DD, Oddone EZ, Hasselblad V, Simel DL, Matchar DB. Noninvasive carotid artery testing. A meta-analytic review. Ann Intern Med. 1995;122(5):360–7.
113. Wardlaw JM, Chappell FM, Best JJ, Wartolowska K, Berry E, NHS Research and Development Health Technology Assessment Carotid Stenosis Imaging Group. Non-invasive imaging compared with intra-arterial angiography in the diagnosis of symptomatic carotid stenosis: a meta-analysis. Lancet. 2006;367(9521):1503–12.
114. Nederkoorn PJ, van der Graaf Y, Hunink MG. Duplex ultrasound and magnetic resonance angiography compared with digital subtraction angiography in carotid artery stenosis: a systematic review. Stroke. 2003;34(5):1324–32.
115. Halliday A, Harrison M, Hayter E, Kong X, Mansfield A, Marro J, et al. 10-year stroke prevention after successful carotid endarterectomy for asymptomatic stenosis (ACST-1): a multicentre randomised trial. Lancet. 2010;376(9746):1074–84.
116. Baker WH, Howard VJ, Howard G, Toole JF. Effect of contralateral occlusion on long-term efficacy of endarterectomy in the asymptomatic carotid atherosclerosis study (ACAS). ACAS Investigators. Stroke. 2000;31(10):2330–4.
117. Hobson 2nd RW, Weiss DG, Fields WS, Goldstone J, Moore WS, Towne JB, et al. Efficacy of carotid endarterectomy for asymptomatic carotid stenosis. The Veterans Affairs Cooperative Study Group. N Engl J Med. 1993;328(4):221–7.
118. Lackland DT, Roccella EJ, Deutsch AF, Fornage M, George MG, Howard G, et al. Factors influencing the decline in stroke mortality: a statement from the American Heart Association/ American Stroke Association. Stroke. 2014;45(1):315–53.
119. Whitty CJ, Sudlow CL, Warlow CP. Investigating individual subjects and screening populations for asymptomatic carotid stenosis can be harmful. J Neurol Neurosurg Psychiatry. 1998;64(5):619–23.
120. Ricotta JJ, Aburahma A, Ascher E, Eskandari M, Faries P, Lal BK, et al. Updated Society for Vascular Surgery guidelines for management of extracranial carotid disease: executive summary. J Vasc Surg. 2011;54(3):832–6.
121. Meschia JF, Bushnell C, Boden-Albala B, Braun LT, Bravata DM, Chaturvedi S, et al. Guidelines for the primary prevention of stroke: a statement for healthcare professionals from the American Heart Association/American Stroke Association. Stroke. 2014;45(12):3754–832.
122. Lloyd-Jones D, Adams R, Carnethon M, De Simone G, Ferguson TB, Flegal K, et al. Heart disease and stroke statistics – 2009 update: a report from the American Heart Association Statistics Committee and Stroke Statistics Subcommittee. Circulation. 2009;119(3):480–6.
123. Lovell M. The peripheral arterial disease coalition and peripheral arterial disease awareness campaign. J Vasc Nurs. 2007;25(4):94–5.
124. Rooke TW, Hirsch AT, Misra S, Sidawy AN, Beckman JA, Findeiss LK, et al. 2011 ACCF/ AHA Focused Update of the Guideline for the Management of Patients With Peripheral Artery Disease (updating the 2005 guideline): a report of the American College of Cardiology Foundation/American Heart Association Task Force on Practice Guidelines. J Am Coll Cardiol. 2011;58(19):2020–45.

125. Moyer VA, U.S. Preventive Services Task Force. Screening for peripheral artery disease and cardiovascular disease risk assessment with the ankle-brachial index in adults: U.S. Preventive Services Task Force recommendation statement. Ann Intern Med. 2013;159(5):342–8.
126. ROSE GA. The diagnosis of ischaemic heart pain and intermittent claudication in field surveys. Bull World Health Organ. 1962;27:645–58.
127. Criqui MH, Denenberg JO, Bird CE, Fronek A, Klauber MR, Langer RD. The correlation between symptoms and non-invasive test results in patients referred for peripheral arterial disease testing. Vasc Med. 1996;1(1):65–71.
128. McDermott MM, Greenland P, Liu K, Guralnik JM, Criqui MH, Dolan NC, et al. Leg symptoms in peripheral arterial disease: associated clinical characteristics and functional impairment. JAMA. 2001;286(13):1599–606.
129. McDermott MM, Liu K, Guralnik JM, Martin GJ, Criqui MH, Greenland P. Measurement of walking endurance and walking velocity with questionnaire: validation of the walking impairment questionnaire in men and women with peripheral arterial disease. J Vasc Surg. 1998;28(6):1072–81.
130. Criqui MH, Fronek A, Klauber MR, Barrett-Connor E, Gabriel S. The sensitivity, specificity, and predictive value of traditional clinical evaluation of peripheral arterial disease: results from noninvasive testing in a defined population. Circulation. 1985;71(3):516–22.
131. Beckman JA, Jaff MR, Creager MA. The United States preventive services task force recommendation statement on screening for peripheral arterial disease: more harm than benefit? Circulation. 2006;114(8):861–6.
132. Fowkes FG, Price JF, Stewart MC, Butcher I, Leng GC, Pell AC, et al. Aspirin for prevention of cardiovascular events in a general population screened for a low ankle brachial index: a randomized controlled trial. JAMA. 2010;303(9):841–8.

Preoperative Optimization of the Elderly Patient Prior to Vascular Surgery

2

Jason M. Johanning, G. Matthew Longo, and Alyson Ashleigh Melin

2.1 General Changes Associated with Aging

In aging, multiple factors including biologic, genetic, environmental, and lifestyle choices effect longevity [1]. Elderly patients exhibit diminished physiologic reserves and often require exhaustion of these reserves to maintain homeostasis. Sarcopenia relates to nutrition and decreased muscle mass in elderly patients compared to age-matched controls. It has been found to correlate with a markedly increased risk of mortality and morbidity [2, 3]. Muscle breakdown and anorexia occur due to an upregulation of IL-1, IL-6, and TNF-alpha [4, 5]. Sarcopenia is observed in more than half of patients over the age of 80 and leads not only to a loss of muscle mass but a decrease in strength and functionality [6, 7]. There is a shift in body mass from muscle to adipose tissue. This is associated with a loss of lean body mass and total body water. This has important implications when prescribing and dosing medications, resulting in higher average and peak plasma concentrations and decreased clearance [8]. Additionally, low albumin levels increase the free levels of drugs usually bound by albumin [9]. Given the patient population a vascular surgeon treats, the presence of sarcopenia should be given consideration when counseling patients as it equates to an approximate two- to threefold risk of complications and mortality compared to the nonsarcopenic patient.

Elderly patients have structural anatomical changes that significantly affect the physiology of individual organ systems. From a cardiopulmonary perspective, decreased chest wall compliance, maximum inspiratory and expiratory force, vital

J.M. Johanning (✉) • G. Matthew Longo
Department of Surgery University of Nebraska Medical Center, Omaha VA Medical Center, The Nebraska Medical Center, Omaha, NE, USA
e-mail: jjohanning@unmc.edu; glongo@unmc.edu

A.A. Melin
Department of Surgery, University of Nebraska Medical Center, Omaha, NE, USA
e-mail: Aly.Melin@unmc.edu

R. Chaer (ed.), *Vascular Disease in Older Adults*,
DOI 10.1007/978-3-319-29285-4_2

capacity, mucociliary clearance, cough reflex, and autonomic response to hypoxia and hypercapnia [10, 11]. Due to changes in pulmonary compliance and incomplete elimination of anesthetics, one must remember respiratory drive may be decreased and aggressive pulmonary toilet must be incorporated. Upright positions and early mobilization must be employed to prevent atelectasis [10].

Cardiac changes include septal thickening, atrial and valvular dilation, and fibrosis of the conduction system [12]. Overall, elderly experience decreased contractility, compliance, and arrhythmias. The most common cause of death in the perioperative elderly patient is cardiac in origin [13]. Myocardial infarction mortality is increased in those over the age of 75 compared with those below 55, 17.8% versus 2.0% [14]. It is vital to recall that a third of patients over 85 will present with classic chest pain during cardiac events, whereas nonspecific complaints are more common heralding a cardiac event [15]. Preoperatively, ECG should be obtained, as well as cardiac clearance should the patient have known underlying cardiac disease. In most vascular procedures, cardiac medications can be continued and case-by-case decisions made regarding anticoagulation or antiplatelet agents given the patient's underlying disease and in conjunction with cardiology recommendations. A multidisciplinary approach is recommended to prevent readmission, improve medication compliance, and improve the functional status of the patient [16].

These changes predispose vascular patients to reduced reserve during open operative cases where cavities are violated, proximal aortic clamping is required, and increased blood loss is expected.

Elderly patients often experience renal dysfunction with reduced glomerular filtration rate and are predisposed to volume overload [17], acute-on-chronic kidney injury, and electrolyte abnormalities [18, 19]. The renal dysfunction in elderly patients should be carefully noted as postoperative renal dysfunction in the elderly is perhaps the single biggest risk factor for increased morbidity and mortality in our surgical elderly population [20, 21]. Knowing renal senescence, irreversible functional and structural changes associated with the kidneys of an aging patient, we must be cognizant of volume overload and electrolyte abnormalities, which are often exacerbated in the perioperative period [21]. Renal failure is not necessary to create a poor postoperative outcome as positive fluid balance alone is an independent risk factor for mortality in critically ill patients with acute kidney injury [22, 23].

The gastrointestinal system remains relatively unchanged in physiology compared to those mentioned previously [24, 25]. Dysphagia is often noted in the perioperative period, but this is more so related to neurologic dysfunction [26]. Postoperative dysphagia, which can lead to aspiration, is often best addressed by a multidisciplinary team of nursing, speech therapy, and the surgical team if identified preoperatively, as aspiration precautions should be mandated in elderly patients who are high risk. H. pylori infection does demonstrate increased incidence with age, thus predisposing patients to gastritis and ulcers, but treatment is similar to that in younger patients. Some studies have noted a shortening of the villi and thus decreased surface area of the intestine with age, which may compound the malnutrition observed in older patients [27]. The presence of malnourishment is observed in 70% of hospitalized elderly patients and is associated with increased morbidity and mortality [28, 29]. Involuntary weight loss is often related to multifactorial risk factors in this patient population [30, 31], but most importantly unintentional weight loss has been repeatedly demonstrated in the literature to be predictive of poor outcomes.

2.2 Preoperative Evaluation of the Surgical Patient: Risk Assessment and Counseling

Consistent with appropriate clinical care, every patient should undergo a thorough history and physical examination, as well as directed evaluation focusing on their underlying comorbidities and extent of necessary operation. Emerging evidence suggests that an objective risk assessment to identify the frail patient can guide decision-making in the preoperative setting, and is important considering 60% of operative interventions performed are done for patients over the age of 65 [32].

Frailty is now a recognized geriatric syndrome that is a strong predictor of postoperative outcomes [33–36]. Frailty, although similar to the previously mentioned sarcopenia, is defined broadly by the presence of one or more of the following: physiological comorbidities, cognitive, physical function, and nutritional and social decline leading to an inability to tolerate physiologic insults. As frailty has become recognized as perhaps the single biggest global risk factor for poor surgical outcomes including mortality, morbidity, length of stay, and readmission rate, it behooves the vascular surgeon to know the basis for assessing frailty in the surgical patient and have the ability to apply frailty identification in surgical practice. Two classic approaches have been utilized to assess the surgical patient for frailty preoperatively. The first is to identify the *frailty phenotype*, which relies heavily on sarcopenic assessment. This is performed using the classic Fried assessment consisting of grip strength, walking speed, exhaustion, and leisure time assessment questionnaires. This approach, although time-consuming taking 20–30 min to complete, has now been clearly documented with markedly increased negative outcomes in surgical patients. The Fried-Hopkins frailty index, when compared to standard risk prediction models, improved the predictive power of associated perioperative risk. Those identified as frail showed increased risk of complications, length of stay, and discharge to facility [35, 36]. The second approach popularized by Rockwood is referred to as the *deficit accumulation index* (DAI). Several DAI tools are available to assess the presurgical patient including the Risk Analysis Index, the FRAIL scale, and mFI. All of the tools rely on simple powerful questions that are nonphysiologic in nature but have high prognostic validity and have been explored in the vascular surgery patient population. Alluding to the strength of this approach, both the Risk Analysis Index (RAI) and Modified Frailty Index (mFI) have been used to assess national outcome databases to demonstrate that poor outcomes in carotid and aneurysm patients, respectively, can be predicted by assessing the frailty status of the preoperative patient. In specific cases such as carotid endarterectomy where outcomes are of utmost importance, recent data suggests it is very important that frail patients are informed of the risk-benefit ratio of the proposed procedure, especially asymptomatic patients. Data suggests that higher RAI or frailty scores were correlated with higher morbidity and mortality than the "acceptable" risk of undergoing CEA Carotid Endarterectomy defined by preceding trials. The utility of this approach is the ease of administration of the tool, which takes less than five min to administer. This simple tool provides the surgeon the ability to identify the patient at marked increased surgical risk in an objective and systematic fashion and provide specific counseling to the patient. This in particular has been used to identify the frail patient in a busy clinic and provides an indicator for an opportunity to refer the patient to the palliative care team for discussions on goals of care to best honor the patient's preferences [32].

Special mention regarding cognitive dysfunction is necessary given our patients' age and prevalence of this condition postoperatively. Surgeons must be mindful of postoperative cognitive impairment in elderly patients. The literature suggests that postoperative delirium, an acute change in cognition characterized by fluctuating attention and consciousness, has an incidence of 36–75% in older adults [37, 38]. Although this is often recognized in our patients, it has been shown to correlate with prolonged length of stay, delayed recovery, and increased morbidity and mortality [39]. Although multiple factors may contribute to postoperative delirium, Inouye et al. have identified five independent risk factors: baseline dementia, vision impairment, physical restraints, functional impairment, and a high number of comorbidities [40]. One may perform the Mini Mental Status Exam, Abbreviated Mental Test, or Confusion Assessment Method to confirm the diagnosis and follow improvement or decline. In an effort to combat delirium, we should monitor and correct dehydration and infectious etiology and return glasses and hearing aids to patients as early as possible. To treat acutely, haloperidol can be used, but if ineffective, lorazepam should be considered [39]. Lastly, normalization of sleep-wake cycle may also be useful. Postoperative cognitive dysfunction may occur later in the postoperative course. It is often more subtle compared with delirium but may be more longstanding. It is characterized by impairment of memory, concentration, and social integration. The literature states that 25% of patients were noted to have postoperative cognitive dysfunction and it remained in 10% at 3 months [41]. Similar to delirium, cognitive dysfunction is also related to increased morbidity and mortality [42]. The use of general anesthesia, multiple comorbidities, and poor functional status is associated with increased risk of cognitive dysfunction [43]. Diagnosis is difficult due to lack of uniform criteria and is often confused with features of Alzheimer's, and even when diagnosed there is no uniform evidence for successful treatment [39, 44].

Those who are identified as frail should ideally undergo a comprehensive geriatric assessment and have a palliative care consultation in conjunction with the standard physiologic workup. This approach will allow the vascular team to incorporate shared decision-making and discussion of increased morbidity and mortality compared to the nonfrail patient; develop a comprehensive treatment plan; provide simple pre-, intra-, and postoperative interventions to improve outcomes; and ultimately increase the communication amongst providers regarding treatment of the high risk patient [40]. An excellent roadmap has been generated by the American College of Surgeons in collaboration with the American Geriatrics Society to create guidelines for the workup of the elderly frail patient. The comprehensive geriatric assessment should not be looked at as an all-or-none endeavor but rather that individual sections of the Comprehensive Geriatric Assessment (CGA) can be chosen a la carte based on the needs of the individual patient [45, 47].

Alluding to the usual sound clinical judgment, mortality rates for elective operations in the elderly are similar to those in younger cohorts; however, this is not applicable in emergent cases. Emergent cases are both more prevalent in elderly patients and carry a much higher morbidity and mortality when compared with younger patients [48–51]. Furthermore, many postoperative elderly patients require discharge to facilities and experience a significant decrease in independence [51, 52]. Taken in total, the data stresses the importance of screening and optimization of elderly patients who must undergo surgical intervention. Additionally, this should encourage us to have appropriate and candid discussions and place emphasis on shared decision-making regarding appropriate risk and end-of-life care.

2.3 Optimization of the Preoperative Patient

Once a surgeon identifies a patient being at higher risk due to physiological comorbidities, and cognitive, social, physical, or nutritional dysfunction, an attempt should be made to address the underlying cause of the dysfunction and ameliorate the perioperative stress. Preoperative patient comorbidities are common, and once identified, the treatment of pulmonary, cardiac, and renal dysfunction should be addressed through appropriate consultations and medical management, the scope of which is beyond this chapter. From a frailty perspective, the ability to reverse or ameliorate the individual aspects of dysfunction is in its infancy, and it is expected over the next decade that intense research and trials will occur to address the ability of interventions to improve the outcomes in this vulnerable population. Current evidence demonstrates that individual interventions can improve the underlying dysfunction if given adequate time. Given that many vascular surgery patients are elderly and many are frail, the obvious question to ask is whether preoperative frailty is a modifiable risk factor. Data in community-dwelling patients suggests that frailty in fact is a syndrome where a patient can fall in and out of frailty over time. Thus, it would appear that frailty can be modified. What remains to be seen is whether the modification can be made for the vascular surgery patient who is often in a situation where delaying elective procedures is not an option, such as symptomatic carotid disease or rest pain. However, there are situations where a person who is frail may benefit from preoperative intervention, including elective abdominal aortic aneurysm repair depending on aneurysm size and asymptomatic carotid artery. Individually, the frailty domains of social, cognitive, nutritional, and physical function have not been widely studied in frailty specific populations. Perhaps the easiest and most promising route of intervention is that of nutrition. A recent pilot randomized study in colon cancer patients has shown the ability of nutrition counseling plus whey protein to significantly improve physical function in the form of walking. A similar pilot study combining nutritional counseling with anxiety reduction demonstrated postoperative walking to be significantly improved in the intervention arm. Thus, it seems nutritional intervention may be a likely target for patients that is relatively easy to administer, but it is yet unknown whether improvements in surgical outcome will occur. In contrast to nutrition, where human intervention is well accepted and reasonable, postoperative cognitive dysfunction is thought to be associated with a neuroinflammatory state with upregulation of IL1-Beta, IL-6, and TNFalpha. Several substances including lithium and candesartan in the aged rat model have proven to be neuroprotective after laparotomy, and suggest a potential avenue for tackling this vexing problem. Socially, little has been done in the way of intervention, but data from cardiac surgery suggests those patients with high levels of social deprivation are expected to have worse outcomes. Although frailty itself is reflective of systemic dysfunction by multiple systems, it is perhaps the best treatment preoperatively, being a wide and diverse approach as advocated by the Proactive care of older people undergoing surgery (POPS) study by Harari et al. [52]. Using multidisciplinary preoperative CGA service with postoperative follow-through, the authors demonstrated marked improvements in surgical outcomes including delirium, pneumonia, and pain control. These findings were repeated in both Scotland and Nebraska, where coordination of preoperative care among a diverse and collaborative team resulted in markedly improved outcomes for frail elderly patients. Thus, as the literature stands there is no magic pill to reverse frailty or single interventions to markedly improve outcomes. However, growing evidence suggests that multimodal intervention through increased communication and use of geriatric or palliative care consultations holds promise to significantly improve surgical outcomes.

Key Points

- Vascular surgery is a challenging specialty, with the average age of our patients being >65 years. Thus, a knowledge of the physiological changes in the arterial system is of significant importance to the vascular surgeon.
- Given the multiple comorbidities present, it is crucial for the vascular surgeon to be able to identify the frail vascular patient with comorbidities and improve the outcomes of operations by optimizing the comorbid conditions.
- Vascular surgery broadly encompasses interventions related to arterial, venous, and lymphatic pathophysiology. The vascular surgeon establishes a diagnosis and a therapeutic plan and then must determine whether elective, urgent (24–72 h), or emergent intervention is warranted. In the case of urgent or elective interventions, time may allow for a more extensive preoperative evaluation.

- Vascular patients by default due to multiple comorbidities often require extensive workup. When coupled with the average age of the vascular patient, it becomes clear that vascular surgeons are often intervening on the multiple chronic condition elderly patient, and thus the recognition of changes associated with aging is paramount in our specialty.

References

1. Hjelmbor V, Iachine I, Skytthe A, Vaupel J, McGue M, Koskenvuo M, et al. Genetic influence on human lifespan and longevity. Hum Genet. 2006;11(3):312–21.
2. Malafarina V, Uriz-Otano F, Iniesta R, Gil-Guerrero L. Sarcopenia in the elderly: diagnosis, physiopathology and treatment. Maturitas. 2012;71:109–14.
3. Pahor M, Kritchevsky S. Research hypotheses on muscle wasting, aging, loss of function and disability. J Nutr Health Aging. 1998;2:97–100.
4. Evans WJ, Morley JE, Argilés J, Bales C, Baracos V, Guttridge D, et al. Cachexia: a new definition. Clin Nutr. 2008;27:793–9.
5. Martinez M, Arnalich F, Hernanz A. Alterations of anorectic cytokine levels from plasma and cerebrospinal fluid in idiopathic senile anorexia. Mech Ageing Dev. 1993;72:145–53.
6. Roubenoff R. Origins and clinical relevance of sarcopenia. Can J Appl Physiol. 2001;26:78–89.
7. Janssen I. The epidemiology of sarcopenia. Clin Geriatr Med. 2011;27:355–63.
8. Aymanns C, Keller F, Maus S, Hartmann B, Czock D. Review on pharmacokinetics and pharmacodynamics and the aging kidney. Clin J Am Soc Nephrol. 2010;5:314–27.
9. White PF, White LM, Monk T, Jakobsson J, Raeder J, Mulroy MF, et al. Perioperative care for older outpatient undergoing ambulatory surgery. Anesth Analg. 2012;114:1190–215.
10. Sprung J, Gajic O, Warner DO. Review article: age related alteration in respiratory function – anesthetic considerations. Can J Anesth. 2006;53:1244–57.
11. Antonelli M, Conti G, Moro ML, Esquinas A, Gonzalez-Diaz G, Confalonieri M, et al. Predictors of failure of noninvasive positive pressure ventilation in patients with acute hypoxemic respiratory failure: a multi-center study. Intensive Care Med. 2001;27:1718–28.
12. Priebe HJ. The aged cardiovascular risk patient. Br J Anaesth. 2000;85:763.
13. Rosenthal RA, Perkal MF. Physiologic considerations in the elderly surgical patient. In: Miller TA, editor. Modern surgical care: physiologic foundations and clinical applications. 1st ed. New York: Informa; 2006.
14. Weaver WD, Litwin PE, Martin JS, Kudenchuk PJ, Maynard C, Eisenberg MS, et al. Effect of age on use of thrombolytic therapy and mortality in acute myocardial infarction. The MITI Project Group. J Am Coll Cardiol. 1991;18:657–62.
15. Wenger NK. Cardiovascular disease. In: Cassell CK, Leipzig RM, Cohen HJ, Larson EB, Meier DE, editors. Geriatric medicine. 4th ed. New York: Springer; 2003.
16. Rich MW, Beckham V, Wittenberg C, Leven CL, Freedland KE, Carney RM. A multidisciplinary intervention to prevent the readmission of elderly patients with congestive heart failure. N Engl J Med. 1995;333:1190–5.
17. Lindeman RD, Tobin J, Shock NW. Longitudinal studies on the rate of decline in renal function with age. J Am Geriatr Soc. 1985;33:278–85.
18. Schlanger LE, Bailey JL, Sands JM. Electrolytes in the aging. Adv Chronic Kidney Dis. 2010;17:308.
19. Melk A. Senescence of renal cells: molecular basis and clinical implications. Nephrol Dial Transplant. 2003;18:2474–8.
20. Allison SP, Lobo DN. Fluid and electrolytes in the elderly. Curr Opin Clin Nutr Metab Care. 2004;7:27–33.

21. Khan MA, Hossain FS, Dashti Z, Muthukumar N. Causes and predictors of early re-admission after surgery for a fracture of the hip. J Bone Joint Surg Br. 2012;94:690–7.
22. Bagshaw SM, Brophy PD, Cruz D, et al. Fluid balance as a biomarker: impact of fluid overload on outcome in critically ill patients with acute kidney injury. Crit Care. 2008;12:169.
23. Payen D, de Pont AC, Sakr Y, et al. A positive fluid balance is associated with a worse outcome in patients with acute renal failure. Crit Care. 2008;12:R74.
24. Shamburek RD, Farrar J. Disorders of the digestive system in the elderly. N Engl J Med. 1990;322:438.
25. Holt PR. Gastrointestinal system: changes in morphology and cell proliferation. Aging. 1991;3:392; Russell RM. Change in gastrointestinal function attributed to aging. Am J Clin Nutr. 1992;55:1203.
26. Wilson JAP. Gastroenterologic disorders. In: Cassell CK, Leipzig RM, Cohen HJ, Larson EB, Meier DE, editors. Geriatric medicine. 4th ed. New York: Springer; 2003.
27. Holt PR. Gastrointestinal disorders in the elderly: the small intestine. Clin Gastroenterol. 1985;14:689.
28. de Luis D, Lopez GA. Nutritional status of adult patients admitted to internal medicine departments in public hospitals in Castilla y Leon, Spain: a multi-center study. Eur J Intern Med. 2006;17:556.
29. Wallace JI, Schwartz RS, LaCroix AZ, et al. Involuntary weight loss in older outpatients: incidence and clinical significance. J Am Geriatr Soc. 1995;43:329.
30. Skipper A, Ferguson M, Thompson K, et al. Nutrition screening tools: an analysis of the evidence. JPEN J Parenter Enteral Nutr. 2012;36:292.
31. Locher JL, Robinson CO, Roth DL, et al. The effect of the presence of others on caloric intake in homebound older adults. J Gerontol A Biol Sci Med Sci. 2005;60:1475.
32. Etzioni DA, Liu JH, Maggard MA, et al. The aging population and its impact on the surgery workforce. Ann Surg. 2003;238:170.
33. Rockwood K, Mitnitski A. Frailty defined by deficit accumulation and geriatric medicine defined by frailty. Clin Geriatr Med. 2011;27:17.
34. Fried LP, Ferrucci L, Darer J, et al. Untangling the concepts of disability, frailty, and comorbidity: implications for improved targeting and care. J Gerontol A Biol Sci Med Sci. 2004;59:255.
35. Fried LP, Tangen CM, Walston J, et al. Frailty in older adults: evidence for a phenotype. J Gerontol A Biol Sci Med Sci. 2001;56(3):M146.
36. Makary MA, Segev DL, Pronovost PJ, et al. Frailty as a predictor of surgical outcomes in older patients. J Am Coll Surg. 2010;210:901–8.
37. Dyer CB, Aston CM, Teasdale TA. Postoperative delirium: a review of 80 primary data-collection studies. Arch Intern Med. 1995;155:461.
38. American Psychiatric Association. Practice guidelines for the treatment of patients with delirium. Am J Psychiatry. 1999;156S:1.
39. Bekker AY, Weeks EJ. Cognitive function after anaesthesia in the elderly. Best Pract Res Clin Anaesthesiol. 2003;17:259.
40. Inouye SK, Zhang Y, Jones RN, et al. Risk factors for delirium at discharge: development and validation of a predictive model. Arch Intern Med. 2007;167:1406.
41. Moller JT, Cluitmans P, Raqssmussen LS, et al. Long-term postoperative cognitive dysfunction in the elderly ISPOCD1 study. ISPOCD investigators. International Study of Post-Operative Cognitive Dysfunction. Lancet. 1998;351:857.
42. Steinmetz J, Christensen KB, Lund T, et al. Long-term consequences of postoperative cognitive dysfunction. Anesthesiology. 2009;110:548.
43. Mason SE, Noel-Storr A, Ritchie CW. The impact of general and regional anesthesia on the incidence of post-operative cognitive dysfunction and post-operative delirium: a systematic review with meta-analysis. J Alzheimers Dis. 2010;22:67.
44. Hussain M, Berger M, Eckenhoff RG, et al. General anesthetic and the risk of dementia in the elderly: current insight. Clin Interv Aging. 2014;4:1619.
45. Chow WB, Rosenthal RA, Merkow RP, et al. Optimal preoperative assessment of the geriatric surgical patient: a best practices guideline from the American College of Surgeons National

Surgical Quality Improvement Program and the American Geriatrics Society. J Am Coll Surg. 2012;215:453.
46. Barlow AP, Zarifa Z, Shillito RG, et al. Surgery in a geriatric population. Ann R Coll Surg Engl. 1989;71:110.
47. Rigberg D, Cole M, Hiyama D, et al. Surgery in the nineties. Am Surg. 2000;66:813.
48. Edwards AE, Seymour DG, McCarthy JM, Crumplin MK. A 5-year survival study of general surgical patients aged 65 years and over. Anaesthesia. 1996;51:3–10.
49. Keller SM, Markovitz LJ, Wilder JR, Aufses Jr AH. Emergency surgery in patients aged over 70 years. Mt Sinai J Med. 1987;54:25–8.
50. Monk TG, Weldon BC, Garvan CW, Dede DE, van der Aa MT, Heilman KM, Gravenstein JS. Predictors of cognitive dysfunction after major noncardiac surgery. Anesthesiology. 2008;108:18–30.
51. Lamont CT, Sampson S, Matthias R, Kane R. The outcome of hospitalization for acute illness in the elderly. J Am Geriatr Soc. 1983;31:282–8.
52. Harari D, Hopper A, Dhesi J, Babic-Illman G, Lockwood L, Martin E. Proactive care of older people undergoing surgery ('POPS'): designing, embedding, evaluating and funding a comprehensive geriatric assessment service for older elective surgical patients. Age Ageing. 2007;36:190–6.

Anesthetic Considerations for Elderly Patients Undergoing Vascular Surgery

3

Shashank Saxena

By 2030, one in five Americans will be aged 65 or older, nearly double the 12% in 2000 [1]. Lower extremity peripheral arterial disease (PAD) is now known to be associated with equal morbidity and mortality and comparable (or higher) health economic costs as coronary heart disease (CHD) and ischemic stroke [2, 3].

In contrast to coronary heart disease, relatively few genetic variants that influence susceptibility to PAD have been discovered due to greater clinical and genetic heterogeneity in PAD [4]. However, prolonged longevity will reveal physiologic strength, clinical variability, and genetic differences among individuals. Studies have revealed the prevalence of PAD to be 4.7% between the ages of 60 and 69 years, and 14.5% for the ages of 70 years and older [5]. In age- and gender-adjusted logistic regression analyses, black race/ethnicity, current smoking, diabetes, and poor kidney function were positively associated with prevalent PAD [5]. More than 95% of persons with PAD had one or more cardiovascular disease risk factors.

Modifiable risk factors in PAD include smoking, high blood pressure, hyperlipidemia, physical inactivity, obesity, diabetes, increased homocysteine levels [6], and hypothyroidism [7]. Judicious use of beta blockers, antiplatelet therapy, angiotensin-converting enzyme (ACE) inhibitors, statins is recommended for all patients with peripheral vascular disease. Decision to hold Acetylsalicylic Acid (Aspirin) (ASA), statins, ACE inhibitors should be made in conjunction with the surgical team on a case-to-case basis.

The prevalence of coronary artery disease (CAD) in PAD patients ranges from 14% to 90%, which clearly reflects differences in sensitivity of the detection technique for CAD [8]. In another study, 30% of all patients scheduled for aortic aneurysm resection, lower extremity revascularization, or extracranial reconstruction have severe CAD [9].

S. Saxena MD (✉)
Department of Anesthesiology, VA Pittsburgh Health Care Center, University of Pittsburgh School of Medicine, Pittsburgh, PA, USA
e-mail: ssaxena@mmchs.org; shank1975@gmail.com

R. Chaer (ed.), *Vascular Disease in Older Adults*,
DOI 10.1007/978-3-319-29285-4_3

Preoperative assessment should take into account all the factors listed above. Preoperative testing should be based on the degree of medical optimization of preexisting diseases, nature of planned surgery, and the likelihood of substantial hemorrhage and disruption of the autonomic homeostasis of hemodynamic and metabolic function. The purpose of this chapter is to make the reader understand the standard preoperative assessment for patients undergoing vascular surgery and to familiarize them with anesthetic considerations for the most common vascular surgery procedures.

3.1 Local Anesthesia and Regional Anesthesia

3.1.1 Pathophysiology and Pharmacology Related to Aging

It is widely accepted that complex interaction in older patients between subtle changes in pharmacodynamics and altered age-related pharmacokinetics are responsible for drug effect.

Densities of myelinated and unmyelinated axons decrease markedly from birth to the end of the eighth decade, due to increasing size and separation of fibers during the first decade, axonal degeneration, and an increase in endoneurial collagen in the older age groups [10]. The conduction velocity in peripheral motor and sensory nerves slows progressively with advancing age. Spinal cord CVs decline sharply after age 60 [11]. These changes lead to increased sensitivity to local anesthetics in the elderly, reflecting changing pharmacodynamics in old age.

Age-related changes in pharmacokinetics of local anesthetics result in reduced clearance of local anesthetics. Free lidocaine concentration is prone to increase in elderly patients during continuous thoracic epidural anesthesia [12]. In a study by Veering et al. [13], pharmacokinetics of aging had minimal, if any, effect on the peak plasma concentration and the corresponding peak time after the epidural administration of bupivacaine. It demonstrated a marked effect of age on the clearance and a moderate effect on the terminal half-life of bupivacaine. However, this did not translate into a higher potential for systemic toxicity, since toxic threshold concentrations may alter with age. This study also showed faster caudad analgesia in older patients.

Elderly patients also have increased cephalad analgesia level than younger patients. This may be related to the decreased lateral escape of the local anesthetic solution due to the sclerotic intervertebral foramina.

A moderate correlation between the maximal cephalad height of analgesia and the age of the patients has been shown in various studies [13, 14].

Age did not influence the rate of regression of analgesia or the total time for recovery from analgesia. Neither could age be shown to affect the degree or time to recovery from motor blockade. However, a recent study by Paqueron et al. [15] showed age is a major determinant of duration of complete motor and sensory blockade with peripheral nerve block, perhaps reflecting increased sensitivity to local anesthetic agents (Fig. 3.1).

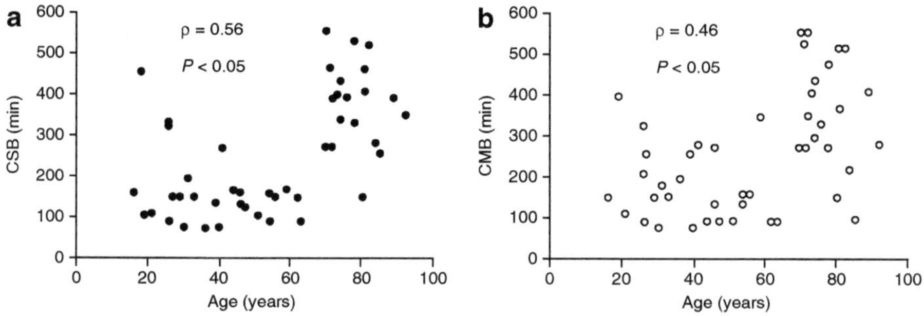

Fig. 3.1 The age of all patients (*x*-axis) in the elderly and young groups and complete sensory (*CSB*, **a**) or motor block (*CMB*, **b**) duration (*y*-axis) are shown. Postoperatively, sensory and motor blocks were assessed hourly for 9 h after time zero. Recovery from sensory and motor blocks was defined as any score greater than zero in any distribution of the radial, median, musculocutaneous, or ulnar nerve. The durations of complete sensory and motor blockade were calculated for each patient as follows: (onset time to a complete sensory or motor block) – (time of recovery from complete sensory or motor block). Durations of complete sensory ($\rho = 0.56$; $P < 0.05$) were significantly correlated with aging (Adapted from Paqueron et al. [15]; with permission)

3.1.2 Procedure-Specific Local and Regional Anesthesia

3.1.2.1 Arteriovenous Access for Hemodialysis and Permanent Vascular Access

Peripheral subcutaneous AV fistula or prosthetic graft is the current procedure of choice for patients requiring permanent hemodialysis access. The procedure is performed in supine position and is usually performed under local anesthesia with intravenous sedations. Elderly patients with chronic renal failure may present a great challenge to the anesthesiologists. Conditions like congestive heart failure, systemic hypertension, electrolyte imbalances, undetermined intravascular fluid volume status are fairly common in this age group. The presence of concomitant dementia, poor baseline cognitive function may make sedation and local anesthesia inadequate choice. In such patients, consideration should be made for brachial plexus block using an ultrasound-guided supraclavicular or infraclavicular approach. In a study by Mizrak et al. [16] when used for Arteriovenous Fistula (AVF) access surgery, infraclavicular brachial plexus block provides higher blood flow in the radial artery and AVF than is achieved with infiltration anesthesia. In another study by Malinzak and Gan [17,] it was also concluded that use of regional blocks may improve the success of vascular access procedures by producing significant vasodilatation, greater fistula blood flow, sympathectomy-like effects, and decreased maturation time. Significant vasodilation after regional block administration is seen in both the cephalic and basilic veins. These vasodilatory properties may assist with AVF site selection.

3.1.2.2 Minimally Invasive Vascular Surgery: Peripheral Arterial Stent Placement and Carotid Stent Placement

Anesthesia for peripheral arterial stent placement can be administered with intravenous moderate sedation and local anesthetic at the puncture site. A common combination for sedation is 1–2 mg of midazolam (Versed) and 25–50 mcg of fentanyl, depending on the patient's size and response. Standard ASA monitoring with Monitored Anesthesia care is used for these procedures.

The anesthetic technique for Carotid artery stent involves minimal sedation with minimal or no midazolam as excessive sedation may contribute to hypotension in the post stent placement phase. Activated clotting time (ACT) is measured. After a baseline ACT, a small heparin bolus is administered IV to achieve an ACT of approximately twice as normal (250–300 s) to prevent thromboembolic complications. Protamine should be immediately available to treat hemorrhage, although it is not routinely used for the reversal of anticoagulation at the end of the case. Often an oral antiplatelet drug (ticlopidine, clopidogrel, or abciximab) is also given.

The anesthesiology team should also anticipate excessive bradycardia with carotid balloon angioplasty necessitating the pre-emptive use of Atropine 0.4–0.8 mg or Glycopyrollate 0.2–0.4 mg.

3.1.2.3 Lower Extremity Vascular Procedures Including Vein Stripping and Perforator Ligation, Lower Extremity Vascular Bypass, Amputation Procedures of the Lower Extremity

The lower extremity vascular procedures can be ideally performed under regional anesthesia. Regional anesthesia involves spinal, epidural anesthesia, lumbar plexus anesthesia, and regional nerve blocks involving the sciatic, femoral, popliteal fossa nerve blocks, and ankle blocks.

Vascular operations for the lower extremity constitute infrainguinal arterial bypass procedures. Use of an autogenous vein provides the best conduit for infrainguinal arterial bypass procedures. The principle is to have an inflow target that has no significant disease proximal to it that can interfere with the inflow into the bypass. The inflow vessel is usually the common femoral artery, profunda femoris artery, the superficial femoral artery, the popliteal artery, and, in some less common instances, one of the tibial vessels. The target recipient artery is either the popliteal artery or tibial, peroneal, or pedal vessel. These can be approached at the level of the knee or below with a medial incision or at mid tibial/malleolus level depending on the target. It requires administration of 10,000 units of heparin prior to distal anastomosis, followed by proximal anastomosis, arteriogram, partial reversal of heparin, and closure.

Spinal anesthesia provides excellent analgesia but since surgery can be unpredictable in complexity and duration, it may be beneficial to either perform a continuous spinal anesthesia [18, 19] with an intrathecal catheter or perform a combined spinal/epidural or just lumbar epidural catheter [20]. This allows the duration of anesthesia to be extended and may also provide postoperative analgesia. Surgical anesthesia involves L1–4 dermatomes, and a dermatomal level of T10-T12 is required. Hoff et al. [21] showed that spinal anesthesia using bupivacaine and tetracaine mixed in a single-injection technique can last 5 h at the T_{12} level without added untoward effects when compared with lower dose spinal anesthetics. Cautious fluid administration and vasoconstrictors use will limit fluid overload in elderly patients especially after sympathectomy resolves. Strict adherence to American Society of Regional Anesthesia (ASRA) anticoagulation guidelines as mentioned in the previous section should be practiced before performing spinal anesthesia and prior to removal of the epidural catheter.

Yazigi et al. [22] showed in a series of 25 patients that infrainguinal bypass can be safely performed with combination femoral and sciatic nerve blockade without conversion to general anesthesia (GA). They [23] further did a prospective, randomized study comparing peripheral nerve blockade with general anesthesia for infrainguinal bypass and showed a statistically significant reduction in intraoperative myocardial ischemia in the group randomized to peripheral nerve blockade. Local anesthesia [24] and a combination [25] of a psoas compartment block, sciatic nerve block, and ipsilateral T12-L1 paravertebral block has also been shown to be successful in performing lower limb vascularization surgeries.

Thus local anesthesia and regional nerve blocks can be safely used for lower extremity vascularization procedures but larger randomized trials are needed to confirm the benefits over spinal and general anesthesia. The regional nerve blocks, neuraxial anesthesia, and local anesthesia are limited in their benefits in patients with moderate to severe chronic low back pain and in elderly patients with dementia, as such patients may be difficult to sedate and may require general anesthesia to perform the surgical procedures safely.

Considerable controversy exists over benefits of regional anesthesia over general anesthesia and many institutions have established different standards of care in managing anesthetic care for patients undergoing the above procedures. The goal of the following section is to clearly state the benefits of regional anesthesia in vascular surgery and specifically to geriatric population.

The advantages of spinal and epidural anesthesia using local anesthetic and/or opioids include avoidance of airway manipulation and pulmonary morbidity, and lower blood loss, which leads to reduction of the surgical stress response [26–28]. Urinary cortisol excretion, a marker of the stress response, was significantly diminished during the first 24 postoperative hours in the group receiving epidural anesthesia in a landmark study by Yeager et al. [29]. Reduction of surgical stress response leads to stable hemodynamics, reduced hypercoagulability, better wound healing, and less immunosuppression.

Further, vasodilation, secondary to sympathetic blockade, should be particularly helpful in sustaining graft patency.

In the Perioperative Ischemia Randomized Anesthesia Trial (PIRAT) [30], 100 patients were randomized to undergo lower extremity grafts under either epidural or general anesthesia found that revascularization rate was high in the GA group. Rosenfeld et al. [31], using patients from the PIRAT study, reported an increase in plasminogen activator inhibitor (PAI-1) in the general anesthesia patients but not in the regional anesthesia patients on the morning after surgery (Fig. 3.2).

A review of retrospective, prospective, and meta-analysis studies by Moraca et al. [32] showed significant reduction in perioperative cardiac morbidity (30%), pulmonary infections (40%), pulmonary embolism (50%), ileus (2 days), acute renal failure (30%), and blood loss (30%). Potential complications related to epidural anesthesia/analgesia ranged from minor issues like transient paresthesias (10%) to rare potentially devastating epidural hematomas (0.0006%).

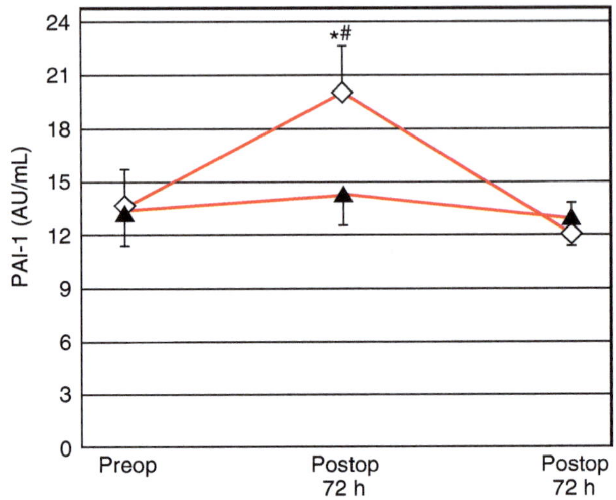

Fig. 3.2 Plasminogen activator inhibitor-1 levels in activity units per milliliter for general and regional anesthesia groups over time. Values are mean ± SEM. #*P*, 0.001 compared to preoperative and 72 h. **P* = 0.05 general anesthesia (GA) compared to regional anesthesia (RA) (From Rosenfeld et al. [31]; with permission; Source: Longnecker et al. [112], Copyright © The McGraw-Hill Companies, Inc. All rights reserved)

Thoracic epidural analgesia can enhance bowel motility not only by producing pain relief and lessening the systemic stress response, but also by creating a sympathectomy, resulting in unopposed parasympathetic innervations to the gut. Sympathetic stimulation, pain, opioids, nitrous oxide, inhalation anesthetics, and increased endogenous catecholamines all contribute to postoperative ileus, and all are blunted in patients treated with perioperative thoracic epidural analgesia [33].

Chery et al. [34] showed in a retrospective review of 407 consecutive patients who underwent above- or below-knee amputations at a single center. The study showed that regional anesthesia group which has older patients (76.6 vs.71.6) was associated with a lower incidence of overall postoperative pulmonary complications and postoperative arrhythmia. Duration of stay in the intensive care unit and hospital was significantly longer in the group receiving general anesthesia. No significant differences in postoperative myocardial infarction, venous thromboembolism, or mortality were seen between groups. Regional anesthesia included either spinal or combined spinal and epidural anesthesia. Nerve blocks were not used.

Singh et al. [35] did an analysis of a prospectively collected database by the National Surgical Quality Improvement Program (NSQIP) of the Veterans Affairs Medical Centers of all patients from 1995 to 2003 in the NSQIP database who underwent infrainguinal arterial bypass. Their results revealed that compared with general endotracheal tube anesthesia, spinal anesthesia (SA) was associated with superior 30-day graft patency, fewer cardiac events in patients without congestive heart failure but with normal functional status, less postoperative pneumonia, and decreased odds of returning to the operating room. In contrast, SA was significantly better than epidural anesthesia only in the incidence of return to the OR. There was no significant difference in 30-day mortality among the three groups with univariate or multivariate analyses.

The use of neuraxial regional anesthesia (epidural) has shown to decrease incidence of elevated intraoperative blood pressure and variability in heart rate and blood pressure when compared to general anesthesia [36].

However, later Ghanami et al. [37] did observational analysis of 5642 patients to evaluate the effects of regional versus general anesthesia for infrainguinal bypass. The study showed no evidence to support the systematic avoidance of general anesthesia for lower extremity bypass procedures. In particular, graft thrombosis was found in 7.3% of patients, with an equal rate in both groups. Pulmonary morbidity occurred in 4% of patients and the rate of cardiovascular complications was 2.8% of general anesthesia patients and 2.2% of regional anesthesia patients. Venous thromboembolism rates were similar. These data suggest that anesthetic choice should be governed by local expertise and practice patterns.

Although neuraxial techniques confer some protection in the reduction in the rate of thromboprophylaxis as eluded in the PIRAT trial and large study by Singh et al., anticoagulant therapy has a major role in the in the maintenance of vascular graft patency in the perioperative period. Since anticoagulation has an important role in the decision making for neuraxial anesthesia, it is important to review the 2010 American Society of Regional Anesthesia and Pain Medicine Evidence-Based Guidelines (Third Edition) on regional anesthesia in patient receiving anticoagulant therapy and compare them with the latest guidelines published in Regional Anesthesia Pain Medicine 2015 [38]:

1. Combining neuraxial techniques with intraoperative anticoagulation with heparin during vascular surgery is acceptable with the following recommendations (Grade 1A):
   (a) Avoid the technique in patients with other coagulopathies.
   (b) Delay heparin administration for 1 h after needle placement.
   (c) Remove indwelling neuraxial catheters 2–4 h after the last heparin dose and assess the patient's coagulation status; re-heparin 1 h after catheter removal.
   (d) Monitor the patient postoperatively to provide early detection of motor blockade and consider use of minimal concentration of local anesthetics to enhance the early detection of a spinal hematoma.
   (e) Currently, insufficient data and experience are available to determine if the risk of neuraxial hematoma is increased when combining neuraxial techniques with the full anticoagulation of cardiac surgery. We suggest postoperative monitoring of neurologic function and selection of neuraxial solutions that minimize sensory and motor block to facilitate detection of new/progressive neurodeficits.

   Although the occurrence of a bloody or difficult neuraxial needle placement may increase risk, there are no data to support mandatory cancelation of a case. Direct communication with the surgeon and a specific risk-benefit decision about proceeding in each case is warranted.

2. There are no current contraindications to using neuraxial techniques in patients on subcutaneous heparin prophylaxis twice daily. Since there is no apparent difference between twice-daily subcutaneous unfractionated Heparin (UFH) with concurrent use of compression devices and thrice-daily subcutaneous UFH, it is advised that patients *not* receive three times a day of subcutaneous UFH while epidural analgesia is maintained. Rather, such patients can continue to be treated with twice-daily subcutaneous UFH and the use of compression devices.
3. Because heparin-induced thrombocytopenia may occur during heparin administration, we recommend that patients receiving heparin for more than 4 days have a platelet count assessed before neuraxial block and catheter removal.
4. For patients on low-molecular-weight heparin (LMWH), needle placement should occur at least 12 h after the last thromboprophylactic dose of LMWH and at least 24 h after the last therapeutic dose (enoxaparin 1 mg/kg every 12 h, enoxaparin 1.5 mg/kg daily, dalteparin 120 U/kg every 12 h, dalteparin 200 U/kg daily, or tinzaparin 175 U/kg daily).
5. In patients administered a dose of LMWH 2 h preoperatively (general surgery patients), we recommend against neuraxial techniques because needle placement would occur during peak anticoagulant activity.
6. The presence of blood during needle and catheter placement does not necessitate postponement of surgery. We suggest that initiation of LMWH therapy in this setting should be delayed for 24 h postoperatively and that this consideration be discussed with the surgeon.
7. Warfarin therapy should be discontinued 4–5 days before block placement, and coagulation status should be checked.
8. Clopidogrel should be discontinued for 7 days and ticlopidine for 14 days prior to neuraxial anesthesia.
9. In a patient on oral anticoagulation with warfarin, discontinue oral anticoagulation and verify PT normalization before neuraxial block. Monitor the PT and INR daily. Remove indwelling neuraxial catheters when the INR is <1.5 in order to assure that adequate levels of all vitamin-K-dependent factors are present.
10. In a patient on Fondaparinux, until additional clinical information is obtained, neuraxial techniques should be performed and managed under conditions utilized in clinical trials (single needle pass, atraumatic needle placement, and avoidance of indwelling neuraxial catheters). If this is not feasible, an alternate method of prophylaxis should be utilized.
11. While ASRA guidelines from 2010 provide no contraindication to performance of neuraxial blocks in patients taking ASA and NSAIDs, there are specific guidelines for high-risk (interventional pain) procedures as per guidelines published in 2015 in Regional Anesthesia and Pain Medicine. At our institution we perform neuraxial blocks routinely on patients taking ASA and NSAIDs without stopping either of them. Please examine recommendations from 2015 closely and refer to Table 3.1.

Although regional anesthesia (spinal and epidural anesthesia) has desirable effects, there is no sufficient data to recommend regional anesthesia over general anesthesia. With the advent of new anesthetic agents, general anesthesia can be

Table 3.1 Recommended time intervals for commonly prescribed anticoagulants

Drug	Half-life	Time of discontinuation	Time of resumption after pain procedure (h)
Coumadin	36–42 h	5 days and NR normalization	24
IV heparin	60–90 min	4 h	2
Subcutaneous heparin BID/TID	60–90 min	8–10 h	2
LMWH	4.5 h, but prolonged in renal failure	24 h	24
Fondaparinux	21 h	4 days	24
Darbigatron	8–17 h	4–5 days	24
Rivaroxaban	9–13 h	9–13 h	24
Apixaban	15 ± 8.5 h	3–5 days	24
Clopidogrel	6 h	7 days	24
Prasugrel	2–15 h	7–10 days	24
Acenocoumarol	11 h	3 days and INR normalization	24
ASA	6–20 h	6 days (primary prophylaxis) for high-risk procedure	24
NSAIDS	Variable	5 half-lives for high-risk procedures	24

Adapted from Ref. [39]

safely used with attention to detail throughout the perioperative period and aggressive management of hemodynamic changes.

It is clearly evident that severe pain after amputation is clearly associated with a higher prevalence of post-amputation pain [39, 40]. While there are numerous studies available showing decrease in incidence of phantom limb pain (PLP) [41, 42] with perioperative epidural analgesia, there are studies [43] which refute this observation. In a recent study by Karanikolas et al. [44,] optimized epidural analgesia or intravenous PCA, starting 48 h preoperatively and continuing for 48 h postoperatively, decreases PLP at 6 months.

3.2 General Anesthesia

All other major vascular procedures are performed under general anesthesia. In this section we will discuss preoperative assessment, pathophysiology, and pharmacology relevant to geriatric anesthesia and then in various subsections we will discuss vascular surgery-specific anesthesia management.

3.2.1 Preoperative Assessment

Patients undergoing peripheral and major vascular surgery constitute a particular challenge, as these patients have high prevalence of significant coronary artery disease. The usual symptomatic presentation for coronary artery disease in geriatric patients with vascular disease may be obscured by exercise limitations imposed by advanced age, intermittent claudication, or both. Perioperative hemodynamic changes like increases in blood pressure and heart rate, elevated preload, increased contractility, hypotension, tachycardia, anemia, and hypoxemia can predispose to myocardial ischemia, which is more pronounced in patients with underlying coronary disease.

The current standards for preoperative cardiac evaluation of these patients are the guidelines published by the American College of Cardiology (ACC) and these were revised in 2007 [45] and again in 2014 [46].

The 2007 Guidelines defined cardiac risk as combined incidence of cardiac death and nonfatal myocardial infarction and stratified it into low, intermediate (including carotid endarterectomy), and high risk (surgery for peripheral vascular diseases, aortic and other major vascular surgeries). In the absence of active cardiac conditions in a patient undergoing low-risk surgery, there was no indication for any further testing. The 2007 guidelines recommended that in patients undergoing intermediate risk or vascular surgery procedure, the presence of clinical risk factors determine further approach if their functional capacity was unknown or less than 4METS. Further invasive testing in patients undergoing vascular surgery should be considered only if it will change management.

The 2014 ACC guideline states that because recommendations for intermediate- and high-risk procedures are similar, classification into two categories, namely, low and elevated risk, simplifies the recommendations without loss of fidelity. A low-risk procedure is one in which the combined surgical and patient characteristics predict a risk of a major adverse cardiac event (MACE) of death or myocardial infarction (MI) of <1%. The lowest-risk operations are generally those without significant fluid shifts and stress. Plastic surgery and cataract surgery are associated with a very low risk of MACE. Procedures with a risk of MACE of >1% are considered elevated risk. Operations for peripheral vascular disease and aortic surgeries are generally performed among those with the highest perioperative risk. Some operations can have their risk lowered by taking a less invasive approach. For example, open aortic aneurysm repair has a high risk of MACE that is lowered when the procedure is performed endovascularly. In addition, performing an operation in an emergency situation is understood to increase risk.

A risk calculator has been developed that allows more precise calculation of surgical risk, which can be incorporated into perioperative decision making. The three most commonly used tools to calculate MACE risk are Revised Cardiac Risk Index (RCRI), American College of Surgeons National Surgical Quality Improvement Program (NSQIP), Myocardial Infarction and Cardiac Arrest (MICA), and American College of Surgeons NSQIP Surgical Risk Calculator.

The RCRI is a simple, validated, and accepted tool to assess perioperative risk of major cardiac complications (MI, pulmonary edema, ventricular fibrillation or primary cardiac arrest, and complete heart block). It has six predictors of risk for major cardiac complications, only one of which is based on the procedure—namely, "Undergoing suprainguinal vascular, intraperitoneal, or intra thoracic surgery". A patient with zero or one predictor(s) of risk would have a low risk of MACE. Patients with >2 predictors of risk would have an elevated risk for adverse major cardiac events (MACE).

In a nutshell, 2014 ACC guidelines recommend that in a patient with known clinical risk factors for CAD scheduled for nonemergent elevated risk surgery (MACE > 1) and with poo r(<4METS) or unknown functional capacity, further pharmacological cardiac testing should be ordered if it will impact decision making or perioperative care. This follows a similar theme as 2007 guidelines.

It is also very important to note that implementation of the American College of Cardiology/American Heart Association guidelines has been associated with better perioperative outcomes.

Preoperative testing should not be determined by patient age alone [47]. Clinical yield of undirected or "routine" preoperative testing protocols is extremely low [48, 49]. Undirected or routine preoperative chest radiographs are unnecessary in elderly surgical patients.

Since older surgical patients are slightly more likely to be anemic, a complete blood count is mandatory for all vascular surgeries.

The prothrombin time (PT) and partial thromboplastin time (PTT) appear to have no value as screening tests in asymptomatic patients of any age with no evidence of liver disease and not taking anticoagulants. However, since most vascular surgery patients are on anticoagulants, a baseline measure of PT/PTT is required especially if planning spinal or epidural anesthesia.

Since many elderly patients may have concomitant renal dysfunction and diastolic dysfunction, a basic blood chemistry is prudent in the management of intraoperative fluid therapy.

ECG appears to be sufficiently cost-effective to warrant routine application in a geriatric population [50]. As per ACC guidelines of 2014, routine preoperative resting 12-lead ECG is not useful for asymptomatic patients undergoing low-risk surgical procedures. Since EG carries baseline information and is a prognostic standard, it is reasonable for patients with known coronary heart disease, significant arrhythmia, peripheral arterial disease, cerebrovascular disease, or other significant structural heart disease. There is poor concordance across different observational studies as to which abnormalities have prognostic significance including arrhythmias, pathological Q-waves, LV hypertrophy, ST depressions, QTc interval prolongation, and bundle-branch blocks. Likewise, the optimal time interval between obtaining a 12-lead ECG and elective surgery is unknown. General consensus suggests that an interval of 1–3 months is adequate for stable patients.

As per AHA guidelines it is reasonable to get an ECHO in the following patients:

Class IIa, dyspnea of unknown origin; Class IIa, known Congestive heart failure (CHF) with worsening dyspnea or other change in clinical status. Echo may be considered (Class IIb), reassessment in stable patients with previously documented LV dysfunction if not assessed within 1 year.

Exercise testing for ischemia may be considered (Class IIb) for patients with elevated risk and unknown or poor (<4METS) functional capacity if it will change management. However, it is to be noted that vascular surgery patients may not be able to do exercise testing due to concomitant claudication. Patients able to achieve approximately 7 METs to 10 METs have a low risk of perioperative cardiovascular events, and those achieving <4 METs to 5 METs have an increased risk of perioperative cardiovascular events. Electrocardiographic changes with exercise are not as predictive.

Noninvasive pharmacological testing may be reasonable (Class IIa) for patients at elevated risk and have poor (<4 METs) functional capacity to undergo noninvasive pharmacological stress testing (either dobutamine stress echocardiogram (DSE) or pharmacological stress (MPI) if it will change management (Level of Evidence: B) The authors identified a slight superiority of stress echocardiography relative to nongated MPI with thallium in predicting postoperative cardiac events. In patients with abnormalities on their resting ECG for example: left bundle-branch block, LV hypertrophy with "strain" pattern, digitalis effect, concomitant stress imaging with echocardiography or MPI may be an appropriate alternative.

As per AHA guidelines consistent and clear associations exist between beta blocker administration and adverse outcomes, such as bradycardia and stroke. Beta blockers should be continued in patients undergoing surgery who have been on beta blockers chronically. In patients with intermediate- or high-risk myocardial ischemia noted in preoperative risk stratification test for instance three or more RCRI risk factors (e.g., diabetes mellitus, HF, CAD, renal insufficiency, and cerebrovascular accident), it may be reasonable to begin perioperative beta blockers 2–7 days before surgery. They recommend against starting beta blockers on the day of surgery in beta–blocker-naïve patients.

Perioperative initiation of statin use is reasonable in patients undergoing vascular surgery and statins should be continued in patients currently taking them.

The risk of coronary stent thrombosis in the perioperative period for both bare metal stent (BMS) and drug-eluting stent (DES) is highest in the first 4–6 weeks after stent implantation. Discontinuation of dual antiplatelet therapy (DAPT), particularly in this early period, is a strong risk factor for stent thrombosis. In patients undergoing urgent noncardiac surgery during the first 4–6 weeks after BMS or DES implantation, DAPT should be continued unless the relative risk of bleeding outweighs the benefit of the prevention of stent thrombosis. As such, use of DAPT or aspirin alone should be individualized on the basis of the considered potential benefits and risks. All elective surgeries should be delayed for minimum 30 days for BMS and 365 days for DES.

3.2.2 Geriatric Physiology

3.2.2.1 Cardiac Physiology

Changes in the cardiovascular system that accompany aging include decreased vascular and myocardial compliance due to fibrotic replacement of elastic tissues of the arteries and the ventricle. This leads to hypertension and diastolic dysfunction.

Due to hypertension there is progressive and sustained increase in left ventricular wall tension and myocardial workload resulting in symmetrical ventricular hypertrophy and increased ventricular mass. This can further complicate diastolic dysfunction.

The phases of diastole are isovolumic relaxation and the filling phase. The filling phase is divided into early rapid filling which is passive(70–80%), diastasis(5%), and atrial systole(15–25%).Early diastolic filling is driven by the left atrial (LA) to left ventricular (LV) pressure gradient.

The cause of diastolic dysfunction is that the stiffer ventricle and atrium do not permit complete chamber relaxation until relatively late in diastole. In elderly there is decreased early diastolic filling because of decreased LA-LV pressure gradient caused by impaired LV relaxation.

Consequently, passive ventricular filling, which occurs during the early phase of diastole, is significantly reduced in older adults. As a result, the elderly are particularly dependent on the synchronous atrial contraction of sinus rhythm for late ventricular filling and this also explains why cardiac rhythm other than sinus is often poorly tolerated in elderly individuals.

There is decrease in autonomic responsiveness namely there is increased vagal tone, and decreased sensitivity of adrenergic receptors leads to a decline in heart rate. Fibrosis of the conduction system and loss of sinoatrial node cells increase the incidence of dysrhythmias, particularly atrial fibrillation and flutter. In the absence of co-existing disease, resting systolic cardiac function seems to be preserved. The stiffer ventricle and atrium do not permit complete chamber relaxation until relatively late in diastole. Consequently, passive ventricular filling, which occurs during the early phase of diastole, is significantly reduced in older adults, producing a form of diastolic dysfunction. As a result, the elderly are particularly dependent on the synchronous atrial contraction of sinus rhythm for complete ventricular filling.

The elderly patient with diastolic dysfunction may poorly tolerate perioperative fluid administration, resulting in elevated left ventricular end-diastolic pressure and pulmonary congestion. Decrease venous capacitance due to stiffening reduces its ability to buffer changes in intravascular volume leading to exaggerated hypotension especially during induction of general anesthesia or spinal anesthesia.

Moderate hypotension can cause intolerable reduction in coronary, cerebral, and renal blood flow. Decreased β-receptor response in the elderly during exercise/stress cause the increased peripheral flow demand to be met primarily by preload reserve, thereby making the heart more susceptible to cardiac failure. As baseline and maximal achieved heart rate is limited, elderly patients will rely on alpha agonists to maintain blood pressure during moments of hypotension.

In older individuals, exercise-induced increases in cardiac output are achieved with a lower heart rate, higher EDV, and higher stroke volume.

3.2.2.2 Respiratory Physiology

Aging decreases the elasticity of lung tissue, allowing overdistention of alveoli and collapse of small airways. Residual volume, functional residual capacity increase with aging along with increased anatomic dead space, increased closing capacity, decreased diffusing capacity all leading to impaired gas exchange. Elderly have less complaint chest wall. The elderly are more prone to respiratory impairment in the recovery after general anesthesia.

3.2.2.3 Nervous System Physiology

With aging there is gray and white matter atrophy, synaptic degeneration. The synthesis of neurotransmitters like acetylcholine and dopamine is reduced. Serotonergic, adrenergic, and gamma-aminobutyric acid-binding sites are also reduced. These changes may be responsible for increased sensitivity of elderly to general anesthetic and local anesthetics.

Such changes may also lead to age-related cognitive and behavioral deficits, and contribute to postoperative cognitive dysfunction in the elderly.

3.2.2.4 Renal and Hepatic Physiology

With normal aging there is progressive decrease in creatinine clearance but since muscle mass also decreases, serum creatinine remains relatively unchanged with aging. Therefore, serum creatinine is a poor predictor of renal function in elderly. Calculated creatinine clearance remains the most sensitive marker of renal function in the elderly.

Critical attention should be placed to perioperative fluid balance and electrolyte imbalance. As renal function declines with aging, the kidney's ability to excrete drugs also declines. The decreased capacity to handle water and electrolyte loads makes proper fluid management more critical during major vascular surgery.

Hepatic blood flow decreases by 10% per decade. Liver's ability to metabolize certain drugs also decreases with age. The rate of biotransformation and albumin production decreases. Plasma cholinesterase levels are reduced in elderly men.

3.2.3 Geriatric Pharmacology

Pharmacokinetic implies the relationship between drug dose and plasma concentration Pharmacodynamics implies the relationship between plasma concentration and clinical effect.

In older patients subtle changes in *pharmacodynamics* and altered age-related alpha phase redistribution *pharmacokinetics* are responsible for varied drug effect.

With aging [1], lean body mass decreases [2], body fat increases [3], and total body water decreases.

The reduced volume of distribution for water-soluble drugs can lead to greater plasma concentrations after rapid bolus or infusions. Conversely, an increased volume of distribution (due to increase in body fat) for lipid-soluble drugs could reduce their plasma concentration but lead to larger volume of distribution after prolonged infusions leading to increased drug effect. It is interesting to note that the decreased dose requirement of fentanyl in the elderly has a pharmacodynamic explanation, that is, elderly brain is more sensitive to opioids [51].Thus pharmacodynamics basis, increased brain sensitivity explains decreased minimum alveolar concentration (MAC) of volatile anesthetics [52, 53], decreased dosing requirement of opioids [54] and benzodiazepines [55].

The prolonged duration of action of vecuronium [56] and rocuronium [57] in the elderly surgical patients is related to altered pharmacokinetics consistent with an age-related decrease in renal and hepatic functions. Recovery from pancuronium that depends on renal excretion may be delayed due to decreased drug clearance. Hofmann elimination, an organ-independent elimination pathway, occurs in plasma and tissue, and is responsible for approximately 77% of the overall elimination of cisatracurium besilate. Therefore, it provides most consistent clinical effects in the elderly. Proper neuromuscular monitoring with meticulous attention to train of four and reversal of neuromuscular blockade along with adherence to clinical criteria for extubation must be met prior to extubation of elderly patients. Complete recovery of neuromuscular function is more likely when anticholinesterases are administered early (>15–20 min before tracheal extubation) and at a shallower depth of block (train-of-four [TOF] count, 4) [58].

3.2.4 Anesthetic Management of Abdominal Aortic Aneurysm Repair

In a large US Veterans Affairs screening study, the prevalence of abdominal aortic aneurysm (AAA) was 1.4% [59].

Abdominal aortic aneurysms were the primary cause of *10,597 deaths* and a contributing cause in more than *17,215 deaths* in the United States in 2009 [60]. AAA repair involves the replacement or bypass of an aneurysmal section of abdominal aorta. There are two primary methods of AAA repair, open repair and endovascular repair (EVAR). Open AAA repair is well established as a definitive treatment, having been in use for over 50 years. Generally, EVAR is advocated for patients who are at increased risk with open repair.

3.2.4.1 Anesthetic Technique for Endovascular Repair

Many institutions initially performed endovascular surgery under general anesthesia. For both the surgeons and anesthesiologists, this was a natural choice due to the uncertain outcomes and possible complications related to the new procedure.

For the transfemoral approach, local anesthesia is well tolerated and provides greater hemodynamic stability than other anesthetic techniques. Henretta et al. [61] reported the first ever series that described the use of local anesthesia for the endovascular repair of infrarenal AAAs in patients with significant co-morbidities. They showed that the advantages of local anesthesia include decreased cardiopulmonary morbidity rates, shorter hospital stays, and lower hospital costs. Multiple other reports have shown decreased procedure times [62, 63], shorter hospital stays [62, 63], and fewer pulmonary complications [64] when local anesthesia is used in place of general anesthesia.

Spinal, epidural, and combined spinal–epidural techniques have been used for endovascular surgery especially with an iliac approach to EVAR. The sensory level at which anesthetic blockade is needed is T10 dermatome. The level of sensory anesthesia required for endovascular surgery has fewer hemodynamic side effects than the high thoracic level needed for open surgical repair.

Aadahl et al. [65] showed that a single dose of spinal anesthesia combined with epidural anesthesia was effective for EVAR with no clinically significant period of hypotension in any case.

EVAR requires brief periods of intermittent apnea to obtain optimal imaging quality in digital subtraction angiography. Therefore, patient cooperation is essential, and a fine balance between optimal sedation and alertness when needed is essential. In patients with back pain or dementia, it may not be possible to maintain such a response, leading to anesthesiologist and surgical preference for general anesthesia.

The key elements in anesthetic management of EVAR include adequate hemodynamic monitoring with arterial line along with standard ASA monitors. Large-bore intravenous access should be obtained given the potential for significant blood loss and especially if a conversion to open surgery is indicated. Central venous access is not routinely required unless indicated by a patient's cardiac function or if a lengthy procedure is planned. General anesthesia typically consists of a balanced technique with a low-dose inhalational agent and opioids. Neuromuscular blocking agents are typically not necessary. A Foley catheter is required as a measure of volume status. Temperature should be closely monitored as patient is exposed and prepped for an open procedure if needed.

Blood loss during a simple infrarenal EVAR is usually minimal approximately 200–600 ml, and intraoperative transfusion is rare. Prolonged procedures and complex repairs have potential for ongoing blood loss from the access sites. Cell salvage should be available and should be used in long procedures due to propensity of extended blood loss. The occurrence of sudden hypotension should prompt immediate evaluation of access sites, followed by angiography to identify any possible causes of bleeding. It should be realized that blood loss can be difficult to quantify, as it is often lost around the sheaths and catheters, and can be retroperitoneal in the case of injury to femoral or iliac vessels. Since the incidence of renal failure is about 6.7% with EVAR [66], close intraoperative fluid management with early replacement of preoperative deficits and maintenance of intravascular volume is extremely essential during surgery especially because the surgery involves extensive use of iodinated contrast. Proper fluoroscopic protection should be provided to all personnel involved in the care of the patient during the procedure.

Postoperative patients can be discharged to a monitored bed but typically do not need intensive care. Analgesic requirements are minimal and rarely require intravenous opioids.

3.2.4.2 Anesthetic Management for Open AAA Repair

The key elements in anesthetic management of open AAA repair include adequate hemodynamic monitoring with arterial line along with standard ASA monitors (ECG, noninvasive blood pressure, pulse oximetry, capnography, and temperature). Arterial line is usually placed pre-induction in the radial artery of the arm which records he highest blood pressure via sphygmomanometer. At our institution we also place a T8-10 thoracic epidural catheter for postoperative pain control. Nishimori et al. [67] found epidural superior to intravenous analgesia, with improved postoperative pain scores as well as a reduction in postoperative intubation times, acute respiratory failure rates, intensive care unit stay duration, and rates of cardiac, gastrointestinal, and renal complications. Central venous catheterization is performed after induction general anesthesia unless needed pre induction, as dictated by patient's cardiovascular status. Pulmonary artery catheterization (PAC) is preferred over Central venous catheterization (CVC) in patients with LV dysfunction (ejection fraction < 30%) and pulmonary hypertension. PACs with capability to monitor mixed venous oxygen saturation and continuous cardiac output may be helpful in hemodynamically unstable patients or patients with ruptured AAA.

Transesophageal echocardiography (TEE) can be used to evaluate regional wall motion abnormalities which may be indicative of ischemia. TEE also helps to accurately assess volume status in a hypotensive patient. Cardiac output measured by TEE correlates very well with thermodilution cardiac output derived from PAC in the absence of significant mitral regurgitation. TEE can be placed quickly if patients become hemodynamically unstable and can immediately provide information about ventricular function (acute myocardial infarction or pulmonary embolus), volume status (hypovolemia), or obstructive flow patterns (cardiac tamponade, LVOT). Rapid rescue [68] TEE has shown to improve outcomes after hemodynamic instability in noncardiac surgical patients and also provides additional diagnostic information in patients with intraoperative cardiac arrest which may directly guide specific, potentially life-saving therapy [69].

Anesthetic technique consists of a balanced technique with inhalational anesthetics and opioids. Agents available for blunting hemodynamic response, such as esmolol, sodium nitroprusside, nitroglycerin, and short-acting b-blockers such as esmolol, should be available for bolus and continuous infusion administration, as needed. Also a vasopressor like phenyepherine or norepinephrine should be available to counteract hypotension especially during unclamping. Since an epidural catheter is placed pre-induction, we typically avoid using long-acting opioids and activate the epidural catheter at the end of the procedure to avoid any hemodynamic consequences for epidural local anesthetic during the surgery. Depending on the location of the lesion, the cross-clamp can be applied to the supraceliac, suprarenal, or infrarenal aorta. Heparin is usually administered prior to aortic clamping. The effects of cross-clamping depend on the level of the clamp, patient's fluid status and baseline myocardial function. Patients with preexisting left ventricular dysfunction manifest more hemodynamic consequences than those with normal LV function.

The primary hemodynamic response [70] to aortic cross-clamping is an increase in mean arterial pressure due to an increase in afterload. Cardiac output often decreases in response to aortic cross-clamping. Preload changes as per the location of the clamp. If the aorta is clamped above the celiac artery, blood volume is shifted proximally to the clamp, the thereby increasing preload and blood flow to the lungs and the cranium.

During infraceliac clamping, the change in preload depends upon the tone of the splanchnic veins. If the splanchnic vascular tone is high, venous return to the heart increases. Alternatively, if splanchnic venous tone is low, a decrease in preload occurs as blood volume shifts into the compliant splanchnic vasculature. Due to increase in preload and after load, left ventricular decompensation can occur in patients with CAD and LV dysfunction. The blood flow to organs distal to the clamp depends on the flow from collateral vessels which depends on the perfusion pressure dictated by the proximal aortic pressure. Therefore, proximal hypotension should be avoided.

It has been shown [71] that infraceliac clamping produces minimal mean arterial pressure, ventricular filling pressures, and ejection fraction. In contrast, supraceliac clamping produces significant increases in proximal mean arterial pressure and filling pressures, and a decrease in cardiac ejection fraction and segmental left ventricular wall motion abnormalities.

The hemodynamic response to clamping and unclamping is less prominent in patients with aortic occlusive disease than in patients getting AAA repair [72].

Before aortic unclamping, the patient should be prepared for the side effects of reperfusion. The primary hemodynamic response to unclamping of the aorta is significant hypotension. The causes include significant decrease in afterload after clamp release, accumulation and release of vasodilating and myocardial depressant metabolites from the ischemic lower extremities, peripheral redistribution of blood volume into a vascular bed that is often vasodilated by hypoxia resulting in central hypovolemia.

Blood and fluid loss should be replaced before unclamping and patient's volume status should be optimized with blood, albumin, or crystalloid, based on patient's hemodynamics which will take in to consideration their CVP, BP, and TEE (if placed) to identify hypovolemia vs LV dysfunction as cause of hypotension. Epinephrine, phenylephrine, sodium bicarbonate, and calcium chloride should be available just before the release of the cross-clamp. The aortic cross- clamp can be gradually released and reapplied if significant hypotension occurs. Correction of metabolic acidosis with sodium may be required. Small boluses of neosynephrine, nor-epinephrine, or even epinephrine may be needed to correct significant hypotension but it should be remembered that correction of hypovolemia takes precedence as using vasopressors to increase the blood pressure without restoring blood volume may further decrease blood flow to coronary, renal, and hepatic circulations.

The incidence of renal failure is approximately 13% after suprarenal (SR) aortic cross-clamping and 5% after infrarenal (IR) clamping [73]. In a review of 1020 patients who underwent elective AAA repair, postoperative decline in renal function was 17.0% in SR vs 9.5% in IR ($P = .003$), however, new-onset dialysis was rare (0.6% SR, 0.8% IR, P = NS) [74]. The reason for the above changes is that aortic cross-clamping increases renal vascular resistance and decreases renal cortical blood flow. The degree of change does not correlate with changes in blood pressure or cardiac output. Gamulin et al. [75] showed an increase of 75% in renal vascular resistance and a decrease of 38% in renal blood flow after IR clamping, whereas systemic cardiovascular measurements did not change appreciably.

Anesthetic drugs including mannitol, ventilator parameters, pre-clamp blood volume were maintained in all. Suprarenal cross-clamping has been shown to reduce renal blood flow by 80%.

Urine output is routinely monitored intraoperatively; however, it does not predict the development of postoperative renal failure. A Cochrane database [76] review showed that there is not enough evidence to show the best fluid replacement to use during and following surgery on the abdominal aorta. Fluid replacement is needed to replace tissue fluids lost during surgery. Blood products, nonblood products, or combinations including crystalloid solutions and colloids are used. Combination therapy is most common. The incidence of postoperative renal insufficiency may be decreased by adequate volume loading, maintaining cardiac output, and aggressively treating hypovolemia based on hemodynamic parameters like CVP, cardiac output, or TEE imaging and reduce cross-clamp timing (<30 min [77] associated with minimal risk).

The incidence of spinal cord injury due to hypoperfusion or ischemia is rare in AAA repair, the incidence being higher in ruptured AAA repair. Three spinal arteries, one anterior and a pair of posterior spinal arteries from the vertebral arteries, supply the cord. The anterior spinal artery is the principal artery of the three [78], supplying the anterior two-thirds of the cord, including the critical motor area. Segmental arteries from subclavian, intercostal, upper lumbar, and branches from the internal iliac and middle sacral arteries regularly feed the anterior spinal artery. The largest of these segmental arteries is the great radicular artery of Adamkiewicz or arteria radicularis magna, which originates as a branch from a left intercostal artery between T9 andT12 in 75% of patients, T5 and T8 in 15%, and L1 and L2 in 10%. The injury to the anterior 2/3rd of the cord results in bilateral flaccid paraplegia and loss of pain and temperature sensation; proprioception and vibratory sensation is maintained.

The incidence of spinal cord damage was reported as 0.25% after abdominal aortic operations and the variation in origin of the artery of Adamkiewicz may explain the incidence of this complication [79].

Epidural opioids decrease incidence of atelectasis and epidural local anesthetics increase PaO2, decrease the incidence of pulmonary infections, pulmonary complications overall compared with systemic opioids [80]. Pain management at our institution is usually via a thoracic epidural catheter which is activated at the end of the procedure to avoid hemodynamic consequences from epidural bupivacaine. We use a dilute concentration of bupivacaine 0.0625% or 0.125% mixed with fentanyl 5 mcg/cc.

The other options for pain management include bilateral paravertebral catheters and bilateral transversus abdominis plane block.

3.3 Surgery on the Ascending Aorta and the Arch of Aorta

Surgery on the ascending aorta and the arch of the aorta uses median sternotomy and cardiopulmonary bypass. The conduct of anesthesia is similar to that for cardiac surgery involving cardiopulmonary bypass which is beyond the scope of this chapter.

3.4 Surgery Involving Thoracic Aortic Abdominal Aneurysm

Aneurysms of the TAAA aorta are primarily caused by atherosclerotic degenerative disease. The remainder can be caused by trauma or connective tissue diseases disorders such as Marfan syndrome, cystic medial degeneration, Takayasu arteritis, syphilitic aortitis, Turner's syndrome, polycystic kidney disease, and Loeys-Dietz syndrome.

The prevalence of TAAA is much less than that of infrarenal AAA. TAAAs have a much lower incidence of CAD, often cited as less than 30%.

The Crawford classification defines aneurysms as types I, II, III, and IV. Type I aneurysms involve all or most of the descending thoracic aorta and the upper abdominal aorta. Type II aneurysms involve all or most of the descending thoracic aorta and all or most of the abdominal aorta. Type III aneurysms involve the lower portion of the descending thoracic aorta and most of the abdominal aorta. Type IV aneurysms involve all or most of the abdominal aorta, including the visceral segment. Types II and III are the most difficult to repair because they involve both the thoracic and the abdominal segments of the aorta.

The anesthesia for open thoracoabdominal aneurysm (TAA) repair involves placement of cerebrospinal fluid drain, thoracic epidural catheter insertion for postoperative analgesia, general anesthesia with lung isolation (double lumen tube or bronchial blocker), placement of multiple large-bore (14 gage or smaller) IV catheters, arterial lines in the upper (radial artery) and lower (femoral artery) extremities, double lumen central venous catheter insertion, pulmonary artery catheterization, and transesophageal echocardiography for monitoring of hemodynamics. TEE is used to evaluate ventricular volumes, ventricular function, valvular abnormalities (regurgitation and stenosis), and optimize cardiac function during clamping and unclamping. Temperature monitoring at multiple sites using PA catheter, urinary catheter, and nasopharyngeal probe is advised.

A lumbar spinal drain is inserted before the procedure to monitor and control cerebrospinal pressure thereby maintaining spinal cord perfusion pressure during aortic occlusion and after the procedure. Moderate systemic hypothermia (34 °C or lower) is used to prolong spinal cord and organ ischemic tolerance.

One-lung anesthesia greatly facilitates surgical exposure. A left-sided double lumen tube (DLT) is usually preferred but endobronchial blocker is ideal in patients with difficult airway, as manipulation of the airway to exchange the endotracheal tube toward the end of the surgical procedure can be avoided. Placement of left-sided DLT or blocker on the left side should be avoided in patients with aneurysm compressing on the left bronchus with distortion of the anatomy. A right-sided DLT should be used in such situations.

If assisted circulation is required, a left heart bypass (LHB) [81] is needed. The goal of LHB, is to divert a portion of saturated blood from the patient's left atrium (LA) to a section of the arterial vasculature distal to the portion of the aorta that is being reconstructed (Fig. 3.1). The most common proximal cannulation site is the left inferior pulmonary vein, although the LA appendage, left ventricular (LV) apex, ascending aorta, or subclavian artery may be used. Distal cannulation is accomplished with cannulation of the femoral artery. TEE is useful in confirming cannulae position. Once the proximal aorta is cross-clamped, the institution of LHB creates two parallel circulations, an upper and a lower. The "upper" consists of native flow from the LV and thence to the great vessels and heart. The "lower" consists of flow from the LA to the centrifugal pump, and then to the distal cannulation site (femoral artery or distal aorta) and/or any visceral vessels that have been selectively cannulated (Fig. 3.1). Lower body circulation also provides blood flow to the spinal cord anastomotic network through sacral vessels. Blood in the "lower" circulation will return to the right side of the heart primarily via the inferior vena cava (IVC). The upper circulation is dependent on the patient's underlying LV function. The lower circulation is dependent on LHB flows, which are typically 1.5–2.5 L/min. The adequacy of upper circulation is measured by the radial artery catheter and that of lower circulation by the femoral

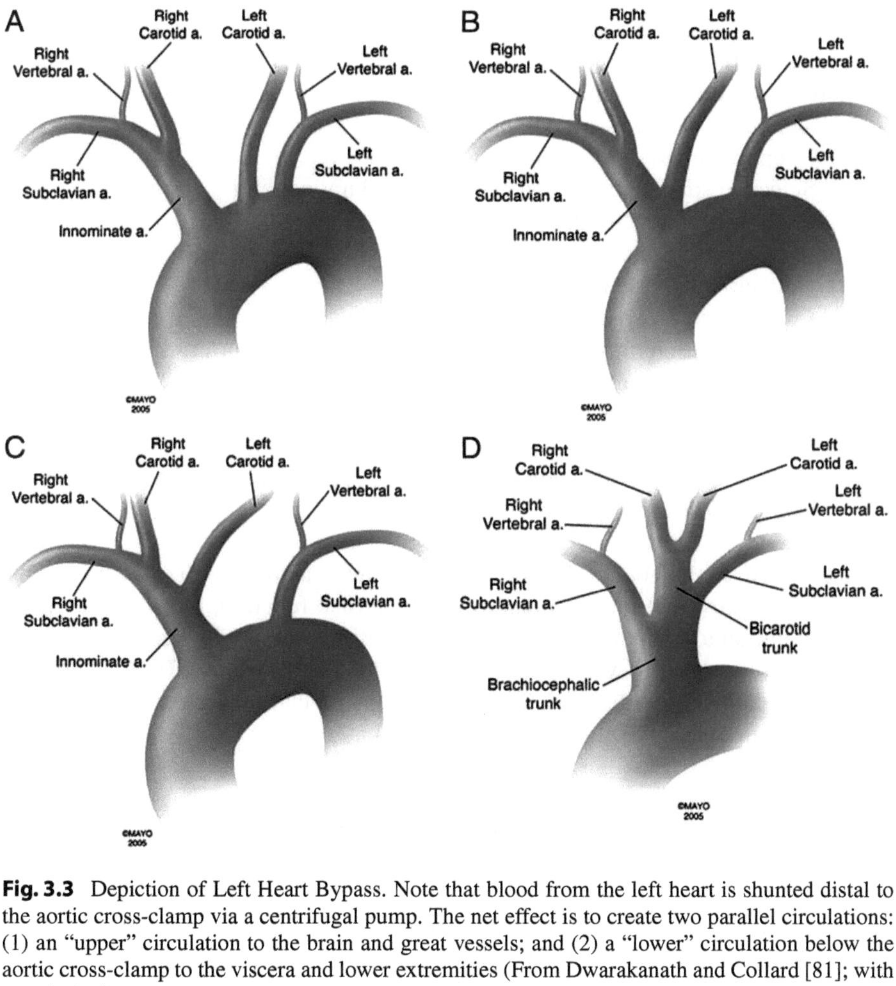

Fig. 3.3 Depiction of Left Heart Bypass. Note that blood from the left heart is shunted distal to the aortic cross-clamp via a centrifugal pump. The net effect is to create two parallel circulations: (1) an "upper" circulation to the brain and great vessels; and (2) a "lower" circulation below the aortic cross-clamp to the viscera and lower extremities (From Dwarakanath and Collard [81]; with permission)

artery catheter. Prior to LHB cannulation, the patient is first heparinized (100–150 units/kg) to achieve an activated clotting time of 200–250 s (Fig. 3.3).

Manipulation of intravascular volume, cardiac contractility, vascular tome proximal to cross- clamp and pump flows is done to optimize the upper and lower body circulation. For example, low flows in the upper circulation can be corrected by (1) volume loading the patient or (2) by decreasing flow to the lower circulation by reducing the rate of LHB flow assuming normal ventricular function. Excessive surgical bleeding and coagulopathy are not uncommon and volume resuscitation using cell saver, rapid infuser, and blood products are necessary in these patients.

Spinal cord protection during thoracic aortic surgery has been well described by Sinha and Cheung [82]. They recommend the following strategy:

1. Minimize spinal cord ischemia time:
   (a) Segmental reconstruction of the descending aorta
   (b) Distal aortic perfusion with a passive shunt (Gott shunt)
   (c) Partial left heart bypass
2. Increase tolerance to ischemia:
   (a) Deliberate mild systemic hypothermia
   (b) Deep hypothermic circulatory arrest
   (c) Selective spinal cord hypothermia by epidural cooling
   (d) Pharmacologic neuroprotection
3. Augmentation of spinal cord perfusion:
   (a) Deliberate hypertension
   (b) Lumbar cerebrospinal fluid (CSF) drainage
   (c) Reimplantation of intercostals and lumbar segmental arteries
   (d) Preservation of subclavian artery flow
4. Early detection of spinal cord ischemia:
   (a) Intraoperative motor evoked potential (MEP)
   (b) Intraoperative SEP monitoring, and serial postoperative neurologic examination

In conclusion, the goal of the anesthesiology team is to maximize tissue oxygen delivery by controlling intravascular volume, cardiac function, mean arterial pressure, in addition to maintaining spinal cord perfusion pressure by keeping adequate mean arterial pressure (MAP) and CSF pressure (below 10 cm H_2O). Transesophageal echocardiography provides real-time assessment of cardiovascular status and is vital to the intraoperative management of these patients.

3.5 Anesthesia for Carotid Endarterectomy

Atherosclerosis can involve the origins of both the internal and external carotid arteries as well as the bifurcation of the common carotid artery. The bifurcation of the common carotid artery is the most common site of atherosclerotic plaques that may lead to transient ischemic attacks (TIAs) or stroke.

The brain receives its blood supply from four major arteries. Eighty to ninety percent of the cerebral blood supply is delivered via the two internal carotid arteries with the majority of the remainder coming from the vertebrobasilar system. The carotid arteries and basilar artery unite to form the Circle of Willis at the base of the brain. This ring of arteries offers the brain considerable protection against the occlusion of one or another vessel; however, in patients with cerebrovascular disease one or more of the vessels within the circle maybe occluded by atheromatous plaque.

Carotid Endartrectomy (CEA) can reduce the risk of stroke in subgroup of patients. As per the guidelines published in the *Journal of Vascular Surgery* in 2011, CEA should be the first-line treatment for most symptomatic patients with stenosis of 50–99%. Symptomatic patients with 50–99% stenosis that are at high risk for CEA from anatomic (like prior neck surgery or radiation injury) or medical reasons should be offered carotid artery stenting.

CEA is first-line treatment for asymptomatic patients with stenosis of 60–99%. Asymptomatic patients at high risk for intervention or with <3 years' life expectancy should be considered for medical management as the first-line therapy.

According to the American Association of Neurological Surgeons and the American Stroke Association, treatment with CEA within 2 weeks of presentation for acute stroke is reasonable and appropriate.

The perioperative risk of stroke and death in asymptomatic patients must be <3% and for symptomatic patients <6%.

The risks associated with CEA involve neurological complications, hypertension, hypotension, hemorrhage, acute arterial occlusion, stroke, MI, venous thromboembolism, cranial nerve palsy, infection, arterial restenosis, and death. Risk is related mainly to the patient's preoperative clinical status. Symptomatic patients have a higher risk than asymptomatic patients, as do those with hemispheric versus retinal symptoms. Intracerebral hemorrhage may occur as a consequence of the hyperperfusion syndrome despite control of blood pressure. Cardiovascular instability has been reported in 20% of patients undergoing CEA, with hypertension reported in 20%, hypotension in 5%, and perioperative MI in 1% [83].

Most patients needing CEA are elderly with hypertension and associated CAD. Patient should be medically optimized with regard to their CAD, DM, and HTN. The patient should receive their blood pressure medications in the morning of surgery and their blood sugar should be well controlled. Standard cardiovascular monitoring should include continuous ECG with Lead II and V5 and arterial blood pressure. At our institution we prefer to place an arterial line pre-induction to keep tight control on blood pressure. Two large-bore IV catheters are placed and one of them is dedicated to running a vasodilator like nitroprusside or nitroglycerine and a vasoconstrictor like phenylephrine or norepinephrine. This surgery does not involve major fluid shifts and a central venous catheter or a pulmonary artery catheter is rarely needed. Patient's "baseline" mean arterial pressure (MAP) should be estimated from the preoperative visit, the patient's records, and the blood pressure in both arms should be measured. We aim to maintain MAP at, or up to 20% above, the documented baseline MAP during carotid cross-clamping using fluids, vasopressors, and hypotensive drugs as required The MAP are also regulated based on the information available from EEG, other cerebral monitoring or neurological symptoms in awake patients. EEG monitoring is used during every CEA.

The carotid artery is temporarily completely occluded by a cross-clamp in order to perform the CEA. A temporary shunt may be inserted through the arteriotomy distally in the internal carotid artery and proximally in the common carotid artery to prevent cerebral hypoperfusion and impending ischemia during the cross-clamping of the carotid artery. Acute complications of shunt insertion include air or plaque embolization, intimal tears, and carotid dissection. There is an associated risk of local complications including hematoma, nerve injury, infection, and late carotid restenosis. Various modalities are used to monitor the need for shunting including EEG monitoring, SSEP, and carotid stump pressure monitoring.

In a study in 2002, it was shown that intraoperative EEG monitoring accurately (99.92%) identified patients who may safely have carotid endarterectomy without the need of a shunt. A statistically significant increase in intraoperative stroke rate was associated with the development of an abnormal EEG (1.1%), contralateral internal carotid artery occlusion (1.8%), and the combination of both abnormal EEG and contralateral internal carotid occlusion (3.3%) [84]. EEG was an excellent detector of cerebral ischemia and a valuable tool in guiding the need for shunting [85].

CEA performed with routine EEG monitoring and selective shunt placement is associated with a low risk of perioperative stroke. Identified predictors of significant EEG changes were anatomic factors including degree of contralateral carotid artery disease and moderate ipsilateral carotid artery stenosis (50–79%) [86].

Anesthetic agents and changes in temperature and blood pressure affect EEG. EEG monitoring is limited by the fact that most neurologic deficits after CEA is caused by thromboembolism rather than occlusion of blood flow during carotid clamping.

Somatosensory-evoked potentials reflect presence of intact sensory pathways from stimulated peripheral nerve to the cortex where the electrical activity is being recorded. There is evidence that distortion of these waveforms reflect ischemia, although these Somatosensory evoked potential (SSEP) changes may not reflect ischemia and may overestimate the need for shunting. SSEP may be superior in patients whose baseline EEG is not easily interpretable because of a previous stroke. Also SSEP may be affected by volatile anesthetics. In a recent study by Nwachuku et al. it was stated that patients with perioperative neurological deficits are 14 times more likely to have had changes in SSEPs during the procedure and intraoperative SSEP is a highly specific test in predicting neurological outcome following CEA [87].

The internal carotid stump pressure (pressure cephalad to the clamp) presumably reflects the pressure transmitted around the Circle of Willis. Studies have shown stump pressure to be specific but not sensitive at identifying patients who develop EEG changes consistent with cerebral ischemia upon carotid cross-clamping [88].

Transcranial Doppler (TCD) provides noninvasive assessment of the middle cerebral artery (MCA) by insonating the MCA through the thin petrous temporal bone using a specially designed Doppler probe. This helps to monitor both cerebral hemodynamics and the occurrence of emboli. However, the probe has to be placed near the surgical site and may need constant adjustment. TCD may be used as a complement to EEG; it is to be realized that it is operator-dependent. TCD may be useful in predicting patients with cerebral hyperperfusion syndrome following CEA or CAS.

Near infrared spectroscopy (NIRS) allows continuous monitoring of regional cerebral oxygenation (rSO2) in the frontal lobe. It is not as reliable as other monitors of cerebral ischemia.

General anesthesia is the most commonly used technique at our institution. It allows reliable airway control, prevents hypoxemia and hypo- or hypercapnia, and provides optimal operating conditions for our surgical team. Induction of anesthesia should be slow with gradual titration of anesthetic drugs. Airway control should be expeditious with minimal hemodynamic alteration and avoidance of hypo or hypertension during induction and laryngoscopy. Hypercarbia causes vasodilation in normally reactive nonischemic areas of the brain and "steals" the blood away from the maximally vasodilated vessels in the territory of the occluded carotid. Hypocarbia may cause vasoconstriction of vessels in normally perfused areas of the brain and divert blood to the maximally vasodilated, unreactive areas of the brain but clinical trials have failed to show any benefit as leftward shift of oxyhemoglobin dissociation curve by hypocarbia decreases oxygen delivery to tissues. The current recommendation is to maintain normocarbia in CEA.

Maintenance of general anesthesia can be achieved with various agents as long as there is hemodynamic stability, cerebral ischemia is not enhanced and consideration is made for rapid emergence at the conclusion of surgery.

In general, volatile anesthetics are vasodilators and intravenous anesthetics are vasoconstrictors of the cerebral vasculature. Hence volatile anesthetics have the potential to cause vasodilation of normally perfused areas of brain and hence steal blood from ischemic areas. The risk of cerebral ischemia will be lessened by agents that cause decrease in cerebral metabolic oxygen consumption (CMRO2). Sevoflurane, desflurane, and isoflurane decrease CMRO2.

In a study, it was shown that times to extubation, movement on command, and consciousness were shorter after desflurane and sevoflurane than after isoflurane anesthesia; it was also noted that desflurane was associated with more hypertension and tachycardia [89].

Michenfelder et al. [90] defined the critical regional cerebral blood flow (rCBF) as the rCBF below which more than 50% of patients developed ipsilateral EEG changes of ischemia within 3 min of carotid occlusion. The critical rCBF varies depending on the volatile anesthetic used.

EEG monitoring for cerebral ischemia is feasible with 0.6–1.2% sevoflurane administered in 50% nitrous oxide, and it is similar to that determined with isoflurane and it may facilitate more rapid emergence [91].

Due to the advantages of the rapid emergence with sevoflurane, it appears to be a good alternative to isoflurane in CEA. We prefer to use remifentanil (0.05–2 mcg/kg/min) with sevoflurne or isoflurane in 0.5–1.0 MAC. There is evidence that cerebral autoregulation is impaired even with concentrations of volatile anesthetic agents <1.0 MAC, although this effect is more marked with isoflurane than with sevoflurane. Which is another potential advantage of sevoflurane. Some centers avoid nitrous oxide as it increases the cerebral metabolic rate, increases cerebral blood flow and decreases the neuroprotective effect of other drugs. Anesthesia can be maintained using a combination of propofol and remifentanil. Propofol and sevoflurane at a concentration up to 1.0 minimum alveolar concentration produce comparable reductions in both the cerebral blood flow and the metabolic rate. Observations also indicate a hemodynamic advantage of propofol anesthesia during carotid clamping [92]. However, at a higher cost of propofol-remifentanil anesthetic it may offer little advantage over inhalational anesthesia for carotid endarterectomy [93]. It is to be noted that both propofol and volatile anesthetics afford neuroprotection during CEA, and anesthetic-induced neuroprotection [94] is an important research topic currently.

Surgical manipulation, traction of the carotid sinus or traction on the carotid artery can cause bradycardia and hypotension due to activation of the baroreceptor reflexes. Cessation of stimulus or infiltration of the carotid bifurcation with 1% lidocaine usually prevents further episodes. Episodes of hypotension during other phases of surgery can be handled by either decreasing depth of anesthesia, or giving vasopressors like phenylepherine or ephedrine. The goal is to maintain the MAP at or 20% above patient's baseline MAP. Hypertension can be treated by either deepening anesthesia or using antihypertensives like esmolol or labetalol.

Patients are extubated after neurologic integrity is confirmed. Emergence may be associated with marked hypertension and tachycardia, which may require aggressive pharmacologic intervention. If patient develops rapidly expanding hematoma at the site of surgery, consideration should be made to immediately intubate the trachea, as stridor is a late sign of airway compromise [95].

Neurologic deficits on emergence may necessitate angiography, reoperation, or both as determined by surgery team. Therefore, the key elements in anesthetic management of CEA involve maintaining normocarbia, controlling blood sugar [96], maintaining MAP equal to or greater that 20% baseline MAPs during clamping, and using neurologic monitoring as a guide to shunting. A controlled induction and emergence being critical to the success of the anesthetic and surgical course.

There is considerable debate on the efficacy of regional anesthesia over general anesthesia in CEA. Regional anesthesia is accomplished by blocking the C2 to C4 dermatomes by use of a superficial, intermediate, or deep cervical plexus block. Pandit et al. [97] showed that a superficial/intermediate block is safer than any method that employs a deep injection. The higher rate of conversion to general anesthesia with the deep/combined block may have been influenced by the higher incidence of direct complications.

A regional anesthesia audit for CEA showed that cervical plexus block is associated with a significantly lower frequency of anesthesia-related complications and should therefore be considered the regional anesthetic of choice. Cervical epidural anesthesia should not be performed except in extenuating circumstances [98].

The GALA (General Anesthetic Versus Local Anesthetic for Carotid Surgery) trial, failed to show a statistically significant improvement in stroke, MI, or death with combined superficial and deep cervical plexus block versus general anesthesia (GA) [99].

Studies comparing CEA under local anesthesia (LA) Vs GA showed a higher rate of shunt usage after GA compared with LA CEA. LA may protect the patient from early postoperative cognitive dysfunction and appears to be more cost-effective [100].

3.6 Postoperative Cognitive Dysfunction (POCD)

Decline in cognitive function after surgery in the elderly is becoming increasingly recognized with an increase in our aging population. The earliest recognition was associated with cardiac surgery but research has shown that cognitive dysfunction is seen after other major noncardiac surgeries. The diagnosis of POCD requires pre- and postoperative neuropsychological testing. The testing is diverse and includes learning and memory, verbal abilities, perception, attention, executive functions, and abstract thinking.

In a recent study, POCD was observed in 15.9% of adults 65 year or older 3 months after major noncardiac surgery [101]. This is similar to the findings of International study of postoperative cognitive dysfunction 1 (ISPOCD1) study of 1218 patients which found that the incidence of POCD after 3 months in age > 70 was 14% [102].

Monk et al. [103] reported that cognitive dysfunction is common in adult patients of all ages at hospital discharge after major noncardiac surgery, but only the elderly (aged 60 years or older) are at significant risk (12.7%) for long-term cognitive problems. They confirmed the findings of ISPOCD1, which found that advancing age and lower educational levels are risk factors for the development of cognitive decline after noncardiac surgery. They also found that asymptomatic patients with a history of stroke with no residual impairment, and POCD at hospital discharge had a higher incidence of late (3 months after surgery) POCD.

No significant difference was found in the incidence of cognitive dysfunction 3 months after either general or regional anesthesia in elderly patients [104].

Russo et al. also found that the type of anesthesia (general or epidural) does not affect the magnitude or pattern of postoperative cognitive dysfunction in older adults undergoing total knee arthroplasty [105].

ISPOCD1 also found no relation between different degrees and durations of hypoxemia or hypotension and early and late postoperative cognitive dysfunction.

The goal of future research should be to incorporate standard psychometric tests in pre anesthesia clinic especially for the elderly patient and follow up testing at 3 months to identify POCD. Currently no preventative strategies have been developed for POCD and proper identification and rehabilitation is the key to successful recovery.

3.6.1 Postoperative Delirium

Postoperative delirium can clearly be distinguished from POCD as the key characteristics are a change in mental status characterized by a reduced awareness of the environment and a disturbance in attention. This may be accompanied by other, more florid, perceptual symptoms (hallucinations) or cognitive symptoms including disorientation or temporary memory dysfunction.

In elderly hip fracture patients, the incidence of delirium was reported to be between 28 and 41% [106, 107].

In a study by Litaker et al., delirium was detected in 11.4% patients aged 70 years or older, pre-existing cognitive impairment, greater preoperative functional limitations, and history of prior delirium [108].

Perioperative hypoxemia, hypotension, sepsis, hypoglycemia, electrolyte disturbances, administration of certain drugs like anticholinergics, barbiturates, benzodiazepines are believed to be risk factors for post-op delirium. There appears to be no difference in the incidence of postoperative delirium with either neuraxial or general anesthesia [109].

Treatment of post-op delirium relies on identifying the reversible medical causes, reassuring and re-orienting the patient to their current hospital environment [110].

Brief postoperative delirium lasting more than 6 weeks is a determining factor for poor long-term functional outcome after hip fracture repair, because it significantly impacts the ability to live independently [111].

Key Points

- Preoperative testing should not be determined by patient's age only.
- Goal of preoperative testing is to determine the functional reserve of each organ system and to identify need for optimization. The new ACC guidelines are helpful in performing a good preoperative evaluation.
- Regional anesthesia (spinal and epidural) and peripheral nerve blocks should be considered strongly in perioperative management as they will help improve postoperative pain control and decrease incidence of postoperative delirium in the elderly.
- Careful consideration should be made to anticoagulation guidelines published by ASRA before performing regional anesthesia/analgesia.
- Diastolic dysfunction and decreased autonomic responsiveness are important causes of perioperative cardiac dysfunction in the elderly.
- Transesophageal echocardiography is an important tool in identifying hypovolemia vs LV dysfunction as the cause of persistent hypotension during major vascular surgery.
- Key elements in anesthetic management of carotid endarterectomy involve maintaining normocarbia, controlling blood sugar, maintaining MAP equal to or greater that 20% baseline MAPs during clamping, and using neurologic monitoring as a guide to shunting.

References

1. Centers for Disease Control and Prevention. The state of aging and health in America, vol. 2013. Atlanta: Centers for Disease Control and Prevention/US Dept. of Health and Human Services; 2013.
2. Mahoney EM, Wang K, Cohen DJ, Hirsch AT, Alberts MJ, Eagle K, et al. REACH registry investigators. One-year costs in patients with a history of or at risk for atherothrombosis in the United States. Circ Cardiovasc Qual Outcomes. 2008;1:38–45.
3. Hirsch AT, Hartman L, Town RJ, Virnig BA. National health care costs of peripheral arterial disease in the Medicare population. Vasc Med. 2008;13(3):209–15.
4. Kullo IJ, Leeper NJ. The genetic basis of peripheral arterial disease: current knowledge, challenges, and future directions. Circ Res. 2015;116:1551–60.
5. Selvin E, Erlinger TP. Prevalence of and risk factors for peripheral arterial disease in the United States: results from the National Health and nutrition examination survey, 1999-2000. Circulation. 2004;110(6):738–43.
6. Aronow WS, Ahn C. Association between plasma homocysteine and peripheral arterial disease in older persons. Coron Artery Dis. 1998;9:49–50.
7. Mya MM, Aronow WS. Increased prevalence of peripheral arterial disease in older men and women with subclinical hypothyroidism. J Gerontol A Biol Sci Med Sci. 2003;58:68–9.
8. Golomb BA, Dang TT, Criqui MH. Peripheral arterial disease morbidity and mortality implications. Circulation. 2006;114:688–99.
9. Hertzer NR, Beven EG, Young JR, O'Hara PJ, Ruschhaupt 3rd WF, et al. Coronary artery disease in peripheral vascular patients: a classification of 1000 coronary angiograms and results of surgical management. Ann Surg. 1984;199(2):223–33.
10. Jacobs JM, Love S. Qualitative and quantitative morphology of human sural nerve at different ages. Brain. 1985;08(Pt 4):897–924.
11. Dorfman LJ, Bosley TM. Age-related changes in peripheral and central nerve conduction in man. Neurology. 1979;29:38–44.
12. Fukuda T, Kakiuchi Y, Miyabe M, Kihara S, Kohda Y, Toyooka H. Free lidocaine concentrations during continuous epidural anesthesia in geriatric patients. Reg Anesth Pain Med. 2003;28:215.
13. Veering BT, Burm AG, Gladines MP, Spierdijk J. Age does not influence the serum protein binding of bupivacaine. Br J Clin Pharmacol. 1991;32:501–3.
14. Simon MJ, Veering BT, Stienstra R, van Kleef JW, Burm AG. Effect of age on the clinical profile and systemic absorption and disposition of levobupivacaine after epidural administration. Br J Anaesth. 2004;93(4):512–20.
15. Paqueron X, Boccara G, Bendahou M, Coriat P, Bruno R. Brachial plexus nerve block exhibits prolonged duration in the elderly. Anesthesiology. 2002;97(5):1245–9.
16. Sahin L, Gul R, Mizrak A, et al. Ultrasound-guided infraclavicular brachial plexus block enhances postoperative blood flow in arteriovenous fistulas. J Vasc Surg. 2011;2011(54):749–53.
17. Malinzak EB, Gan TJ. Regional anesthesia for vascular access surgery. Anesth Analg. 2009;109(3):976–80.
18. Denny NM, Selander DE. Continuous spinal anesthesia. Br J Anaesth. 1998;81(4):590–7.
19. Aksoy M, Dostbil A, Ince I, Ahiskalioglu A, Alici HA, Aydin A, Kilinc OO. Continuous spinal anaesthesia versus ultrasound-guided combined psoas compartment-sciatic nerve block for hip replacement surgery in elderly high-risk patients: a prospective randomised study. BMC Anesthesiol. 2014;14:99.
20. Damask MC, Weissman C, Todd G. General versus epidural anesthesia for femoral-popliteal bypass surgery. J Clin Anesth. 1990;2:71–5.
21. Hoff BH, Fletcher SJ, Rickford WJ, Matjasko MJ. Spinal anesthesia using a 1:1 mixture of bupivacaine and tetracaine for peripheral vascular surgery. J Clin Anesth. 1994 Jan-Feb;6(1):18–22.
22. Yazigi A, Madi-Gebara S, Haddad F, Hayeck G, Tabet G. Combined sciatic and femoral nerve blocks for infrainguinal arterial bypass surgery: a case series. J Cardiothorac Vasc Anesth. 2005;19(2):220–1.

23. Yazigi A, Madi-Gebara S, Haddad F, Hayeck G, Tabet G. Intraoperative myocardial ischemia inperipheral vascular surgery: general anesthesia vs combined sciatic and femoral nerve blocks. J Clin Anesth. 2005;17:499–503.
24. Mackay CA, Razik W, Simms MH. Local anaesthetic for lower-limb revascularization in high-risk patients. Br J Surg. 1997;84:1096–8.
25. Basagan-Mogol E, Turker G, Yilmaz M, Goren S. Combination of a psoas compartment, sciatic nerve, and T12-L1 paravertebral blocks for femoropopliteal bypass surgery in a high-risk patient. J Cardiothorac Vasc Anesth. 2008;22(2):337–9.
26. Liu S, Carpenter RL, Neal JM. Epidural anesthesia and analgesia. Anesthesiology. 1995;82:1474–506.
27. Grass JA. The role of epidural anesthesia and analgesia in postoperative outcome. Anesthesiol Clin North Am. 2000;18:407–28.
28. Park WY, Thompson JS, Lee KK. Effect of epidural anesthesia and analgesia on perioperative outcome. Ann Surg. 2001;234:560–71.
29. Yeager MP, Glass DD, Neff RK, Brinck-Johnsen T. Epidural anesthesia and analgesia in high-risk surgical patients. Anesthesiology. 1987;66:729–36.
30. Christopherson R, Beattie C, Frank SM, Norris EJ, Meinert CL, Gottlieb SO, et al. Perioperative morbidity in patients randomized to epidural or general anesthesia for lower extremity vascular surgery. Perioperative ischemia randomized anesthesia trial study group. Anesthesiology. 1993;79:422–34.
31. Rosenfeld BA, Beattie C, Christopherson R, Norris EJ, Frank SM, Breslow MJ, et al. The effects of different anesthetic regimens on fibrinolysis and the development of postoperative arterial thrombosis. Perioperative ischemia randomized anesthesia trial study group. Anesthesiology. 1993;79:435–43.
32. Moraca RJ, Sheldon DG, Thirlby RC. The role of epidural anesthesia and analgesia in surgical practice. Ann Surg. 2003;238:663–73.
33. Carpenter RL. Gastrointestinal benefits of regional anesthesia/analgesia. Reg Anesth. 1996;21:13–7.
34. Chery J, Semaan E, Darji S, Briggs WT, Yarmush J, D'Ayala M. Impact of regional versus general anesthesia on the clinical outcomes of patients undergoing major lower extremity amputation. Ann Vasc Surg. 2014;28(5):1149–56.
35. Singh N, Sidawy AN, Dezee K, Neville RF, Weiswasser J, Arora S, et al. The effects of the type of anesthesia on outcomes of lower extremity infrainguinal bypass. J Vasc Surg. 2006;44(5):964–8. discussion 968–70.
36. Christopherson R, Glavan NJ, Norris EJ, Beattie C, Rock P, Frank SM, Gottlieb SO. Control of blood pressure and heart rate in patients randomized to epidural or general anesthesia for lower extremity vascular surgery. J Clin Anesth. 1996;8:578–84.
37. Ghanami RJ, Hurie J, Andrews JS, Harrington RN, Corriere MA, Goodney PP, et al. Anesthesia-based evaluation of outcomes of lower-extremity vascular bypass procedures. Ann Vasc Surg. 2013;27(2):199–207.
38. Horlocker TT, Wedel DJ, Rowlingson JC, Enneking FK, Kopp SL, Benzon HT, et al. Regional anesthesia in the patient receiving antithrombotic or thrombolytic therapy: American Society of Regional Anesthesia and Pain Medicine evidence-based guidelines (third edition). Reg Anesth Pain Med. 2010;35(1):64–101.
39. Narouze S, Benzon HT, Provenzano DA, Buvanendran A, De Andres J, Deer TR, et al. Interventional spine and pain procedures in patients on antiplatelet and anticoagulant medications: guidelines from the American Society of Regional Anesthesia and Pain Medicine, the European Society of Regional Anaesthesia and Pain Therapy, the American Academy of Pain Medicine, the International Neuromodulation Society, the North American Neuromodulation Society, and the World Institute of Pain. Reg Anesth Pain Med. 2015;40(3):182–212.
40. Jensen TS, Krebs B, Nielsen J, Rasmussen P. Immediate and long-term phantom limb pain in amputees: incidence, clinical characteristics and relationship to pre-amputation limb pain. Pain. 1985;21:267–78.

41. Nikolajsen L, Ilkjaer S, Kroner K, Christensen JH, Jensen TS. The influence of preamputation pain on postamputation stump and phantom pain. Pain. 1997;72:393–405.
42. Bach S, Noreng MF, Tjéllden NU. Phantom limb pain in amputees during the first 12 months following limb amputation, after preoperative lumbar epidural blockade. Pain. 1988;33: 297–301.
43. Jahangiri M, Jayatunga AP, Bradley JW, Dark CH. Prevention of phantom pain after major lower limb amputation by epidural infusion of diamorphine, clonidine and bupivacaine. Ann R Coll Surg Engl. 1994;76:324–6.
44. Nikolajsen L, Ilkjaer S, Christensen JH, Krøner K, Jensen TS. Randomised trial of epidural bupivacaine and morphine in prevention of stump and phantom pain in lower-limb amputation. Lancet. 1997;350:1353–7.
45. Karanikolas M, Aretha D, Tsolakis I, Monantera G, Kiekkas P, Papadoulas S, et al. Optimized perioperative analgesia reduces chronic phantom limb pain intensity, prevalence, and frequency: a prospective, randomized, clinical trial. Anesthesiology. 2011;114:1144–54.
46. Fleisher LA, Beckman JA, Brown KA, Calkins H, Chaikof E, Fleischmann KE, et al. ACC/AHA 2007 guidelines on perioperative cardiovascular evaluation and care for noncardiac surgery: executive summary: a report of the American College of Cardiology/American Heart Association task force on practice guidelines (writing committee to revise the 2002 guidelines on perioperative cardiovascular evaluation for noncardiac surgery) developed in collaboration with the American Society of Echocardiography, American Society of Nuclear Cardiology, Heart Rhythm Society, Society of Cardiovascular Anesthesiologists, Society for Cardiovascular Angiography and Interventions, Society for Vascular Medicine and Biology, and Society for Vascular Surgery. J Am Coll Cardiol. 2007;50:1707–32.
47. Fleisher LA, Fleischmann KE, Auerbach AD, Barnason SA, Beckman JA, Bozkurt B, et al. 2014 ACC/AHA guideline on perioperative cardiovascular evaluation and management of patients undergoing noncardiac surgery: a report of the American College of Cardiology/American Heart Association task force on practice guidelines. American College of Cardiology; American Heart Association. J Am Coll Cardiol. 2014;64(22):e77–137.
48. Disbrow E, Lichtor JL, Binstock W, et al. Is age a predictor of preoperative test requirements in asymptomatic patients? Anesthesiology. 1993;79(suppl 3A):A44.
49. Domoto K, Ben R, Wei JY, Pass TM, Komaroff AL. Yield of routine annual laboratory screening in the institutionalized elderly. Am J Public Health. 1985;75:243–5.
50. Golub R, Cantu R, Sorrento JJ, Stein HD. Efficacy of preadmission testing in ambulatory surgical patients. Am J Surg. 1992;163:565–70.
51. Gold BS, Young ML, Kinman JL, Kitz DS, Berlin J, Schwartz JS. The utility of preoperative electrocardiograms in the ambulatory surgical patient. Arch Intern Med. 1992;152:301–5.
52. Scott JC, Stanski DR. Decreased fentanyl and alfentanil dose requirements with age. A simultaneous pharmacokinetic and pharmacodynamic evaluation. J Pharmacol Exp Ther. 1987;240(1):159–66.
53. Gold MI, Abello D, Herrington C. Minimum Alveolar concentration of desflurane in patients older than 65 years. Anesthesiology. 1993;79:710–4.
54. Nakajima R, Nakajima Y, Ikeda K. Minimum alveolar concentration of sevoflurane in elderly patients. Br J Anaesth. 1993;70:273–5.
55. Matteo RS, Schwartz AE, Ornstein E, Young WL, Chang WJ. Pharmacokinetics of sufentanil in the elderly surgical patient. Can J Anaesth. 1990;37:852–6.
56. Bell GD, Spickett GP, Reeve PA, Morden A, Logan RF. Intravenous midazolam for upper gastrointestinal endoscopy: a study of 800 consecutive cases relating dose to age and sex of patient. Br J Clin Pharmacol. 1987;23:241–3.
57. Lien CA, Matteo RS, Ornstein E, Schwartz AE, Diaz J. Distribution, elimination, and action of vecuronium in the elderly. Anesth Analg. 1991;73(1):39–42.
58. Matteo RS, Ornstein E, Schwartz AE, et al. Pharmacokinetics and pharmacodynamics of rocuronium (org 9426) in elderly surgical patients. Anesth Analg. 1993;77:1193.
59. Brull SJ, Murphy GS. Residual neuromuscular block: lessons unlearned. Part II: methods to reduce the risk of residual weakness. Anesth Analg. 2010;111:129–40.

60. Lederle FA, Johnson GR, Wilson SE, Chute EP, Littooy FN, Bandyk D, et al. Prevalence and associations of abdominal aortic aneurysm detected through screening. Aneurysm detection and management (ADAM) veterans affairs cooperative study group. Ann Intern Med. 1997;126(6):441–9.
61. Kochanek KD, Xu JQ, Murphy SL, Miniño AM, Kung HC. Deaths: final data for 2009. Natl Vital Stat Rep. 2011;60:1–116.
62. Henretta JP, Hodgson KJ, Mattos MA, Karch LA, Hurlbert SN, Sternbach Y, et al. Feasibility of endovascular repair of abdominal aortic aneurysms with local anesthesia with intravenous sedation. J Vasc Surg. 1999;29:793–8.
63. Asakura Y, Ishibashi H, Ishiguchi T, Kandatsu N, Akashi M, Komatsu T. General versus locoregional anesthesia for endovascular aortic aneurysm repair: influences of the type of anesthesia on its outcome. J Anesth. 2009;23:158–61.
64. Karthikesalingam A, Thrumurthy SG, Young EL, et al. Locoregional anesthesia for endovascular aneurysm repair. J Vasc Surg. 2012;56:510–9.
65. Edwards MS, Andrews JS, Edwards AF, Ghanami RJ, Corriere MA, Goodney PP, et al. Results of endovascular aortic aneurysm repair with general, regional, and local/monitored anesthesia care in the American College of Surgeons National Surgical Quality Improvement Program database. J Vasc Surg. 2011;54:1273–82; Aadahl P, Lundbom J, Hatlinghus S, Myhre HO. Regional anesthesia for endovascular treatment of abdominal aortic aneurysms. J Endovasc Surg. 1997;4:56–61.
66. Wald R, Waikar SS, Liangos O, Pereira BJ, Chertow GM, Jaber BL. Acute renal failure after endovascular vs open repair of abdominal aortic aneurysm. J Vasc Surg. 2006;43:460–6.
67. Nishimori M, Low JH. Epidural pain relief versus systemic opioid-based pain relief for abdominal aortic surgery. Cochrane Database Syst Rev. 2012;7:CD005059.
68. Shillcutt SK, Markin NW, Montzingo CR, Brakke TR. Use of rapid "rescue" perioperative echocardiography to improve outcomes after hemodynamic instability in noncardiac surgical patients. J Cardiothorac Vasc Anesth. 2012;26(3):362–70.
69. Memtsoudis SG, Rosenberger P, Loffler M, Eltzschig HK, Mizuguchi A, Shernan SK, Fox JA. The usefulness of transesophageal echocardiography during intraoperative cardiac arrest in noncardiac surgery. Anesth Analg. 2006;102(6):1653–7.
70. Gelman S. The pathophysiology of aortic cross-clamping and unclamping. Anesthesiology. 1995;82:1026–60.
71. Roizen MF, Beaupre PN, Alpert RA, Kremer P, Cahalan MK, Shiller N, et al. Monitoring with two-dimensional transesophageal echocardiography: comparison of myocardial function in patients undergoing supraceliac, suprarenal-infraceliac, or infrarenal aortic occlusion. J Vasc Surg. 1984;1:300–5.
72. Johnston WE, Balestrieri FJ, Plonk G, D'Souza V, Howard G. The influence of periaortic collateral vessels on the intraoperative hemodynamic effects of acute aortic occlusion in patients with aorto-occlusive disease or abdominal aortic aneurysm. Anesthesiology. 1987;66(3):386–9.
73. Ellis JE, Roizen MF, Mantha S, Schwarze ML, Lubarsky DA, Keenan CA. Anesthesia for vascular surgery. In: Clinical anesthesia. 5th ed. Philadeplhia: Lippincott, Williams and Wilkins; 2006. p. 956.
74. Chong T, Nguyen L, Owens CD, Conte MS, Belkin M. Suprarenal aortic cross-clamp position: a reappraisal of its effects on outcomes for open abdominal aortic aneurysm repair. J Vasc Surg. 2009;49(4):873–80.
75. Gamulin Z, Forster A, Morel D, Simonet F, Aymon E, Favre H. Effects of infrarenal aortic cross-clamping on renal hemodynamics in humans. Anesthesiology. 1984;61(4):394–9.
76. Zavrakidis N. Intravenous fluids for abdominal aortic surgery. Cochrane Database Syst Rev. 2000; (3):CD000991. doi:10.1002/14651858.CD000991.
77. Cunningham JN, Laschinger JC, Spencer FC. Monitoring of somatosensory evoked potentials during surgical procedures on the thoracoabdominal aorta. IV. Clinical observations and results. J Thorac Cardiovasc Surg. 1987;94:275–85.
78. Mallick IH, Kumar S, Samy A. Paraplegia after elective repair of an infrarenal aortic aneurysm. J R Soc Med. 2003;96:501–3.

79. Szilagyi DE, Hageman JH, Smith RF, Elliott JP. Spinal cord damage in surgery of the abdominal aorta. Surgery. 1978;83(1):38–56.
80. Ballantyne JC, Carr DB, de Ferranti S, Suarez T, Lau J, Chalmers TC, et al. The comparative effects of postoperative analgesic therapies on pulmonary outcome: cumulative meta-analyses of randomized, controlled trials. Anesth Analg. 1998;86(3):598–612.
81. Dwarakanath K, Collard CD. Anesthetic considerations for left heart bypass during aortic repair surgery. www.scahq.org/sca3/events/2013/annual/wpsyllabus/Submissions/Workshops.
82. Sinha AC, Cheung AT. Spinal cord protection and thoracic aortic surgery. Curr Opin Anaesthesiol. 2010;23:95–102.
83. Brott TG, Halperin JL, Abbara S, Bacharach JM, Barr JD, Bush RL, et al. AJSA/ACCF/AHA/AANN/AANS/ACR/ASNR/CNS/SAIP/SCAI/SIR/SNIS/SVM/SVS guideline on the Management of Patients with Extracranial Carotid and Vertebral Artery Disease: executive summary. J Am Coll Cardiol. 2011;57(8):1002–44.
84. Pinkerton Jr JA. EEG as a criterion for shunt need in carotid endarterectomy. Ann Vasc Surg. 2002;16(6):756–61.
85. Ballotta E, Saladini M, Gruppo M, Mazzalai F, Da Giau G, Baracchini C. Predictors of electroencephalographic changes needing shunting during carotid endarterectomy. Ann Vasc Surg. 2010;24(8):1045–52.
86. Tan TW, Garcia-Toca M, Marcaccio Jr EJ, Carney Jr WI, Machan JT, Slaiby JM. Predictors of shunt during carotid endarterectomy with routine electroencephalography monitoring. J Vasc Surg. 2009 Jun;49(6):1374–8.
87. Nwachuku EL, Balzer JR, Yabes JG, Habeych ME, Crammond DJ, Thirumala PD. Diagnostic value of somatosensory evoked potential changes during carotid endarterectomy: a systematic review and meta-analysis. JAMA Neurol. 2015;72(1):73–80.
88. Harada RN, Comerota AJ, Good GM, Hashemi HA, Hulihan JF. Stump pressure, electroencephalographic changes, and the contralateral carotid artery: another look at selective shunting. Am J Surg. 1995;170:148–53.
89. Umbrain V, Keeris J, D'Haese J, et al. Isoflurane, desflurane and sevoflurane for carotid endarterectomy. Anaesthesia. 2000;55:1052–7.
90. Michenfelder JD, Sundt TM, Fode N, Sharbrough FW. Isoflurane when compared to enflurane and halothane decreases the frequency of cerebral ischemia during carotid endarterectomy. Anesthesiology. 1987;67:336–40.
91. Grady RE, Weglinski MR, Sharbrough FW, Perkins WJ. Correlation of regional cerebral blood flow with ischemic electroencephalographic changes during sevoflurane-nitrous oxide anesthesia for carotid endarterectomy. Anesthesiology. 1998;88:892–7.
92. McCulloch TJ, Thompson CL, Turner MJ. A randomized crossover comparison of the effects of propofol and sevoflurane on cerebral hemodynamics during carotid endarterectomy. Anesthesiology. 2007;106(1):56–64.
93. Jellish WS, Sheikh T, Baker WH, Louie EK, Slogoff S. Hemodynamic stability, myocardial ischemia, and perioperative outcome after carotid surgery with remifentanil/propofol or isoflurane/fentanyl anesthesia. J Neurosurg Anesthesiol. 2003;15(3):176–84.
94. Jovic M, Unic-Stojanovic D, Isenovic E, Manfredi R, Cekic O, Ilijevski N, et al. Anesthetics and cerebral protection in patients undergoing carotid endarterectomy. J Cardiothorac Vasc Anesth. 2015;29:178–84.
95. Munro FJ, Makin AP, Reid J. Airway problems after carotid endarterectomy. Br J Anaesth. 1996;76(1):156–9.
96. McGirt MJ, Woodworth GF, Brooke BS, Coon AL, Jain S, Buck D, et al. Hyperglycemia independently increases the risk of perioperative stroke, myocardial infarction, and death after carotid endarterectomy. Neurosurgery. 2006;58(6):1066–73.
97. Pandit JJ, Satya-Krishna R, Gration P. Superficial or deep cervical plexus block for carotid endarterectomy: a systematic review of complications. Br J Anaesth. 2007;99(2):159–69.
98. Hakl M, Michalek P, Sevcík P, Pavlíková J, Stern M. Regional anaesthesia for carotid endarterectomy: an audit over 10 years. Br J Anaesth. 2007;99:415–20.

99. Lewis SC, Warlow CP, Bodenham AR, et al. General anaesthesia versus local anaesthesia for carotid surgery (GALA): a multicentre, randomised controlled trial. Lancet. 2008;372:2132–42.
100. Unic-Stojanovic D, Babic S, Neskovic V. General versus regional anesthesia for carotid endarterectomy. J Cardiothorac Vasc Anesth. 2013;27(6):1379–83.
101. Shoair OA, Grasso Ii MP, Lahaye LA, Daniel R, Biddle CJ, Slattum PW. Incidence and risk factors for postoperative cognitive dysfunction in older adults undergoing major noncardiac surgery: a prospective study. J Anaesthesiol Clin Pharmacol. 2015;31(1):30–6.
102. Moller JT, Cluitmans P, Rasmussen LS, Houx P, Rasmussen H, Canet J, et al. Long-term postoperative cognitive dysfunction in the elderly ISPOCD1 study. ISPOCD investigators. International study of post-operative cognitive dysfunction. Lancet. 1998;351(9106):857–61.
103. Monk TG, Weldon BC, Garvan CW, Dede DE, van der Aa MT, Heilman KM, Gravenstein JS. Predictors of cognitive dysfunction after major noncardiac surgery. Anesthesiology. 2008;108:18–30.
104. Rasmussen LS, Johnson T, Kuipers HM, Kristensen D, Siersma VD, Vila P, et al. Does anaesthesia cause postoperative cognitive dysfunction? A randomised study of regional versus general anaesthesia in 438 elderly patients. Acta Anaesthesiol Scand. 2003;47:260–6.
105. Williams-Russo P, Sharrock NE, Mattis S, Szatrowski TP, Charlson ME. Cognitive effects after epidural vs. general anesthesia in older adults. JAMA. 1995;274:44–50.
106. Edlund A, Lundstrom M, Lundstrom G, Hedqvist B, Gustafson Y. Clinical profile of delirium in patients treated for femoral neck fractures. Dement Geriatr Cogn Disord. 1999;10:325–9.
107. Marcantonio ER, Flacker JM, Michaels M, Resnick NM. Delirium is independently associated with poor functional recovery after hip fracture. J Am Geriatr Soc. 2000;48:618–24.
108. Litaker D, Locala J, Franco K, Bronson DL, Tannous Z. Preoperative risk factors for postoperative delirium. Gen Hosp Psychiatry. 2001;23:84–9.
109. Bryson GL, Wyand A. Evidence-based clinical update: general anesthesia and the risk of delirium and postoperative cognitive dysfunction. Can J Anaesth. 2006;53:669–77.
110. Rudoph J, Marcantonio E. Postoperative delirium: acute change with long term implications. Anesth Analg. 2011;112:1202.
111. Zakriya K, Sieber FE, Christmas C, Wenz JF Sr, Franckowiak S. Brief postoperative delirium in hip fracture patients affects functional outcome at three months. Anesth Anal. 2004;98:1798–802, table of contents.
112. Longnecker DE, Brown DL, Newman MF, Zapol WM. Anesthesiology. 2nd ed. New York: McGraw Hill; 2012. www.accessanesthesiology.com

4 Deep Vein Thrombosis in the Elderly

Anthony J. Comerota

4.1 Introduction

Venous thromboembolism (VTE) is a major global health problem. Additionally, pulmonary embolism (PE) is recognized as the most common cause of preventable death in hospitalized patients in the United States and other developed countries. While it has been estimated that VTE affects over 900,000 patients [1, 2] and causes up to 300,000 deaths annually in the United States, these estimates may understate the problem as the US population has grown and may have more patients at risk since those observations were made.

Aging is one of the strongest and most prevalent risk factors for venous thromboembolic disease. The overall incidence of the first symptomatic venous thromboembolic event in the general population is usually reported as 1/1000 person years. However, in the age group 25–30 years old, it is 1/10,000 person years compared to individuals 85 years or older, where it is 8/1000 person years. This is an 80-fold increased risk [3]. The cumulative incidence of VTE in persons aged 90 is 15%. Sixty percent of all VTE events occur in those aged 70 and older. The population attributable risk of aging for venous thromboembolism is 90%, indicating that 90% of the overall incidence of thromboembolism in the population can be attributed to increased age [3]. Therefore, physicians caring for patients with VTE are well served to be familiar with the age-related risk of VTE, its diagnosis, and treatment.

A.J. Comerota (✉)
Jobst Vascular Institute, Toledo, OH, USA

University of Michigan, Ann Arbor, MI, USA
e-mail: shakela.watkins@promedica.org

R. Chaer (ed.), *Vascular Disease in Older Adults*,
DOI 10.1007/978-3-319-29285-4_4

4.2 Risk Factors for Age-Related Venous Thromboembolism

4.2.1 Genetic Risk Factors

While enthusiasm for testing for hereditary thrombophilia is diminishing, it is known that the most common genetic risk factors for venous thromboembolism are factor V Leiden and the Prothrombin G20210A mutation. Since these are relatively weak prothrombotic risk factors one would expect their prevalence to be similar in young and older patients presenting with VTE, which is indeed the case [4, 5].

4.2.2 Medical Comorbidities

A host of medical diseases have been identified as risk factors for venous thromboembolism. These include chronic obstructive pulmonary disease, diabetes, stroke, and congestive heart failure. The severity of each of these has been shown to positively correlate with the risk of thrombosis [6–8].

Increasing age is directly associated with the prevalence of chronic diseases [9]. The prevalence of multiple chronic diseases has been estimated in 35% of patients aged 40–59, compared to 80% in patients 80 years or greater. Therefore, elderly patients who have multiple comorbidities are increasingly vulnerable to venous thromboembolism.

4.2.3 Malignancy

Patients with malignancy have a sevenfold increased risk of venous thromboembolism compared to those without a malignancy. The risk differs according to cancer type, with ovarian cancer, pancreatic cancer, and brain tumors associated most strongly with venous thromboembolism. This is true in elderly patients as well as young patients. However, cancer-associated venous thromboembolism appears to be more prevalent in patients 70 years of age and older than in younger patients. This can, in part, be explained by the increased incidence of malignancy with age. There is a threefold increased incidence of cancer in patients over the age of 65 compared to those younger than 65.

4.2.4 Sex

There is no apparent sex difference in the risk of venous thromboembolism in the general population. Since women have a longer life expectancy than men, this will lead to a higher proportion of women having venous thromboembolism in the elderly population.

4.2.5 Age-Specific Risk Factors

4.2.5.1 Alterations in Vein Wall Anatomy and Physiology

Age-related changes in the anatomy of vein walls have been demonstrated. Atrophy of muscle fibers and vein valve thickening as a result of increased collagen deposition have been reported [10]. It appears there is re-modeling of the vein wall as individuals age, which may contribute to the increased risk of thrombosis in the elderly.

Endothelial function has been shown to be altered in patients with spontaneous venous thromboembolism. Migliacci et al. [11] demonstrated that flow-mediated vasodilatation was significantly reduced in patients with spontaneous venous thromboembolism, compared to age- and gender similar controls. As risk factors for endothelial dysfunction increase with associated medical comorbidities, one can recognize that endothelial dysfunction will be more prevalent in the aged, as they have more comorbidities.

Findings associated with vein wall re-modeling lead to functional venous disease. It has been shown that chronic venous disease associated with valvular incompetence increases with age [12].

4.2.5.2 Physical Functioning

The strength and physical activity of the aging patient can have a substantial effect on risk for venous thrombosis and the effectiveness and safety of treatment (Table 4.1). Specific to the lower extremities, Olsen et al. [14] demonstrated a reduction in compliance in the veins of the lower limbs of aging individuals and its relative importance for the capacitance function of the central circulation. A reduction in calf muscle pump function, most likely due to restricted ankle motion, further accentuates the vein wall anatomic changes occurring over time as discussed above.

Table 4.1 Cumulative 2-year incidence of bleeding versus physical activity in elderly patients taking long-term vitamin K antagonists

	Physical activity			
Characteristic	Low ($N = 367$)	Moderate ($N = 310$)	High ($N = 311$)	p-value
Age	78	76	71	NA[a]
TTR[b]	55%	57%	63%	<0.001
Bleeding				
Major	18.8%	11.4%	6.2%	<0.001
Clinically Relevant	22.1%	18.1%	13.4%	<0.001
Fall Related(non-major)	9.9%	3.9%	4.1%	<0.001

Data from Frey et al. [13]
[a]Not Available
[b]Time in Therapeutic Range (INR 2–3)

Frailty is increasingly recognized as an important comorbid condition. Defined as loss of physiologic reserve, which increases the risk of disability, frailty has been associated with restricted activity, reduction in activities of daily life, and a reduction in cognition and physical performance. It has been shown that frailty increases with age, from less than 4% in individuals 65–74 years old to 25% in individuals 85 years and older. Frail individuals have a 30% increased risk of developing venous thromboembolism compared to nonfrail individuals [11].

4.3 Testing for Venous Thromboembolism

A detailed review of imaging tests for pulmonary embolism and deep venous thrombosis is beyond the scope of this chapter. However, a brief review of the pretest probability model (PTP) and d-Dimer testing to exclude patients from deep vein thrombosis (DVT) is worthwhile.

Deep vein thrombosis (DVT) can be safely and reliably excluded in patients with a low clinical probability and a negative d-Dimer test [14].The d-Dimer is the final fragment of the plasmin-mediated degradation of cross-linked fibrin. d-Dimers are sensitive indicators of the presence of acute thrombus and can be measured with a simple blood test. d-Dimer is the most frequently used laboratory marker of coagulation and endogenous fibrinolytic breakdown of thrombus.

Carrier et al. [15] demonstrated in a review of 2696 patients that the negative predictive values of a low or unlikely PTP score in combination with a negative d-Dimer was 99% for all groups of patients, including the elderly. However, it has been demonstrated that d-Dimer concentration increases with age, thereby reducing the potential clinical value of the d-Dimer assay in the elderly [16].

Recently, Andro et al. [17] performed a review with the intent of improving the performance of d-Dimer in elderly patients. They concluded that an age-adjusted cut-off was appropriate and could be applied to all d-Dimer tests. They recommended that the optimal cut-off value (in mg/L) was equal to the patients' age in years multiplied by ten in those over 50 years of age who had a low pretest clinical risk of DVT. This age-adjusted cut-off value was externally validated in retrospective studies applied mostly to outpatients with suspected DVT or PE. Various quantitative d-Dimer assays were used. Although their review confirmed the improved usefulness of the age-adjusted cut-off, prospective evaluations are necessary before definitive recommendations can be made.

4.4 Special Considerations in the Elderly

There are numerous age-related problems making the management of the elderly patient with venous thromboembolism more challenging. Elderly patients more often have multiple underlying comorbidities and take medications which alter the monitoring of vitamin K antagonists. The elderly population has a greater percentage of patients that weigh less than 65 kg, a higher percent use platelet inhibitor drugs, and renal dysfunction is more prevalent.

Elderly patients frequently have illnesses and are often immobilized prior to hospitalization. In a prospective study, Oger et al. [18] performed venous ultrasound examinations within 48 h of admission in medically ill patients. Asymptomatic DVT was found in 18% of patients older than 80 years of age, whereas no DVT was found in patients less than 55 years of age [19].

Renal dysfunction is an important risk factor for bleeding in patients receiving anticoagulation [15]. Elderly patients frequently can have normal creatinine levels, which are misleading, since their muscle mass diminishes and, therefore, serum creatinine diminishes. Hence, a serum creatinine within the normal range can exist despite abnormal renal function. Estimating the creatinine clearance is a more effective way to assess renal function. When properly evaluated, creatinine clearance alone has identified approximately 60% of critically ill medical patients aged 70 years and greater as having some degree of renal impairment [20].

4.5 Specific Anticoagulants

Despite the increased risk of thromboembolism in elderly patients, physicians in the real world environment are often reluctant to treat the elderly with anticoagulants because of concerns about bleeding. Recognizing the appropriate balance of risk of thrombosis versus bleeding and how to modify treatment offers patients the best chance of appropriate care

4.5.1 Unfractionated Heparin

Unfractionated heparin is the most commonly recommended anticoagulant for initial therapy in patients with acute VTE. Unfractionated heparin is affected by renal dysfunction. It has been shown that the elderly have an increased risk of bleeding with higher heparin levels after standard heparin doses [17] and that lower doses of unfractionated heparin are required to maintain therapeutic anticoagulation [21]. Since unfractionated heparin has a short half-life, can be rapidly adjusted, and can be fully reversed, it is usually recommended as the initial therapy in patients with renal dysfunction.

4.5.2 Enoxaparin

A number of studies have been performed evaluating the use of enoxaparin at therapeutic doses, adjusted doses, and prophylactic doses in patients with renal dysfunction. Lin et al. [18] published a meta-analysis of patients receiving enoxaparin with compromised renal function (creatinine clearance <30 ml/min). They found that when enoxaparin was administered at routine therapeutic doses, it was associated with a supratherapeutic anti-Xa level and a two to threefold increased risk of major bleeding. When the enoxaparin dose was adjusted, a therapeutic anti-Xa level was maintained without an increased risk of major bleeding. Patients with renal dysfunction accumulated enoxaparin even at prophylactic doses if they were not adjusted.

The manufacturer of enoxaparin recommends that in patients with a creatinine clearance of less than 30, prophylactic doses be reduced to 30 mg once daily and therapeutic doses be reduced to 1 mg/kg once daily.

4.5.3 Dalteparin

A small number of studies in patients of older age and renal impairment have been performed. Data suggest that the administration of prophylactic doses of dalteparin in patients with renal dysfunction is not associated with accumulation, and dose reduction is not recommended [22–24].

Limited data are available to guide therapeutic doses of dalteparin in patients with renal dysfunction [22–25]. These studies demonstrated that when peak anti-Xa levels were measured 4 h after dosing, no bioaccumulation of dalteparin was observed. The use of dalteparin reduced VTE events and was not associated with an increased risk of major hemorrhage. However, patients with profound renal dysfunction were excluded.

The manufacturer of dalteparin does not provide any information about dose adjustment in the elderly or renally impaired patients.

4.5.4 Tinzaparin

Evidence exists that the low-molecular-weight heparin tinzaparin may have a better safety profile in elderly patients with renal dysfunction. Tinzaparin is a larger molecule than other low-molecular-weight heparins, with an average molecular weight of 5500–7500 Da. A small study by Siguret et al. [26] evaluated patients with acute thromboembolic disease with a mean age of 87 years using a dose of 175 anti-Xa IU/kg daily for 10 days. The mean anti-Xa activity was measured as no correlation was found between anti-Xa activity and creatinine clearance. There were no major bleeding complications and no heparin induced thrombocytopenia.

A much larger study by Pautas et al. [27] evaluated the safety profile of tinzaparin in elderly patients with compromised renal function. Median age was 85, with mean creatinine clearance of 51. Patients were treated with tinzaparin 175 anti-Xa IU/kg daily. The measured anti-Xa activity did not correlate with age or creatinine clearance. Complications occurred in 1.5%, and heparin-induced thrombocytopenia occurred in 1%.

The results of these studies suggest that the larger molecular weight tinzaparin may be preferable in elderly patients with compromised renal function in whom a low-molecular-weight heparin therapy is preferred.

The manufacturer of tinzaparin does not recommend dose adjustment in elderly renally impaired patients.

4.5.5 Vitamin K Antagonists

Bleeding is the most feared complication of anticoagulation in patients, especially in older patients. The risk of bleeding significantly increases in older individuals. As mentioned earlier, age is a dose-related risk factor, with the elderly facing considerably increased risk. It has become apparent that age is also a major increased risk factor for bleeding complications. Vitamin K antagonists (VKA) belong to the group of medicines that cause the most adverse drug reactions in older patients [28].

Hutten et al. [29] performed a systematic review and concluded that in patients taking Vitamin K antagonists, there was a twofold increased risk of bleeding in patients greater than 60 years of age than those less than 60 years of age.

Across all age categories, the risk of hemorrhage is higher during the first 3 months after the initiation of VKAs. In the ISCOAT trial, major and minor bleeding complications were 11.0 per 100 patient years in the first 3 months compared to 6.3 per 100 patient years, thereafter ($p < 0.001$). Older patients are frequently at higher risk for falls than younger patients and, therefore, are presumed to be at an increased risk of intracranial hemorrhage. Often, the risk for falls and subsequent intracranial bleeds are cited as contraindications to antithrombotic therapy in the elderly. However, there are few data to substantiate this concern. Bond et al. [30] evaluated the risk of hemorrhagic complications in patients who fall. In general there is a 5–10% risk of major hemorrhagic injury due to falls; however, patients who take warfarin were not at higher risk than those not taking an anticoagulant [29]. Man-Son-Hing et al. [31] calculated that patients taking warfarin for atrial fibrillation would have to fall 295 times per year for warfarin not to have a favorable risk-benefit ratio.

The rate of major bleeding of patients of all ages being treated with VKAs ranges from 1.2% to 7.4% per year, depending upon the study. Clinical trials, however, report major bleeding rates between 0.5% and 4.2% per year. The bleeding rates in major trials may underestimate those in broad-based clinical practice, due to patient selection and protocols for careful monitoring.

Table 4.2 summarizes selective studies which reveal information regarding age-related bleeding in patients on Vitamin K antagonists. Many of the patients treated in these trials were those with atrial fibrillation; however, the age distinction is what appears important as related to age-related risk.

Intracranial hemorrhage (ICH) represents a major cause of iatrogenic death in patients treated with VKAs. In the SPAF II trial, advanced age was a predictor of ICH. The rate of ICH was 0.6% per year in patients receiving warfarin who were less than 75 years of age and 1.8% per year in those greater than 75 years of age ($p = 0.05$) [38]. In the ISCOAT study, ICH was significantly more frequent in the elderly (≥75 years vs. <70 years, RR 6.5; $p = 0.047$).

There are numerous factors that put elderly patients at risk of bleeding from VKAs. Comorbidities such as impaired liver function, congestive heart failure, diarrhea, and fever have been identified as risk factors for high international normalized ratios (INRs). Acute illness and deterioration of chronic comorbidities as well as changes in weight, physical activity, dietary intake, and alcohol consumption are all

Table 4.2 Age-related major bleeding on vitamin K antagonists

Clinical trial	INR range	Age categories (years)	Incidence major bleed	Ratio of incidence older: younger
EAFT [32]	2.5–3.9	>75 ≤75	Overall 2.8%	3.6
SPAF [33]	2.0–4.5	>75 ≤75	4.2% 1.7%	2.6 (p = .009)
ISCOAT [34]	2.0–4.5	≥75 <70	2.1% 1.1%	$p = 0.19$
ISCOAT [35]	1.0–3.5	>75 ≤75	5.1% 1.0%	6.6
Copeland et al. [36]	2.0–3.0	≥75 60–69	2.9% 2.8%	$p = 0.96$

Data from Pautas et al. [37]

contributory. Interestingly, poor compliance is not an issue in most elderly patients. These factors are superimposed upon the generally increased risk of ICH with VKAs due to their intrinsic inhibition of tissue-factor/Factor VIIa complexes. Tissue factor/Factor VIIa complexes are present in high concentrations in the brain, which have neuroprotective properties in the event of injury. Inhibition of this neuroprotective pathway by VKAs may account for the differential rates of ICH between direct oral anticoagulants (DOACs) and VKAs.

4.5.6 Direct Oral Anticoagulants

The direct oral anticoagulants are a new class of drugs that are made up of small molecules, nonpeptidic, and orally available and directly inhibit one of two key serine proteases, thrombin (Factor IIa [dabigatran]) and Factor Xa (rivaroxaban, apixaban, edoxaban).

These drugs are efficiently absorbed from the GI tract providing rapid therapeutic anticoagulation (1–3 h). They eliminate the need for monitoring, and there is no dose adjustment. There is minimal, if any, interindividual difference, minimal drug–drug interaction, and minimal food interactions. Each of the above-mentioned compounds has been studied head to head against Vitamin K antagonists in patients presenting with acute DVT and/or acute PE. Sharma et al. [38] performed a systematic review and meta-analysis of randomized controlled trials of the use of DOACs in the management of atrial fibrillation and acute venous thromboembolism, where VKAs were used as a comparator. Their goal was to evaluate the DOACs for efficacy and harms in comparison with VKA in the elderly participants age ≥ 75 years in randomized trials.

Although 19 multicenter randomized controlled trials were performed, 11 reported data on elderly patients which were used for analysis.

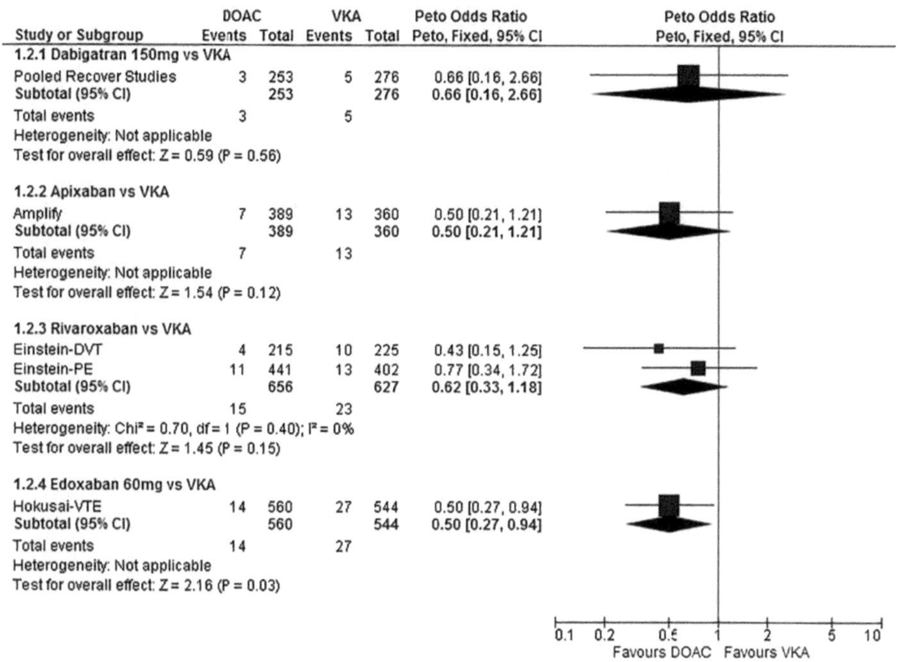

Fig. 4.1 Forest plots for risk of recurrent venous thromboembolism in VTE in Elderly: DOACS vs. VKA (Modified from Sharma et al. [38]; with permission)

A review of the data demonstrates that the DOACs for VTE are at least as effective as VKAs in the overall population, and this observation is preserved in the elderly age ≥ 75 years (Fig. 4.1). The meta-analysis of bleeding risks with DOACs versus VKAs is summarized in Figs. 4.2 and 4.3. The DOACs demonstrated distinct differences in bleeding risks compared to VKAs. The direct thrombin inhibitor, dabigatran, differed for bleeding between the elderly and the total population, and the populations of patients <75. Dabigatraon 150 mg showed a higher risk of major bleeding than VKA in the elderly. However, patients <75 years had a reduced major bleeding risk versus VKAs. Apixaban and Edoxoban showed a lower major bleeding risk than VKA in both the elderly and younger populations.

Elderly patients receiving dabigatran were at a higher risk of gastrointestinal bleeding than those treated with VKAs. All DOACs provided protection against intracranial bleeding compared to VKAs (Fig. 4.3).

This analysis by Sharma et al. [38] provides important information for the prescription of DOACs in elderly populations who may be at higher risk of bleeding from either concomitant comorbidities or other antithrombotic medications. Proper use of this information can favorably alter the risk-benefit ratio when managing elderly VTE patients over the long term.

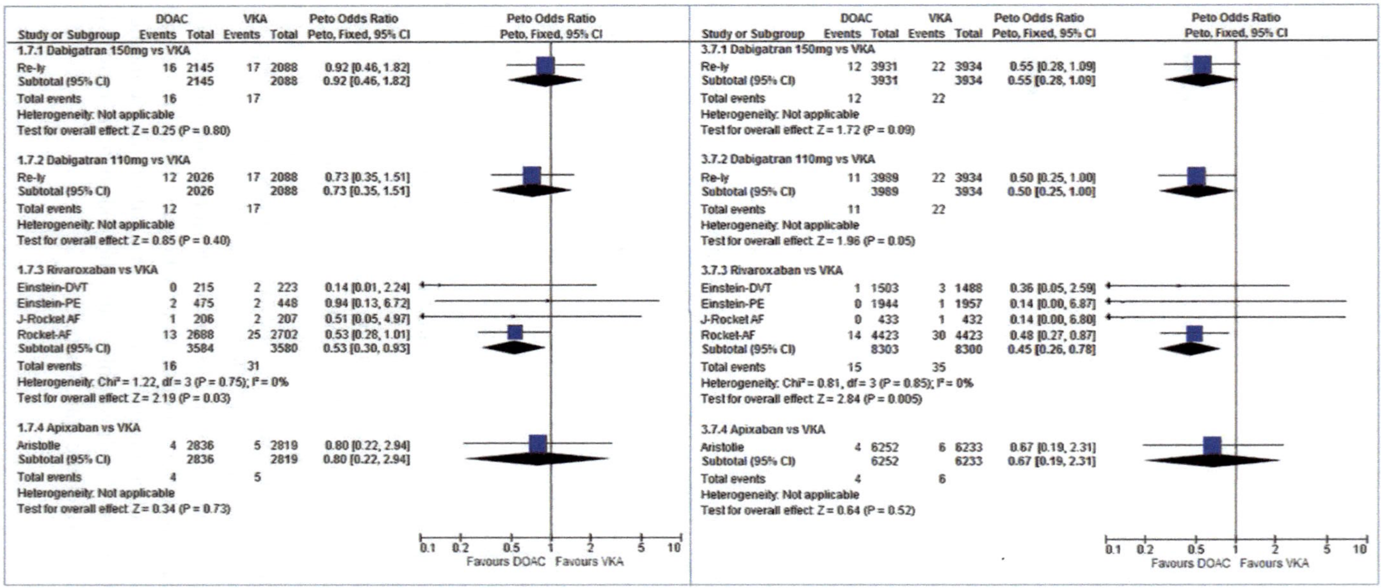

Fig. 4.2 Forest Plots for risk of Fatal Bleeding in Elderly: DOACs vs. VKA (Modified from Sharma et al. [38]; with permission)

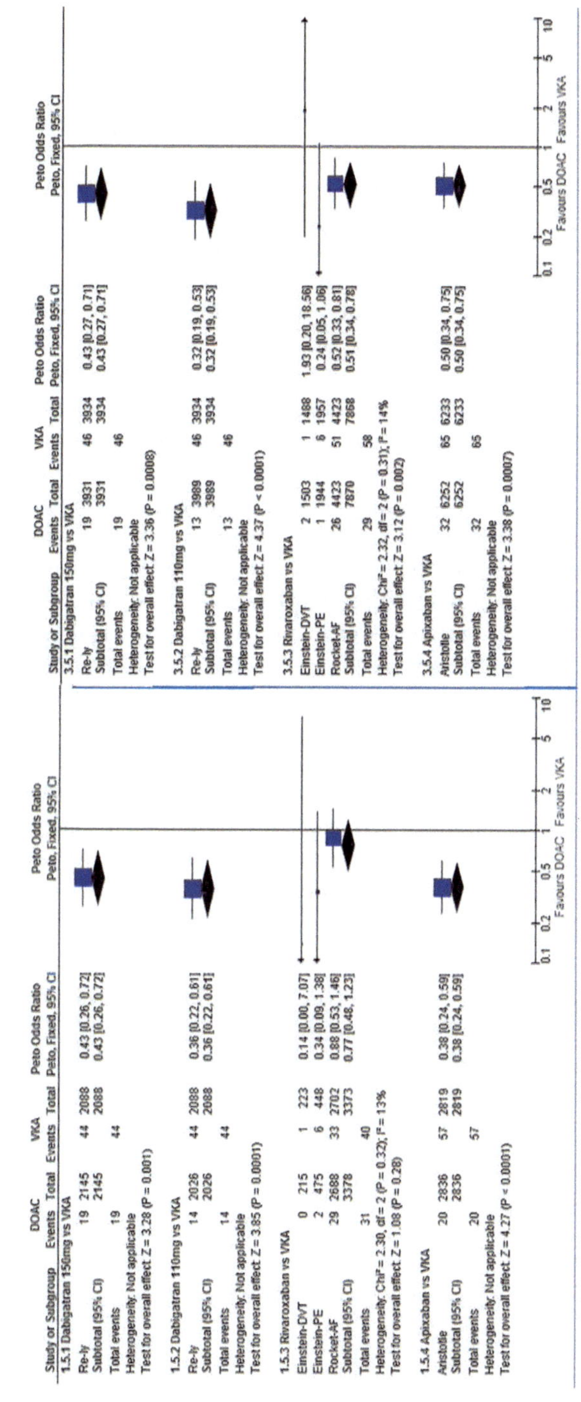

Fig. 4.3 Forest plots for risks of intracranial bleeding in elderly: DOACs vs. VKA (Modified from Sharma et al. [38]; with permission)

4.6 Systemic Thrombolysis

Thrombolytic therapy for acute deep venous thrombosis has evolved to catheter-directed approaches. Systemic thrombolysis for VTE is limited to patients with PE. Low-risk patients are well treated with anticoagulation alone. High-risk patients (massive PE) are those who are hemodynamically unstable and require an intervention to reduce the obstruction in their pulmonary arteries in order to improve upon their 50% mortality. Intermediate-risk PE (submassive) patients are those with right ventricular dilation or those with biomarker evidence of myocardial stretch (elevated pro–B-type natriuretic peptide [BNP]) or myocardial injury (elevated troponins).The use of thrombolytic agents in intermediate-risk patients remains controversial, especially for those in the older age groups.

Chatterjee et al. [39] attempt to put this into proper perspective in recent meta-analysis. They set out to determine the mortality benefit and bleeding risks associated with systemic thrombolytic therapy versus anticoagulation in those patients with intermediate-risk pulmonary embolism. They further analyze the data (where available) in patients 65 years and younger versus those older than 65 years (Table 4.3). They found a significant mortality reduction in patients treated with thrombolytic therapy versus anticoagulation (52% relative risk reduction). Patients of both age groups benefited in terms of reduced mortality when treated with lytic therapy. The younger patients had no increased risk of major bleeds, whereas those over 65 had a significant increased risk of major bleeds ($p < .001$). The differential in risk/benefit would be magnified further if the age cut-off was 75 years versus 65 years.

In elderly patients with high-risk submassive and massive pulmonary embolism, it is now our preference to treat these patients with catheter-based techniques [40]. Catheter-based techniques, which fragment large central pulmonary emboli after a pulse spray of tissue plasminogen activator into the thrombus and with continued low-dose infusion (1 mg tissue plasminogen reactor [rt-PA]/h), are an effective way to manage these patients resulting in a marked risk reduction in major bleeding complications.

Table 4.3 Risk metrics of outcomes for patients treated for pulmonary embolism with thrombolysis or anticoagulation: a meta-analysis

	Absolute event rate (%)			
Outcome	Thrombolytic group (%)	Anticoagulant group (%)	*p*-value	No. needed to treat/harm
Age ≤ 65 yrs				
All-cause mortality	2.3	4.3	.09	NNT-51
Major bleed	2.8	2.3	.09	NNH-176
Age > 65 yrs				
All-cause mortality	2.1	3.7	.07	NNT-64
Major bleed	12.9	4.1	<.001	NNH-11

Data from Chatterjee et al. [39]

4.7 Catheter-Directed Thrombolysis

Patients with symptomatic iliofemoral venous thrombosis who are physically active suffer significant postthrombotic morbidity following iliofemoral DVT treated with anticoagulation alone as do those with thrombotic obliteration of their popliteal and calf veins. In these patients, catheter-directed thrombolysis with intrathrombus infusion of low doses of rt-PA has been shown to effectively reduce postthrombotic morbidity [41–43].

Data do not exist which evaluate the differential risk of older patients versus younger patients who receive catheter-directed thrombolysis. It is unlikely that we will receive any insight from randomized trials, as patients older than 75 years are often excluded from randomization.

I have not excluded elderly patients who have had extensive deep venous thrombosis from catheter-directed thrombolysis if they are physically active, have a negative CT scan of the brain, and have no high-risk factor for bleeding. Maintenance of activity in the elderly population significantly contributes to their quality of life and ongoing good health.

The use of catheter-directed low doses of lytic agents (0.5–1.0 mg/h) and the routine use of adjunctive mechanical techniques have contributed significantly to reductions in the dose of plasminogen activator and the duration of infusion [44]. The use of a high volume (50 cc to 100 cc per h) has accelerated the thrombolytic effect more than increasing the dose of rt-PA. Therefore, one can expect favorable efficacy outcomes with a reduced risk of bleeding complications. Subsequent to thrombolysis, correction of underlying venous stenoses and therapeutic anticoagulation are important for long-term success.

Key Points

- Elderly patients deserve special consideration when they are treated for venous thromboembolic disease.
- Thromboembolic risk significantly increases with age; therefore, proper therapy is important. Bleeding complications likewise increase risk.
- The newer target specific oral anticoagulants are associated with reduced bleeding complications compared to vitamin K antagonists.
- Catheter-based techniques for high-risk pulmonary emboli and extensive symptomatic deep venous thrombosis offer significant advantage with a reduced risk of bleeding complications.

Acknowledgement The author wishes to recognize the expert asssistance of medical writer/editor, Shakela Watkins, MA, in the preperation of this chapter.

References

1. Galson SK. The surgeon general's call to action to prevent deep vein thrombosis and pulmonary embolism. NA.2015.http:///www.surgeiongeneral.gov/topics/deepvein/.

2. National Quality Forum. National Voluntary Consensus Standards for Prevention and Care of Venous Thromboembolism: additonal perfomance measures. Executive Summary 2008. NA.2015.http://www.qualityforum.org/Publications/2008/10/National_Voluntary_Consensus_Standards_for%20Prevention_and_Care_of_Venous_Thromboembolism_Additonal_ Performance_Measures.aspx.
3. Naess IA, Christiansen SC, Romundstad P, Cannegieter SC, Rosendaal FR, Hammerstrom J. Incidence and mortality of venous thrombosis: a population-based study. J Thromb Haemost2007;5:692–9. doi:10.1111/j.1538-7836.2007.02450.x.JTH02450 [pii].
4. Cushman M, Rosendaal FR, Psaty BM, et al. Factor V Leiden is not a risk factor for arterial vascular disease in the elderly: Results from the Cardiovascular Health Study. Thromb Haemost. 1998;79:912–5.
5. Poort SR, Rosendaal FR, Reitsma PH, Bertina RM. A common genetic variation in the 3-untranslated region of the prothrombin gene is associated with elevated plasma prothrombin levels and an increase in venous thrombosis. Blood. 1996;88:3698–703.
6. Mosterd A, Hoes AW, de Bruyne MC, et al. Prevalence of heart failure and left ventricular dysfunction in the general population; The Rotterdam Study. Eur Heart J. 1999;20:447–55. doi:10.1053/euhj.1998.1239.
7. Erelel M, Cuhadaroğlu C, Ece T, Arseven O. The frequency of deep venous thrombosis and pulmonary embolus in acute exacerbation of chronic obstructive pulmonary disease. Respir Med. 96:515–8. doi:10.1053/rmed.2002.1313.
8. Kamphuisen PW, Agnelli G, Sebastianelli M. Prevention of venous thromboembolism after acute ischemic stroke. J Thromb Haemost. 2005;3:1187–94.
9. Ageno W, Agnelli G, Imberti D, et al. Risk factors for venous thromboembolism in the elderly: results of the master registry. Blood Coagul Fibrinolysis. 2008;19:663–7.
10. Paneesha S, McManus A, Arya R, et al. Frequency, demographics and risk (according to tumour type or site) of cancer-associated thrombosis among patients seen at outpatient DVT clinics. Thromb Haemost. 2010;103:338–43.
11. Migliacci R, Becattini C, Pesavento R, et al. Endothelial dysfunction in patients with spontaneous venous thromboembolism. Haematologica. 2007;92:812–8. doi:10.3324/haematol.10872.
12. Chopard RP, Miranda Neto MH, Biazotto W, Molinari SL. Age-related changes in the human renal veins and their valves. Ital J Anat Embryol. 1994;99:91–101.
13. Frey PM, Méan M, Limacher A, Jaeger K, Beer HJ, Frauchiger B, et al. Physical activity and risk of bleeding in elderly patients taking anticoagulants. J Thromb Haemost. 2015;13(2): 197–205.
14. Olsen H, Länne T. Reduced venous compliance in lower limbs of aging humans and its importance for capacitance function. Am J Physiol Heart Circ Physiol. 1998;275:H878–86.
15. Carrier M, Le Gal G, Bates SM, Anderson DR, Wells PS. D-dimer testing is useful to exclude deep vein thrombosis in elderly outpatients. J Thromb Haemost. 2008;6:1072–6.
16. Folsom AR, Boland LL, Cushman M, Heckbert SR, Rosamond WD, Walston JD. Frailty and Risk of Venous Thromboembolism in Older Adults. J Gerontol A Biol Sci Med Sci. 2007;62:79–82.
17. Andro M, Righini M, Le GG. Adapting the D-dimer cutoff for thrombosis detection in elderly outpatients. Expert Rev Cardiovasc Ther. 2013;11:751–9. doi:10.1586/erc.13.51.
18. Oger E, Bressollette L, Nonent M, et al. High prevalence of asymptomatic deep vein thrombosis on admission in a medical unit among elderly patients. Thromb Haemost. 2002;88:592–7.
19. Wells PS, Anderson DR, Rodger M, et al. Evaluation of D-dimer in the diagnosis of suspected deep-veinthrombosis.NEnglJMed.2003;349:1227–35.doi:10.1056/NEJMoa023153.349/13/1227 [pii].
20. Harper PL, Theakston E, Ahmed J, Ockelford P. D-dimer concentration increases with age reducing the clinical value of the D-dimer assay in the elderly. Intern Med J. 2007; 37:607–13.
21. Lopez-Jimenez L, Montero M, Gonzalez-Fajardo JA, et al. Venous thromboembolism in very elderly patients: findings from a prospective registry (RIETE). Haematologica. 2006;91:1046–51.

22. Levine MN, Raskob G, Beyth RJ, Kearon C, Schulman S. Hemorrhagic complications of anticoagulant treatment : The seventh accp conference on antithrombotic and thrombolytic therapy. Chest. 2004;126:287S–310S. doi:10.1378/chest.126.3_suppl.287S.
23. Clase CM, Garg AX, Kiberd BA. Prevalence of Low Glomerular Filtration Rate in Nondiabetic Americans: Third National Health and Nutrition Examination Survey (NHANES III). J Am Soc Nephrol. 2002;13:1338–49.
24. Campbell NC, Hull RD, Brant R, Hogan DB, Pineo GF, Raskob GE. AGing and heparin-related bleeding. Arch Intern Med. 1996;156:857–60. doi:10.1001/archinte.1996.00440080047006.
25. Spinler SA, Evans CM. Update in unfractionated heparin, low-molecular-weight heparins, and heparinoids in the elderly (age >/= 65 years). J Thromb Thrombolysis. 2000;9:117.
26. Lim W, Dentali F, Eikelboom JW, Crowther MA. Meta-Analysis: Low-Molecular-Weight Heparin and Bleeding in Patients with Severe Renal Insufficiency. Ann Intern Med. 2006;144:673–84. doi:10.7326/0003-4819-144-9-200605020-00011.
27. Kucher N, Leizorovicz A, Vaitkus PT. Efficacy and safety of fixed low-dose dalteparin in preventing venous thromboembolism among obese or elderly hospitalized patients: A subgroup analysis of the prevent trial. Arch Intern Med. 2005;165:341–5. doi:10.1001/archinte.165.3.341.
28. Hajjar ER, Hanlon JT, Artz MB, et al. Adverse drug reaction risk factors in older outpatients. Am J Geriatr Pharmacother.2003;1:82–9. doi:S1543594603900043 [pii].
29. Hutten BA, Lensing AW, Kraaijenhagen RA, Prins MH. Safety of treatment with oral anticoagulants in the elderly. A systematic review. Drugs Aging. 1999;14:303–12.
30. Bond AJ, Molnar FJ, Li M, Mackey M, Man-Son-Hing M. The risk of hemorrhagic complications in hospital in-patients who fall while receiving antithrombotic therapy. Thromb J.2005;3:1. doi:10.1186/1477-9560-3-1. 1477–9560–3-1 [pii].
31. Man-Son-Hing M, Nichol G, Lau A, Laupacis A. Choosing antithrombotic therapy for elderly patients with atrial fibrillation who are at risk for falls. Arch Intern Med. 1999;159:677–85.
32. Optimal oral anticoagulant therapy in patients with nonrheumatic atrial fibrillation and recent cerebral ischemia. The European Atrial Fibrillation Trial Study Group. N Engl J Med. 1995;333:5–10. doi:10.1056/NEJM199507063330102
33. Bleeding during antithrombotic therapy in patients with atrial fibrillation. The stroke prevention in atrial fibrillation investigators. Arch Intern Med.1996;156:409–16.
34. Palareti G, Hirsh J, Legnani C, et al. Oral anticoagulation treatment in the elderly: a nested, prospective, case-control study. Arch Intern Med. 2000;160:470–8.
35. Pengo V, Legnani C, Noventa F, Palareti G. Oral anticoagulant therapy in patients with nonrheumatic atrial fibrillation and risk of bleeding. A Multicenter Inception Cohort Study. Thromb Haemost.2001;85:418–22. doi:01030418 [pii].
36. Copland M, Walker ID, Tait RC. Oral anticoagulation and hemorrhagic complications in an elderly population with atrial fibrillation. Arch Intern Med.2001;161:2125–8. doi:ioi00745 [pii].
37. Pautas E, Gouin-Thibault I, Debray M, Gaussem P, Siguret V. Haemorrhagic complications of vitamin k antagonists in the elderly: risk factors and management. Drugs Aging. 2006;23(1): 13–25.
38. Sharma M, Cornelius VR, Patel JP, Davies JG, Molokhia M. Efficacy and harms of direct oral anticoagulants in the elderly for stroke prevention in atrial fibrillation and secondary prevention of venous thromboembolism: systematic review and meta-analysis. Circulation.2015;132:194-204. doi:10.1161/CIRCULATIONAHA.114.013267. CIRCULATIONAHA.114.013267 [pii].
39. Chatterjee S, Chakraborty A, Weinberg I. Thrombolysis for pulmonary embolism and risk of all-cause mortality, major bleeding, and intracranial hemorrhage: A meta-analysis. JAMA. 2014;311:2414–21. doi:10.1001/jama.2014.5990.
40. Akin H, Al-Jubouri M, Assi Z, Acino R, Sepanski D, Comerota AJ. Catheter-directed thrombolytic intervention is effective for patients with massive and submassive pulmonary embolism. Ann Vasc Surg. 2014;28:1589–94.
41. Enden T, Haig Y, Klow NE, et al. Long-term outcome after additional catheter-directed thrombolysis versus standard treatment for acute iliofemoral deep vein thrombosis (the CaVenT study): a randomised controlled trial. Lancet.2012;379:31–8. doi:10.1016/S0140-6736(11)61753-4. S0140–6736(11)61753–4 [pii].

42. Comerota AJ, Throm RC, Mathias SD, Haughton S, Mewissen M. Catheter-directed thrombolysis for iliofemoral deep venous thrombosis improves health-related quality of life. J Vasc Surg.2000;32:130–7. doi:10.1067/mva.2000.105664.S0741–5214(00)81612–2 [pii].
43. Comerota AJ, Grewal N, Martinez JT, et al. Postthrombotic morbidity correlates with residual thrombus following catheter-directed thrombolysis for iliofemoral deep vein thrombosis. J Vasc Surg.2012;55:768–73. doi:10.1016/j.jvs.2011.10.032.S0741–5214(11)02407–4 [pii].
44. Martinez Trabal JL, Comerota AJ, LaPorte FB, Kazanjian S, Disalle R, Sepanski DM. The quantitative benefit of isolated, segmental, pharmacomechanical thrombolysis (ISPMT) for iliofemoral venous thrombosis. J Vasc Surg. 2008;48:1532–7. doi:10.1016/j.jvs.2008.07.013. S0741–5214(08)01148–8 [pii].

Management of Chronic Venous Disease and Varicose Veins in the Elderly

5

Huiting Chen, Bradley Reames, and Thomas W. Wakefield

5.1 Background

Varicose veins in the extremities are a clinical sequela of chronic venous insufficiency (CVI). Previous estimates indicate more than 30 million Americans suffer from CVI, with more than half being women [1, 2]. More recently, Kaplan and colleagues estimated 23% of adults have varicose veins and 6% have even more advanced disease skin changes, healed ulcers, or active ulcers [3]. In addition to being an unwanted cosmetic state, varicose veins substantially lower health-related quality-of-life. Patients with varicose veins frequently suffer from pain and disability with resultant loss of working days and economic disablement. With an aging population and a higher prevalence of chronic venous disease in an older population, understanding how the pathophysiology of chronic venous disease leads to varicosities and applying current evidence-based guidelines to their treatment is of the greatest importance.

5.2 Workup for Leg Edema

Lower extremity edema is a common clinical finding, with an array of vastly different pathologic etiologies. Therefore, the workup for leg edema must include a narrowing of this sizable list of differential diagnoses using clinical insight, as the overuse of multiple radiographic and physiologic studies is neither efficient nor financially practical.

H. Chen (✉)
Section of Vascular Surgery, University of Michigan, Ann Arbor, MI, USA
e-mail: huitingc@med.umich.edu

B. Reames
Department of Surgery, University of Michigan, Ann Arbor, MI, USA

T.W. Wakefield
Section of Vascular Surgery, Samuel and Jean Frankel Cardiovascular Center, University of Michigan, Ann Arbor, MI, USA

R. Chaer (ed.), *Vascular Disease in Older Adults*,
DOI 10.1007/978-3-319-29285-4_5

5.2.1 Special Considerations for the Elderly

For patients of all ages, both intrinsic vascular and systemic causes of leg edema must be considered in the differential diagnoses. While idiopathic edema is the most likely cause of leg edema in women under the age of 50 [4], the considerations are different for the elderly population. Of the vascular causes of edema, chronic venous insufficiency is the most common, with other etiologies to consider being deep venous thromboses and lymphedema. The pathophysiology of CVI is mostly due to reflex, but in certain groups, obstruction plays a larger role. In a study of 163 limbs in 150 postmenopausal women with a mean age of 68 who had leg swelling as the primary complaint and who were unresponsive to conservative therapy, intravascular ultrasound-guided iliac vein stenting of a venous obstruction resulted in significant improvement in swelling and in pain [5]. In as early as 36 months post-stenting, approximately 65% of limbs had complete pain relief, with approximately 70% of limbs with a subjective improvement in swelling.

In elderly patients who often have underlying comorbidities, other principal causes should be entertained. Cardiopulmonary dysfunction may cause chronic bilateral leg edema in the form of heart failure, pulmonary hypertension, and associated obstructive sleep apnea. Other organ dysfunction such as renal disease with glomerulonephritis and liver disease may be considered. As the occurrence of certain malignancies increases with age, the exertion of external pressure from pelvic tumors or lymphomas is a less likely but additional cause of chronic bilateral lower extremity edema not to be ignored. Lastly, medications have been implicated in causing leg edema—most commonly calcium channel blockers (up to 50% of patients) and nonsteroidal anti-inflammatory drugs (approximately 5%) [6–8]. Additional drug considerations include dihydropyridines and hormones [6].

Following a thorough history and physical to narrow the differential diagnosis to chronic venous insufficiency, various diagnostic studies are available for further evaluation and confirmation of CVI. Both noninvasive and invasive techniques may be considered, depending on the complexity of the presentation. Duplex ultrasound is the mainstay of the standard clinical evaluation. This modality is both cost-effective and typically readily available, and can be performed safely on all patients, including pregnant patients. Additional noninvasive studies to consider include air plethysmography (APG) or magnetic resonance venography (MRV). Invasive testing such as phlebography or intravenous ultrasound is performed selectively for operative planning or for patients with suspected or confirmed iliac vein obstruction.

5.2.2 Duplex Ultrasound

The use of duplex ultrasound allows for the evaluation of pathophysiology—reflux or obstruction—along with the assessment of anatomical findings at various levels—superficial, deep, and perforating veins. Additionally, this modality provides information on the chronicity of deep venous thromboses that may be visualized.

Typically, multi-frequency 4–7-MHz linear array transducers are used for assessment of lower extremity venous reflux. Often, the exam is performed while the patient is standing, with manual compression of the calf or thigh to assess reflux. The Valsalva maneuver or automatic rapid inflation/deflation cuffs may also be used. Venous reflux, defined as pathologic retrograde flow due to valvular absence or incompetence, results in prolonged valve closure times. The cutoff values for reflux differ depending on the anatomic location of the vein evaluated: for superficial veins, the value is greater than 500 ms; for deep veins, the value is greater than 1000 ms. For perforating veins, while a recommendation is using a cutoff value of greater than 350 ms, often the convention is 500 ms. Notably, perforating veins, which penetrate between anatomic layers and flow between superficial and deep veins, may have inward and/or outward flow with compression and release of the leg. When bidirectional flow is seen, the net flow from deep to superficial is used for assessment.

While duplex ultrasound of the lower extremity venous system is quick, noninvasive, and inexpensive, its use is limited by the need for an experienced vascular technologist to perform the exam and by inter-operator variability. Additionally, it is unable to provide direct evaluation of the pelvic vasculature due to anatomic limitations. Indirect evidence of obstruction above the inguinal ligament is inferred by lack of venous flow with Valsalva maneuver and loss of respiratory variation.

5.2.3 Air Plethysmography

Air plethysmography (APG) is a noninvasive, physiologic study for the evaluation of venous reflux, calf muscle pump function, and venous obstruction. To measure reflux, a low-pressure cuff is first placed around the calf and a baseline volume is obtained with the patient resting. Upon standing, the volume tracing at plateau reflects the venous volume (VV), with 90% filling time (VFT90) defined as the time required to achieve 90% VV. The venous filling index (VFI) is the ratio between 90% VV and VFT90; normally, it is less than 2 mL/s. APG also evaluates calf muscle pump function. The patient performs a tiptoe maneuver followed by a return to rest, with the amount of venous blood expelled from the leg defined as the ejection fraction (EF). After ten consecutive tiptoe maneuvers with rest in between, the blood remaining in the leg is the residual volume, with residual volume fraction (RVF) expressed as a percentage of the baseline volume of the leg. Lower RVF values indicate better calf pump function, with a normal RVF defined as less than 35%.

Venous obstruction is estimated by APG following an outflow curve obtained from the limb. A thigh cuff is inflated, and the VV is measured. After deflation of the cuff, the outflow curve is recorded, with a lower outflow fraction (the volume expelled after cuff deflation in 1 s divided by VV) reflective of obstruction. Notably, outflow is affected by collaterals and limited by technique, making it difficult to see compensated obstruction. Taking all aspects of APG into account, the most valued aspect of its use is to determine presence and severity of reflux.

5.2.4 CT Venogram

Computed tomography with contrast enhancement timed for venous filling is useful in evaluating centrally located veins that are difficult to image with duplex ultrasound. Extrinsic compression from nearby structures or intrinsic obstruction is easily visualized with this modality, and its use extends to preoperative planning for both open and endovascular procedures. However, it is an expensive modality which exposes the patient to both radiation and contrast and should not be an initial imaging modality to evaluate CVI.

5.2.5 MR Venogram

Magnetic resonance venography, similar to CT venography, allows imaging of the central veins and their surrounding structures. While useful in operative planning, its expensive nature and risk of nephrogenic systemic fibrosis in patients with renal failure preclude it from being a first-line imaging technique.

5.2.6 Phlebography

While once considered the "gold standard" for assessment of chronic venous obstruction, phlebography is now used for specific indications due to innovations in noninvasive assessment modalities. Indications include diagnosis of a deep venous thrombosis when duplex ultrasound is inconclusive or nonfeasible (although this is rare in our experience), venous mapping prior to surgical intervention, and evaluation of venous malformations.

Ascending phlebography can be used to clarify the existence of DVT in the lower extremity. In this procedure, venous access is obtained through a dorsal foot vein, with contrast directed toward the deep system by placing tourniquets at the ankle and at the knee, released prior to image acquisition. A luminal filling defect with a surrounding rim of contrast or an abrupt cessation of intravascular contrast indicates venous thrombosis.

Descending phlebography is used to evaluate incompetent valves in patients with suspected CVI, as it provides more localization of specific incompetent segments than duplex ultrasound. This procedure requires direct injection of contrast material into the deep venous system, often through the common femoral vein. Using a tilt radiographic table and C-arm fluoroscopy, a catheter is placed into common femoral vein of the leg of interest from an internal jugular or contralateral femoral vein access, and the table is elevated to approximately 60°. Contrast is injected in the catheter during quiet respiration and, if the valves are competent, during the Valsalva maneuver. Eccentric reflux through one or two valve levels is within normal limits. This imaging allows reflux to be graded as the following: 0: no reflux, 1: reflux confined to the upper thigh, 2: reflux to femoral but not the popliteal vein, 3: reflux extending to the popliteal vein and extending to the calf veins, and 4: reflux through the calf or ankle.

5.2.7 Special Considerations in the Elderly

Evaluation by duplex ultrasound and APG contain an element of standing for optimal assessment of reflux, although standing is not necessary when evaluating for DVT. However, this segment of the population may have more difficulties with prolonged standing or may lack the musculature required to perform calf muscle pumps. The ultrasound evaluation may be modified by having the patient lie on the examination table. However, the APG results may be suboptimal, as there are no alternative methods to measuring calf pump function if the patient is unable to perform the muscular squeeze.

Phlebography and CT venogram require the administration of iodinated contrast, which must be used with caution in an elderly population predisposed to impaired renal clearance as its administration may worsen preexisting renal insufficiency. MR venogram uses gadolinium, and its administration in patients with compromised renal function places them at a higher risk of nephrogenic systemic fibrosis. All three modalities require patients to lay supine, which may be difficult for patients with heart failure or severe lung dysfunction. In addition, magnetic resonance cannot be used in patients with metal-based implanted devices—a substantial consideration in an elderly population with pacemakers and orthopedic implants.

A degree of malnutrition and dehydration, which may lead to under-distention of the venous system and suboptimal examination, is an additional consideration in the elderly population. When dehydration is suspected either by history or by physical exam (dry mucous membranes or orthostatic hypotension, for example), the assessment would be more accurate by appropriate hydration of the patient prior to performing the evaluation.

5.3 Venous Insufficiency

Chronic venous insufficiency is a venous pathology with resultant clinical sequelae ranging from edema to venous stasis ulcers. Compared to the arterial system, the vessels of the venous system are highly compliant and easily collapsible due to their thin walls and lack of in situ external support. In normal venous physiology, veins in the lower extremity accept venous blood delivered by arterial inflow. Due to the high compliance of veins, increasing the venous volume by over two and one half times results in only a 0–15 mm Hg increment rise in pressure, allowing a significant amount of blood to be sequestered in the lower limb without a substantial buildup of intraluminal pressure [9]. However, capacitance has been met once the vein distends to its full circular shape, such that further increases in volume result in proportional increases in pressure. Normally, contraction of the leg muscles, which act as a pump, will expel the venous blood volume and propel blood cephalad. The closure of valves along the entire venous system—those of the superficial, deep, and perforating veins—prevents reflux of the venous blood and moves the blood centrally to return to the heart and lungs. However, prolonged pooling of the blood in the lower extremity venous system due to valvular incompetence results in sustained venous hypertension manifested as edema.

The underlying dysfunction in chronic venous insufficiency is from obstruction, valvular insufficiency, calf muscle pump malfunction, or a combination of the three. Venous obstruction, which causes venous bloods exiting the lower extremity to meet high resistance, results in elevated intravenous pressure. The role of obstruction is considerable, with reports that suggest venous occlusive disease in combination with venous insufficiency is found in 55% of patients with chronic venous insufficiency, most notably in patients with severe symptoms [10]. Noted findings of deep venous obstruction include left common iliac vein compression by the right common iliac artery (May-Thurner Syndrome); external iliac vein compression from the internal iliac artery on either side [11, 12]; external compression from tumors, infection, fibrosis, femoral hernias (femoral vein), and popliteal aneurysms (popliteal vein); and external vein wall scarring with webs and bands from deep venous thromboses.

While valvular insufficiency is estimated to be the underlying cause in up to 85% of cases of symptomatic chronic venous disease, this figure may not account for the associated role venous obstruction plays in many cases. Nonetheless, valvular insufficiency affects all levels of the venous system. Patients with isolated superficial valvular reflux tend to exhibit minimal symptoms, but those with perforator or deep reflux demonstrate increased risk of progression along higher clinical manifestations in Clinical Etiology Anatomy Pathophysiology (CEAP) classification. In patients with venous ulcers, two vein systems were involved in 50–70% of patients, with all three systems involved in 16–50% of patients [13–16]. The presence of obstruction further compounds the severity of clinical symptoms.

In patients with calf muscle pump dysfunction, the muscle is unable to generate the force needed to propel venous blood centrally. Elderly patients are at higher risk of this dysfunction from muscle disuse or bedridden status. Muscle fibrosis conditions such as muscular dystrophy are additional causes. Often treatment is limited to physical conditioning and muscle rehabilitation.

Correctly diagnosing and classifying chronic venous insufficiency is the foundation to providing accurate treatment and to assessing progress. The CEAP classification is based on clinical signs of venous disease (C), etiology (E), anatomy (A), and the underlying pathophysiology (P) (Table 5.1). However, while the basic CEAP classification allows for a clinical grading and understanding among clinicians, it does not allow longitudinal follow-up nor provide subjective information. The Venous Clinical Severity Score (VCSS) was subsequently developed to reflect clinical changes following treatment (Table 5.2). The VCSS is comprised of ten attributes (pain, varicose veins, edema, pigmentation, inflammation, induration, number of ulcers, duration of ulcers, size of ulcers, compressive therapy) which can be followed longitudinally to reflect developments in a patient's disease state, with both objective and subjective measures.

Table 5.1 CEAP Classification of Chronic Venous Disease

Clinical classification		
C0	No visible or palpable signs of venous disease	
C1	Telangictasias or reticular veins	
C2	Varicose veins	
C3	Edema	
C4a	Pigmentation and/or eczema	
C4b	lipodermatosclerosis and/or atrophie blanche	
C5	Healed venous ulceration	
C6	Active venous ulceration	
Etiologic classification		
E_c	Congenital	
E_P	Primary	
E_S	Secondary	
E_n	No venous etiology identified	
Anatomic classification		
A_s	Superficial veins	
	1	Telangiectasias/reticular veins
	2	Great saphenous vein (above knee)
	3	Great saphenous vein (below knee0)
	4	Small saphenous vein
	5	Nonsaphenous veins
A_d	Deep veins	
	6	Inferior vena cava
	7	Common iliac vein
	8	Internal iliac vein
	9	External iliac vein
	10	Pelvis veins (gonadal, broad ligament, other)
	11	Common femoral vein
	12	Deep femoral vein
	13	Femoral vein
	14	Popliteal vein
	15	Crural vein (anterior tibial, posterior tibial, peroneal)
	16	Muscular vein (gastrocnemial, soleal, other)
A_p	Perforating veins	
	17	Thigh perforator veins
	18	Calf perforator veins
Pathophysiological classification		
P_r	Reflux	
P_o	Obstruction	
$P_{r,o}$	Reflux and obstruction	
P_n	No venous pathophysiology identified	

Table 5.2 Venous Clinical Severity Score (VCSS)

Attribute	Clinical severity			
	Absent = 0	Mild = 1	Moderate = 2	Severe = 3
Pain	None	Occasional, not restricting activity, no analgesics	Daily, moderate activity limits, occasional analgesics	Daily, severe activity limits, regular use of analgesics
Varicose veins	None	Few, isolated branch varices	Multiple, GSV, or SSV varices, calf only	Extensive, GSV or SSV varices, calf and thigh
Venous edema	None	Evening, ankle	Afternoon, above the ankle	Morning, above the ankle, requires activity change, elevation
Skin pigmentation	None or focal, low intensity (tan)	Diffuse, limited in area and old (brown)	Diffuse over gaiter distribution (lower 1/3) or recent pigmentation (purple)	Wider distribution (above lower 1/3) and recent pigmentation
Inflammation	None	Mild cellulitis, limited to marginal area around ulcer	Moderate cellulitis, involves most of gaiter area	Severe cellulitis (lower 1/3 and above) or venous eczema
Induration	None	Focal, circum-malleolar, <5 cm	Medial or lateral, less than lower third of leg	Enter lower greater third of leg or more
No. of active ulcers	0	1	2–4	>4
Ulcer duration	None	<3 month	>3 mo, <1 year	Not healed >1 year
Ulcer size	None	<2 cm diameter	2–4 cm diameter	>4 cm diameter
Compressive therapy	Not used or noncompliant	Intermittent use of stockings	Use most days	Full compliance and elevation

5.3.1 Special Considerations in the Elderly

During the workup of CVI, the physician gathers a patient's full history and physical and weighs the risk and benefits of any therapeutic interventions. An important consideration in the process of weighing operative therapy is the optimal type of anesthesia for the procedure. Common modes of anesthesia for venous procedures include local tumescent anesthesia (LA), regional anesthesia (RA), and general anesthesia. While no dedicated studies exist on the type of optimal anesthesia for CVI procedures in the elderly—indeed, optimal anesthesia is largely patient-specific—one may extrapolate from studies in the elderly population as a whole. In general, anesthesia-associated risks depend on American Society of Anesthesiologists classification (ASA score), comorbidities, the type of surgery, and the emergent nature of the surgery. A recent Cochrane review of LA, RA, and GA in noncardiac surgery for patients >65 years reviewed morbidity and mortality in mostly orthopedic and various surgical disciplines (not vascular-specific) [17]. The review found that in elderly orthopedic patients, RA showed a lower early-term mortality rate, reduced fatal pulmonary embolisms rates, and lessened postoperative confusion compared to GA. However, GA is associated with a lower incidence of hypotension. Nausea and vomiting was observed in a lesser extent with LA compared to RA and GA in elderly patients undergoing hernia surgery. Overall, the authors note that the occurrence of true anesthesia-related complications is rare and that the postoperative complications are often related to the procedure itself, not the anesthetic of choice. While difficult to generalize these findings to vascular patients undergoing procedures for CVI, physicians must work closely with the anesthesia team to optimize the patient's individual anesthetic choice.

5.4 Telangiectasias and Reticular Veins

As previously discussed (Table 5.1), the CEAP classification presents a standardized system by which to catalog the clinical findings of chronic venous insufficiency. As the severity of CVI increases, the patient's concerns typically shift from cosmetic to impaired functional status and discomfort. In the early stage with telangiectasias and reticular veins (C1), however, cosmetic concerns typically drive the request for physician evaluation and potential invasive intervention. In addition to discussing surgical risks and benefits as with all patients, providers must make aware to patients whose clinical severity is C1 that the insurance coverage may not extend to procedures performed for cosmetic indications.

Patients with C1 disease with cosmetic concerns or minimal symptoms may benefit from local ablative therapies [18]. These include chemical-based therapies such as sclerotherapy and heat-based therapies such as thermocoagulation and laser treatments. Sclerotherapy is often used for smaller affected veins, and common sclerosing agents are classified as detergents, hypertonic solutions, or chemical irritants. While the agents act through different mechanisms, the ultimate result is sclerosis through endothelial cell injury. Heat-based therapies also produce endothelial injury, resulting in thrombosis and eventual fibrosis of the treated vein. Regardless of the modality used to treat telangiectasias or reticular veins, posttreatment compression of the lower extremity is recommended for more effective sclerosis and improved cosmetic results. Postoperative bruising and hyper-pigmentation of the treated areas are potential outcomes, which must be discussed specially with patients who are undergoing the procedure for cosmetic purposes. Both bruising and the hyper-pigmentation, caused by deposition of dermal hemosiderin, fade over time.

5.5 Varicose Veins

As CVI continues to progress from reticular veins and telangiectasias, varicose veins develop, marking C2 disease in the CEAP classification. This chronic condition is estimated in more than 20% of adults in the United States [3], and risk factors include older age, female gender, multiparity, family history, obesity, history of thrombophlebitis, or history of thrombosis. As previously discussed in the "Venous

Insufficiency" section, the underlying etiology of the development and progression of CVI is from valvular insufficiency leading to reflux, obstruction, calf muscle pump malfunction, or a combination of these factors. While some patients with varicosities may not present with symptoms, those with more advanced disease may complain of heaviness of the legs, tingling, achiness, prutitis, pain, and fatigue. These symptoms are often exacerbated by prolonged dependency or heat and relieved by leg elevation or compression elastic bandages or stockings. The presence of varicosities is often more than a nuisance or a cosmetic concern—they are a frequent cause of discomfort, disability, and decreased quality of life.

Following a dedicated history and physical and imaging (duplex scanning as the most common noninvasive modality) confirming varicose veins from underlying CVI, treatment options are considered on a patient-specific basis. The clinical practice guidelines of the Society for Vascular Surgery and the American Venous Forum [19] provide recommendations to enhance consistent evidence-based approaches to care for patients with varicose veins and associated chronic venous diseases, and they encompass medical therapy, compression, and surgical interventions.

Medical treatment incorporates venoactive drugs for the treatment of symptoms of varicose veins, though they do not address the underlying etiology. While the exact mechanism of action for most of these agents is unknown and they are unavailable in the United States, their use is intended to improve venous tone and capillary permeability. A recent Cochrane review by Martinez and colleagues analyzed 44 studies and found diosmin, hesperidin, and MPFF were the most effective venoactive drugs [20]. Diosmin and hesperidin also helped with the healing of trophic skin changes and treated cramps and swelling. Cramps and restless legs were also reduced by calcium dobesilate. Rutosides reduced venous edema. Overall, the meta-analysis concluded that evidence was insufficient to support the global use of these agents in the treatment of chronic venous disease.

Compression therapy is the most often used treatment of varicose veins and comes in various forms including elastic compression stockings, multilayer elastic wraps, bandages, and Unna boots. The use of compression is recommended in order to decrease venous hypertension in the lower extremities. While randomized control trials have not suggested definitive compressive pressures for addressing C2 disease, currently, the SVS/AVF Guideline Committee suggests graded prescriptions stockings with an ankle pressure of 20–30 mm Hg (Grade 2C). The use of compression therapy prior to consideration for surgical therapy may be a requirement for some practitioners due to insurance company policies for coverage. The REACTIV trial (Randomized Clinical Trial, Observational Study and assessment of Cost-Effectiveness of the Treatment of Varicose Veins), which randomized 246 patients with C2 disease to conservative management or surgery, demonstrated a significant quality of life benefit for surgery in the first 2 years after treatment, with substantial improvements in symptomatic and anatomic measures [21]. As noted in the SVS/AVF guidelines, there is virtually no scientific evidence to support requiring a trial of compression prior to more aggressive intervention, even though third-party payers often require it. Indeed, the REACTIV trial as described above has demonstrated that surgical treatment to treat superficial reflux is more efficacious and more cost-effective.

5.5.1 Special Considerations in the Elderly

In addition to considering the quality of life improvement from surgical intervention compared to compression alone, one must consider the limited functional ability the elderly population may have in applying elastic stockings. Patients with limited strength, pain from arthritis, chair- or bed-bound status, and obesity will predictably have difficulty with tight elastic stockings or wraps. In these patients, assistive devices, reliable family members, or nursing aides may improve compliance and effectiveness of this conservative approach.

Frequent surgical options include ablation of axial reflux by radiofrequency ablation (RFA) or endovenous laser treatment (EVLT) and phlebectomy by transilluminated powered phlebectomy (TIPP), stab approach, and, when relatively small, with sclerotherapy. Classically, the surgical approach for varicose veins was ligation and stripping, which was associated with large skin incisions and nerve injury. Over the past decade, endovenous thermal ablation has replaced much of the previous approach except in circumstances such as an exceptionally large and tortuous saphenous vein located immediately under the skin or difficult cannulation of the affected vein due to previous thrombophlebitis. Notably though, limited incisions are still made to perform ligations and miniphlebectomies of bulging varicosities of the great and small saphenous vein.

Endovenous thermal ablation is performed on the saphenous veins in place of the previous maximally invasive open surgical technique. This method encompasses both radiofrequency ablation (RFA) and endovenous laser treatment (EVLT): with both, the endothelium of the vein is destroyed by direct thermal energy to the vein wall, ultimately leading to fibrosis and thrombosis of the vein. The percutaneous placement of the radiofrequency or laser ablation catheter is minimally invasive, and the procedure is performed under direct ultrasound visualization to ensure both complete treatment of the saphenous vein and no thrombotic extension into the deep system. This outpatient procedure is then followed by the application of either elastic or nonelastic wraps or graduated compression stockings for at least 1 week, with encouragement to ambulate the same postoperative day to minimize risk of DVT and PE. Thrombosis prophylaxis is routine as well and driven by individual patient thrombosis risk assessment. Postoperative progress may be tracked with VCSS changes. Other new non-heat-inducing techniques to close off incompetent saphenous veins are being developed today, including mechanicochemical and glue.

For the branch varicosities, traditionally stab incision technique and the use of special vein hooks can be employed. Transilluminated powered phlebectomy (TIPP) is another technique used to remove large clusters of varicosities. It is often performed in combination with endothermal ablation to address both the source of reflux in addition to the cluster of varicose veins. In this approach, typically only small incisions are necessary in order to pass the instruments: an illuminator with a fiber optic cable for transillumination under the skin and delivery of tumescence irrigation, a central power until with an irrigation pump and a control of resection oscillation speeds, and a resector hand piece. Additionally, small punch incisions are made to drain the blood following phlebectomy, which is further cleared out with the tumescence fluid.

At our institution, the University of Michigan, 979 limbs from 3/31/2008–6/4/2014 were evaluated who had undergone RFA + TIPP compared to RFA alone. VCSS improved more with RFA + TIPP (3.8 ± 3.4 vs. 3.2 ± 3.1, $p = 0.018$) compared to RFA alone. Postoperative complications assessed were deep venous thrombosis/pulmonary embolism, EHIT (endovenous heat-induced thrombosis), infection, hematoma, and superficial venous thrombosis (SVT). More hematomas ($p < 0.001$) and SVTs ($p = 0.01$) occurred in patients who had undergone RFA + TIPP compared to RFA alone; other differences in complications between the two procedures were not significant. These results suggest RFA + TIPP provides improved VCSS with only incremental increases in morbidity for patients with symptomatic varicose veins and superficial venous insufficiency and should be considered first-line therapy. From the same University of Michigan database, a subset of these patients aged 65 and older who underwent RFA versus RFA + TIPP was analyzed for VCSS changes and the same complications as above, and WAS compared to those under age 65. Notably, with the age 65 and older subset, there was a trend toward a higher percentage of patients who had RFA alone compared to RFA + TIPP. In comparison to the entire group and to those under age 65, VCSS improved more with RFA alone compared to RFA + TIPP, although both groups improved VCSS improvement 4.1 and 3.8 for RFA and RFA + TIPP, respectively. Compared to the all-ages complications, the age 65 and older subset did not have significant differences in complications between the two procedures. In the older patients, thus they appeared to improve more with the lesser procedure. We speculate that this is because the underlying concern with the elderly is addressing their pain rather than the concern of the extent of the varicosities.

5.6 Venous Stasis Ulceration and Therapeutic Interventions

Venous leg ulcers (VLUs) are defined as open skin lesions of the leg or foot which occur in areas affected by venous hypertension and venous stasis. They account for 70% of all leg ulcers and are the most common ulceration of the lower extremity [22]. The Edinburgh study, a cross-sectional study examining 1566 subjects from age 18 to 64, found an estimate of venous leg ulcer prevalence of 1% with increasing prevalence with age [23]. An estimated 20% of the 2.5 million people in the United States who suffer from chronic venous insufficiency develop venous ulcers at some stage of their lives [24], and the estimated direct cost of treating these ulcers has been estimated to be $2500 per month per patient [25]. With such an economic impact and health care burden, it is of utmost importance that the treatment protocols given to patients are effective in maximizing the healing of VLUs and minimizing their recurrence.

The clinical practice guidelines of the Society of Vascular Surgery and the American Venous Forum impart a consistent approach to diagnosing and treating venous leg ulcers [26]. They provide both best practice guidelines for approaches with the strongest level of evidence and, for guidelines with less definitive evidence, recommendations and suggestions for additional approaches to care. Select guidelines and recommendations are presented below for clinical evaluation, wound care, compression, ancillary measures, and primary prevention.

A. *Clinical Evaluation*

Best practice guidelines recommend clinical evaluation performed for evidence of chronic venous disease for all patients with suspected leg ulcers. Additionally, medical conditions that affect ulcer healing and nonvenous causes of ulcer should be identified. All patients with VLUs are recommended to be classified with CEAP, revised Venous Clinical Severity Score, and venous disease-specific quality of life assessment.

Additional suggestions and recommendations include a recommendation for comprehensive venous duplex ultrasound exam of the lower extremity in all patients with suspected VLUs (Grade 1; level of evidence B) and a recommendation for wound biopsy for leg ulcers that do not improve with standard wound and compression therapy after 4–6 weeks (Grade 1; level of evidence C). They also recommend arterial pulse exam and measurement of ankle-brachial index on all patients with VLUs (Grade 1; level of evidence B). The guidelines suggest against routine culture of VLUs, but to obtain when clinical evidence of infection is present (Grade 2; level of evidence C).

B. *Wound Care*

There are no best practice guideline recommendations for wound care.

Additional suggestions and recommendations include a recommendation for VLUs to receive thorough debridement at their initial evaluation to remove obvious necrotic tissue (Grade 1; level of evidence B) and a recommendation that surgical debridement be performed for VLUs with slough, nonviable tissue, or eschar, with serial wound assessment for determining the need for repeated debridement (Grade 1; level of evidence B). The guidelines recommend that cellulitis surrounding the VLU be treated with systemic gram-positive antibiotics (Grade 1; level of evidence B) and suggest against systemic antimicrobial treatment of VLU colonization or biofilm without clinical evidence of infection (Grade 2; level of evidence C). Additionally, they recommend VLUs with clinical evidence of infection to be treated with systemic antibiotics guided by wound culture sensitivities (Grade 1; level of evidence C). Initial preferences are oral antibiotics, with a duration limited to 2 weeks unless there is persistent evidence of infection (Grade 1; level of evidence C).

The guidelines suggest hydrosurgical debridement as an alternative to standard surgical debridement (Grade 1; level of evidence B) and suggest against ultrasonic debridement over surgical debridement (Grade 2; level of evidence C). They suggest application of skin lubricants under compression to reduce dermatitis to surrounding skin (Grade 2; level of evidence C) and suggest cultured allogeneic bilayer skin replacements to increase the chances for healing in patients with difficult to heal VLUs who have not shown signs of healing after standard therapy for 4–6 weeks, in addition to compression therapy (Grade 2; level of evidence A)

C. *Compression*

There are no best practice guideline recommendations for compression.

Additional suggestions and recommendations include a recommendation for compression therapy over none to increase VLU healing rate (Grade 1; level of evidence A) and a suggestion of compression therapy in patients with healed VLUs to decrease risk of ulcer recurrence (Grade 2; level of evidence B). The guidelines recommend ablation of incompetent veins in addition to standard compressive therapy for patients with VLU (C6) and incompetent superficial veins with reflux directed to the bed of ulcer to prevent recurrence (Grade 1; level of evidence B). The guidelines also recommend ablation of the incompetent veins in addition to standard compressive therapy for patients with a healed VLU (C5) and incompetent superficial veins with reflux directed to the bed of the ulcer to prevent recurrence (Grade 1; level of evidence C). Percutaneous techniques over open venous perforator surgery for patients who would benefit from pathologic perforator vein ablation are also recommended (Grade 1; level of evidence C). The guidelines suggest ablation of incompetent veins in addition to standard compressive therapy for patients with VLU (C6) and incompetent superficial veins with reflux directed to the bed of ulcer for improved ulcer healing (Grade 2; level of evidence C). They also suggest ablation of both the incompetent superficial veins with reflux to the ulcer bed and pathologic perforator veins located beneath or associated with the ulcer bed to aid in ulcer healing and to prevent recurrence (Grade 2; level of evidence C).

D. *Ancillary Measures*

Best practice guidelines recommend nutrition assessment to be performed and nutritional supplementation to be provided if malnutrition identified.

Additional suggestions and recommendations include a recommendation for treatment with either pentoxifylline or micronized purified flavonoid fraction in combination with compression therapy for long-standing or large VLU (Grade 2; level of evidence B). They suggest supervised active exercise to improve muscle pump function and to reduce pain and edema in patients with VLUs (Grade 2; level of evidence B) and suggest against use of ultraviolet light for the treatment of VLUs (Grade 2; level of evidence C).

E. *Primary Prevention*

Best practice guidelines suggest patient and family education, regular exercise, leg elevation when at rest, careful skin care, weight control, and appropriately fitting foot wear for patients with C1-4 disease.

Additional suggestions and recommendations incorporate a recommendation for compression 20–30 mm Hg, knee or thigh high, for patients with clinical CEAP C3-4 disease due to primary valvular reflux (Grade 2; level of evidence C). Additionally, they recommend compression 30–40 mm Hg, knee or thigh high, for patients with clinical CEAP C1-4 disease related to prior deep venous thrombosis (DVT) (Grade 1; level of evidence B). Finally, current evidence-based therapies are recommended for acute DVT treatment, as postthrombotic syndrome is a common preceding event for VLUs (Grade 1; level of evidence B). Low-molecular-weight heparin over vitamin K antagonist therapy is suggested for 3 months to decrease postthrombotic syndrome (Grade 2; level of evidence B).

A recent systematic review and meta-analysis of surgical approaches compared to conservative treatment for VLUs evaluated open surgery versus compression, endovascular surgery versus compression, and open versus endovascular surgery. Mauck and colleagues did not uncover superiority of either surgical approach to conservative therapy for ulcer healing or recurrence outcomes in patients with VLUs [27]. However, the SVS/AVF guidelines propose a more aggressive approach to promoting ulcer healing, prevent recurrence of an active ulcer, and address a healed ulcer as indicated above. Due to the ulcer's chronicity and high likelihood of recurrence, this more aggressive method may be the more appropriate approach to improve a patient's ultimate quality of life.

5.6.1 Special Considerations for the Elderly

VLUs are wounds marked by chronicity and a difficulty in achieving healing without recurrence. Elderly patients have a higher prevalence of comorbid conditions that lead to poor wound healing such as malnutrition, diabetes mellitus, and arterial vascular disease. The intrinsic changes in the components of the skin that occur with aging—thinned epithelium, reduction in adnexa such as oil glands and sebaceous glands resulting in drier skin more prone to cracking, deceased angiogenesis, decline in the ability to re-epithelialize—all factor into impaired recovery [28]. These intrinsic factors cannot be altered, but external factors that can be addressed should be optimized to improve the chances of healing. These include maximizing nutritional-balanced intake—including the use of protein supplementation with commercially available shakes for those with dental or digestive difficulties, improving glucose control and compliance with diabetic restrictions, ceasing tobacco use, and improving arterial inflow as appropriate. Decreasing ultraviolet light damage by reducing sun exposure to beneficial levels should also be encouraged.

Key Points

- Chronic venous disease affects millions of patients in the United States, and its prevalence rises with age.
- With an increasing elderly population, practitioners must weigh special considerations specific to caring for all CEAP levels of CVI in this group.
- Special considerations for the care of CVI in the elderly involve unique attention to the effects of multiple comorbidities, limited mobility and ability to tolerate physiologic testing, the choice of various anesthetics when undergoing surgery, and prolonged healing time for skin changes despite medical and surgical interventions.
- Surgical treatment of varicose veins has demonstrated significant quality of life benefit with substantial improvements in symptomatic and anatomic measures compared to conservative treatment alone

- Our institution's experience demonstrated a trend toward a higher percentage of patients who had RFA alone compared to RFA + TIPP in an age 65 and older subset. The VCSS of this subset tended to improve more with RFA alone compared to RFA + TIPP, though compared to the all-ages complications, this subset did not have significant differences in complications between the two procedures.
- The SVS/AVF guidelines are an invaluable approach to evidence-based care in the maintenance, treatment, and prevention of CVI.

References

1. Brand FN, Dannenberg AL, Abbott RD, Kannel WB. The epidemiology of varicose veins: the framingham study. Am J Prev Med. 1988;4:96–101.
2. Coon WW, Willis 3rd PW, Keller JB. Venous thromboembolism and other venous disease in the tecumseh community health study. Circulation. 1973;48:839–46.
3. Kaplan RM, Criqui MH, Denenberg JO, Bergan J, Fronek A. Quality of life in patients with chronic venous disease: San Diego population study. J Vasc Surg. 2003;37:1047–53.
4. Streeten DH. Idiopathic edema. Curr Ther Endocrinol Metab. 1997;6:203–6.
5. Raju S, Oglesbee M, Neglen P. Iliac vein stenting in postmenopausal leg swelling. J Vasc Surg. 2011;53(1):123–30.
6. Cho S, Atwood JE. Peripheral edema. Am J Med. 2002;113:580–6.
7. Topham EJ, Mortimer PS. Chronic lower limb oedema. Clin Med. 2002;2:28–31.
8. Frishman WH. Effects of nonsteroidal anti-inflammatory drug therapy on blood pressure and peripheral edema. Am J Cardiol. 2002;89:18D–25D.
9. Moreno AH, Katz AI, Gold LD, Reddy RV. Mechanics of distension of dog veins and other very thin-walled tubular structures. Circ Res. 1970;27:1069–80.
10. Neglen P, Thrasher TL, Raju S. Venous outflow obstruction: an underestimated contributor to chronic venous disease. J Vasc Surg. 2003;38:879–85.
11. Cockett FB, Thomas ML. The iliac compression syndrome. Br J Surg. 1965;52:816–21.
12. Lalka SG. Management of chronic obstructive venous disease of the lower extermity. In: Rutherford RB, editor. Vascular surgery. 4th ed. Phildelphia: WB Saunders; 1995. p. 1862–82.
13. Labropoulos N, Giannoukas AD, Nicolaides AN, Ramaswami G, Leon M, Burke P. New insights into the pathophysiologic condition of venous ulceration with color-flow duplex imaging: Implications for treatment? J Vasc Surg. 1995;22:45–50.
14. Hanrahan LM, Araki CT, Rodriguez AA, Kechejian GJ, LaMorte WW, Menzoian JO. Distribution of valvular incompetence in patients with venous stasis ulceration. J Vasc Surg. 1991;13:805–11; discussion 811–2.
15. Barwell JR, Davies CE, Deacon J, Harvey K, Minor J, Sassano A, et al. Comparison of surgery and compression with compression alone in chronic venous ulceration (eschar study): randomised controlled trial. Lancet. 2004;363:1854–9.
16. Yamaki T, Nozaki M, Sasaki K. Color duplex ultrasound in the assessment of primary venous leg ulceration. Dermatol Surg. 1998;24:1124–8.
17. Luger TJ, Kammerlander C, Luger MF, Kammerlander-Knauer U, Gosch M. Mode of anesthesia, morality and outcome in geriatric patients. Z Gerontol Geriatr. 2014;47(2):110–24.
18. Weiss MA, Hsu JT, Neuhaus I, Sadick NS, Duffy DM. Consensus for sclerotherapy. Dermatol Surg. 2014;40(12):1309–18.
19. Gloviczki P, Comerota AJ, Dalsing MC, Eklof BG, Gillespie DL, Gloviczki ML, et al.; Society for Vascular Surgery; American Venous Forum. The case of patients with varicose veins and associated chronic venous diseases: clinical practice guidelines of the Society for Vascular Surgery and the American Venous Forum. J Vasc Surg. 2011; 53(5 Suppl):2S–48S.

20. Martinez MJ, Bonfill X, Moreno RM, Vargas E, Capella D. Phlebotonics for venous insufficiency. Cochrane Database Syst Rev. 2005;(3):CD003229.
21. Michaels JA, Brazier JE, Campbell WB, MacIntyre JB, Palfreyman SJ, Ratcliffe J. Randomized clinical trial comparing surgery with conservative treatment for uncomplicated varicose veins. Br J Surg. 2006;93(2):175–81.
22. Tatsioni A, Balk E, O'Donnell Jr TF, Lau J. Usual care in the management of chronic wounds: a review of the recent literature. J Am Coll Surg. 2007;205:617–24.
23. Ruckley CV, Evans CJ, Allan P, Lee AJ, Fowkes GR. Chronic venous insufficiency: Clinical and duplex correlations. The Edinburgh Vein Study of venous disorders in the general population. J Vasc Surg. 2002;36:520–5.
24. Rhodes JR, Gloviczki P, Canton LG, Rooke T, Lewis BD, Lindsey JR. Factors affecting clinical outcome following endoscopic perforator vein ablation. Am J Surg. 1998;176:162–7.
25. Van Gent BW, Wilschut ED, Wittens CW. Management of venous ulcer disease. BMJ. 2010;341:c6045.
26. O'Donnell Jr TF, Passman MA, Marston WA, Ennis WJ, Dalsing M, Kistner RL, et al. Management of venous leg ulcers: clinical practice guidelines of the Society for vascular surgery and the American Venous Forum. J Vasc Surg. 2014;60:3S–59S.
27. Mauck KF, Asi N, Undavalli C, Elraiya TA, Nabham M, Altayar O, Sonbol MB, Prokop LJ, Murad MH. Systematic review and meta-analysis of surgical interventions versus conservative therapy for venous ulcers. J Vasc Surg. 2014;60(2 Suppl):60S–70S.
28. Greenhalgh DG. Management of the skin and soft tissue in the geriatric surgical patient. Surg Clin North Am. 2015;95(1):103–14.

Cerebrovascular Disease in the Elderly

6

Brajesh K. Lal and Rafael S. Cires-Drouet

6.1 Introduction

Stroke is the fifth leading cause of death and the leading cause of disability in the United States [1]. Approximately one third of all strokes are hemorrhagic, while two thirds are ischemic in origin [2].

Risk factors predisposing to stroke are more frequent among elderly (>65 year old) individuals. Consequently stroke is a common affliction of the elderly [3]. Stroke outcome is worse in the elderly. Progressive brain injury from silent infarctions may lead to "reduced cerebrovascular reserve" resulting in more catastrophic deficits for an equivalent ischemic insult. Many traditional carotid trials have excluded octogenarians, and there are few evidence-based guidelines to help determine care in this age group. In this chapter, we will define the characteristics of stroke that are unique in the elderly. We will also describe optimal and pragmatic management approaches to stroke in the elderly as related to carotid atherosclerotic occlusive disease.

6.2 Epidemiology and Rehabilitation of Stroke in the Elderly

Age is an important risk factor for stroke. The elderly, age 65 or older, are at an increased risk for stroke compared to the general population (8.1% vs. 0.8%) [3]. Among 472 stroke events in the Framingham study, risk factors included age,

B.K. Lal (✉)
University of Maryland School of Medicine, University of Maryland Medical Center, Baltimore VA Medical Center, Baltimore, MD, USA
e-mail: blal@smail.umaryland.edu

R.S. Cires-Drouet
Vascular Medicine, University of Maryland Medical Center, Baltimore, MD, USA

R. Chaer (ed.), *Vascular Disease in Older Adults*,
DOI 10.1007/978-3-319-29285-4_6

hypertension, diabetes, cigarette smoking, and atrial fibrillation [4]. The incidence of each of these risk factors is higher in the elderly and therefore explains the higher risk of stroke in this population.

Increasing age is associated with enhanced morbidity and disability after stroke. Fifteen to thirty per cent of the elderly are permanently disabled and 26% require institutionalization into a nursing home [5]. These rates are less in patients <65 suffering a stroke. Advanced age has a negative impact on stroke mortality too [6]. In an analysis of Health Care Financing Administration Medicare Part B patients in four communities in the United States, the 1-month case fatality rate for stroke was 12.6% (8.1% for ischemic strokes, and 44.6% for hemorrhagic strokes) in patients age 65 years or older [7]. In 2002, death certificates showed that the mean age at death from a stroke was 79.6 years [8].

The estimated cost of strokes in 2008 was 65.5 billion dollars [9]. Projected estimates of the total cost of stroke from 2005 to 2050 is thought to be 1.52 trillion dollars for non-Hispanic whites, 313 billion dollars for Hispanics, and $379 billion for African Americans [10].

6.3 Medical Management of Risk Factors for Stroke in the Elderly

While risk factors for stroke may be more prevalent in the elderly, control of these factors results in risk reduction regardless of age. Implementation of an effective and aggressive risk factor reduction program in elderly patients is an essential and oftentimes the best form of therapy for asymptomatic carotid atherosclerosis.

The relationship between elevated blood pressure and the risk of stroke is linear [11]. The Framingham Heart Study and the Atherosclerosis Risk in Communities (ARIC) study both concluded that reduction in blood pressure reduced the risk of future strokes [12]. Medical management with antihypertensive therapy is generally aimed at reducing blood pressure to less than 140/90 for CVA prevention.

Tight serum glucose control in patients with diabetes was traditionally thought to reduce the risk of stroke. The Action in Diabetes and Vascular diseases (ADVANCE) [13], United Kingdom Prospective Diabetes Study (UKPDS) [14], and Action to Control Cardiovascular Risk in Diabetes (ACCORD) [15] study, all tested the hypothesis that tight control of serum glucose levels would reduce their risk of future cerebrovascular events. However, they all found no reduction in stroke risk with hemoglobin A_{1c} levels less than 6.5%. Therefore, only normoglycemic serum levels with a target hemoglobin A_{1c} of less than 7% are now recommended among diabetic patients.

It is well established that smoking increases the risk for coronary and peripheral arterial disease. Similarly, the risk of a stroke is doubled with smoking and an aggressive smoking cessation program reduces this risk, based on results from the Framingham study [16]. Counseling for smoking cessation in conjunction with nicotine replacement therapy are effective approaches to reducing smoking among patients and results in a benefit regardless of age.

Antithrombotic therapy with daily aspirin is recommended by the US Preventive Services Task Force for cardiovascular prophylaxis in patients with anticipated cardiac morbidity [17]. The use of aspirin in asymptomatic carotid atherosclerosis also reduces the incidence of stroke. Similar prophylaxis has been shown to be effective for secondary prevention of recurrent stroke [18]. Based on the cardiovascular and stroke prevention benefits, it is recommended that all individuals above the age of 50–55 years should receive antithrombotic prophylaxis.

In early studies elevated cholesterol levels were associated with an increased incidence of stroke. Subsequently, high LDL levels and high HDL/LDL ratios have all been correlated with an increased risk of stroke and other cardiovascular morbidities. A meta-analysis of randomized, placebo-controlled, double-blind trials with statin therapy reported a greater than 15% reduction in stroke rates [19]. The Education Program-Adult Treatment Panel III guidelines recommend the use of statins toward a target LDL of ≤100 mg/dl for low-risk patients and ≤70 mg/dl for high-risk patients [20]. It has been proposed that statin therapy may result in regression of carotid artery atherosclerosis. The METEOR study found regression in carotid intima-media thickness (IMT) with the use of rosuvastatin [21]. These results were confirmed by the ARBITER trial, comparing the effects of two statins (pravastatin 40 mg/day and atorvastatin 80 mg/day) on carotid IMT [22]. The benefit of statins appears to extend to patients undergoing revascularization for carotid stenosis too. Patients undergoing vascular surgery suffer fewer cerebrovascular adverse events when placed on perioperative statins [23].

6.4 The Role of Carotid Endarterectomy in Stroke Prevention for the Elderly

6.4.1 Carotid Endarterectomy

The era of carotid revascularization began in the 1950s with frequent reports of direct anastomosis between internal and common carotid artery, carotid endarterectomy, eversion endarterectomy and patch angioplasty along with shunting in quick succession. Carotid surgical revascularization experienced rapid expansion over the next four decades as a means to prevent stroke from carotid atherosclerosis.

6.4.2 Asymptomatic Carotid Stenosis

In the early 1990s, the VA Asymptomatic Carotid Stenosis Study, Asymptomatic Carotid Atherosclerosis Study (ACAS) and Asymptomatic Carotid Surgery Trial (ACST) demonstrated a benefit for carotid endarterectomy (CEA) plus best medical therapy over best medical therapy alone in asymptomatic patients that were less than 80 years of age [24–26]. It is important to note that in the era of ACAS and ACST, best medical therapy generally comprised of aspirin 325 mg/day with a very small proportion of patients receiving cholesterol-lowering medications and adequate blood pressure and glucose control. In ACAS, 1662 patients ages 40–79 with

60–99% carotid stenosis were randomized to surgery versus medical therapy alone. Perioperative stroke and death plus post-perioperative stroke were lower in the surgical group as compared to the medical group (5.6% vs. 11.0% over 4 years). The ACST randomized 3120 patients between the ages of 40 and 91 with greater than 60% asymptomatic carotid artery disease to CEA versus best medical therapy. The 5-year rate for stroke and death in CEA versus medical therapy was 6.4% and 11.8%, respectively. Patients did not show a measurable benefit until 2 years after the surgery. This is understandable, since surgery resulted in an up-front elevated risk of stroke and death in the perioperative period.

The general consensus that emerged as a result of these trials was that CEA was an optimal treatment for most patients with high-grade carotid artery stenosis, provided they survived long enough to derive prophylactic benefit (i.e. at least 2 years) and the perioperative stroke/death rate was below 3%.

The recently concluded Carotid Revascularization Endarterectomy versus Stent Trial (CREST) demonstrated the best peri-procedural outcomes associated with CEA that have been reported till date [27]. The primary endpoints were stroke, myocardial infarction (MI), and death, and octogenarians were included in the trial. The surgeons were rigorously credentialed, and this produced a perioperative stroke, death, and MI rate of 1.4% in asymptomatic patients. These excellent results have led to several clinicians proposing that the 3% threshold defining safe CEA be further reduced to 2%. The study also provided reassurance that CEA could be safely offered to octogenarians and that they would derive an equivalent benefit for stroke prevention as compared to younger patients.

6.4.3 Symptomatic Carotid Stenosis

Symptomatic carotid disease is defined based on symptoms such as weakness of the face, arm, leg, or both; sensory deficit or paresthesia of the face, arm, leg, or both; or transient blindness anosognosia, asomatognosia, neglect, visual, or sensory extinction, aphasia, alexia, anomia, and agraphesthesia within 6 months of diagnosis. Results from two landmark studies guide the current management of symptomatic carotid disease, North Atlantic Symptomatic Carotid Endarterectomy Trial (NASCET) and European Carotid Surgery Trial (ECST) [28, 29].

NASCET—a multi-center, randomized, prospective trial, commenced enrollment in the late 1980s to compare the efficacy of CEA versus best medical therapy for patients with symptomatic carotid artery disease. A total of 659 patients with history of carotid territory ischemic events within the previous 120 days were enrolled. The study was prematurely terminated at 18 months since the benefit of CEA was overwhelming. The 30-day risk of stroke and death in CEA versus medical therapy was 5.8% versus 3.3%; at 2 years the differential between the two groups had expanded to 15.8% versus 32.3%. An additional analysis confirmed that CEA also benefited patients with 50–69% symptomatic stenosis [30]. Importantly, patients age 75 and older with 50–99% stenosis benefited from CEA more than younger patients with the same degree of stenosis [31].

ECST—a multi-center, prospective, randomized controlled trial enrolled 2518 patients with symptomatic ischemic strokes to CEA or medical therapy. At 3 years CEA patients had a stroke incidence of 2.8% compared to 16.8% in those treated non-operatively.

Octogenarians were excluded from the ACAS and NASCET studies but were not excluded from ACST and ECST. These patients are now optimized better than ever for operative management and have been shown to be at no increased surgical risk just by virtue of their chronological age [32, 33]. In fact, subgroup analysis of patients older than 75 years was associated with an increased risk of stroke in symptomatic patients managed non-operatively, when compared to the younger-than-65-year-old patient population with similar comorbidities [34].

6.5 Carotid Artery Stenting in the Elderly

Successful endovascular revascularization of carotid disease was first reported in the 1980s [35]. Carotid artery stenting (CAS) has subsequently evolved with the introduction of nitinol stents and embolic protection devices. Several randomized trials comparing CEA to CAS have helped elucidate the potential role for CAS in the management of carotid disease.

In the early stages of its introduction, the percutaneous minimally invasive nature of CAS was thought to be of potential preferential benefit to elderly patients. The Carotid and Vertebral Artery Transluminal Angioplasty Study (CAVATAS) trial randomized 504 symptomatic patients into angioplasty without embolic protection or CEA and achieved stroke or death rates of 10% versus 9.9% in 30-day post-procedural period respectively [36]. The results were critiqued due to the unusually high rate of stroke in the CEA arm of the study. The Stenting and Angioplasty with Protection in Patients at High Risk for Endarterectomy (SAPPHIRE) was the first multi-center randomized trial to use mandatory distal embolic protection [37]. The 30-day peri-procedural adverse event rate for CAS and CEA was 4.8% and 9.8%, respectively. The endpoint in this study included non-Q-wave MI and excluding these events resulted in elimination of the advantage of CAS over CEA. As experience with CAS continued to accumulate in the Carotid Revascularization, Endarterectomy versus Stent Trial (CREST) lead-in registry, it became apparent that while CAS could potentially achieve better results than CEA in certain high-risk patients, elderly patients were not part of that category. In fact, octogenarians were found to have a stroke rate 4 times more than patients less than 60 years of age [38]. The results were so significant that enrollment of octogenarians was halted in the registry. This finding was later confirmed in the CREST randomized trial [39]. While the composite stroke, MI, and death rate were similar in CEA compared to CAS, complications were higher in CAS compared to CEA in patients older than 70 years of age. Increasing age is generally associated with larger deposits of calcium or atheroma in the aortic arch resulting in increased atheroembolization during CAS [40]. The elderly frequently have tortuous vessels that render the procedure more technically challenging and hazardous.

The CREST study also showed that CAS resulted in a lower incidence of cardiac events compared to CEA and would therefore be ideal in patients with severe cardiac comorbidities. In addition, several anatomic conditions may increase the risk for peri-procedural adverse events with CEA and therefore benefit from preferential treatment with CAS. Distal lesions (above C2 cervical vertebral body) [41], prior neck radiation, cervical stoma, or radical neck dissection can increase the risk of wound infection or cranial nerve injury. Conversely, long-segment disease (>15 mm), circumferential heavy calcification and ulceration aortoiliac tortuosity, type III aortic arch, carotid tortuosity are some of the situations where complications from CAS are enhanced [42].

6.5.1 Cognitive Impairment and Its Association with Carotid Stenosis

Carotid artery stenosis is a long-recognized cause of atheroembolic stroke or transient ischemic attacks (TIAs). An under-appreciated but clinically significant consequence of carotid stenosis may be an insidious impairment in cognitive function without associated focal neurologic deficits (stroke, TIA). Cognitive function is the production and control of behavioral and mental processes such as thinking, learning, remembering, problem solving, and consciousness. These processes can be objectively quantified by standardized cognitive measures. Cognitive function has been documented to affect the well-being of patients and their ability to live independent productive lives [43]. As a consequence, cognitive impairment places large demands on societal support systems, hospital resources, and financial resources [44]. It is well-known that cognitive impairment co-exists in patients with stroke from carotid stenosis [45]. However, isolated cognitive deficits in carotid stenosis patients currently labeled as being "asymptomatic" in the absence of a focal neurologic deficit have not traditionally been looked for systematically and have therefore not been reported in any detail [46].

6.5.2 High Socioeconomic Burden of Cognitive Decline in the Elderly

Asymptomatic carotid stenosis has a prevalence of 4.2%, affecting ~12 million people in the United States. Among people ≥70 years, prevalence increases to 12.5% in men and 6.9% in women [47]. Small studies indicate that 34% of patients with carotid may be at risk for cognitive impairment thereby potentially affecting ~3.4 million individuals [48]. The cost of social and medical care for patients with cognitive impairment ranges from $9300 to $21,700/year [44]. Conservatively assuming mild cognitive impairment in this population, at $9300/year we may be incurring a hidden cost of up to $31.6 billion/year in the care of these patients.

6.5.3 Evidence for Cognitive Decline in Patients with Carotid Stenosis

Stroke prevention has been the dominant focus of identifying carotid disease and of carotid artery revascularization. The possibility that carotid stenosis could result in cognitive impairment in the absence of a stroke has only recently received attention [48]. A subset analysis of the Cardiovascular Health Study noted significant cognitive decline in 34% of 32 patients with asymptomatic CS (≥75%) when serially tested with a modified mini-mental state examination (MMSE) over 5 years [49]. A decline was also noted in patients with stenoses ≥50%, even after adjustments for vascular risk factors. Conversely, Martinic et al. observed normal MMSE scores in 26 patients with asymptomatic high-grade carotid stenosis, though they did have reduced Montreal Cognitive Assessment scores [50]. Benke et al. observed reduced mental speed, learning, visuospatial abilities, verbal processing, and deductive reasoning in 20 patients with asymptomatic carotid stenosis compared to unmatched controls [51]. In a subset analysis of the Framingham study, 35 participants with asymptomatic CS ≥50% had significantly worse cognitive performance compared to cohorts with increased intima-media thickness alone [52]. In the Tromso study, subjects with asymptomatic carotid stenosis performed lower in tests of attention, psychomotor speed, memory, and motor function. However, there were no significant differences in tests of speed of information processing, word association, or depression [53]. Conversely, other studies have not been able to demonstrate such associations.

Most broadly accepted cognitive tests have standardized administration procedures with normative comparison groups. Guidelines for cognitive assessment in vascular research have been published, derived largely from cardiac surgery and medical treatment studies [54, 55]. Testing of both composite and domain-specific outcomes, over long follow-up times, has been recommended. The National Institute of Neurologic Disorders (NINDS) has encouraged a harmonization of standards for identifying and describing cognitive function in patients with vascular disease [56]. The makeup of the final test battery must also accommodate practicality of testing. We have targeted this issue in a recently completed American Heart Association-funded investigation contrasting cognitive outcome after CEA versus CAS [57]. Our unique test battery was guided by NINDS recommendations and previous literature that has documented effects on motor speed, information processing, attention, and memory. It was sensitive enough to identify clinically relevant impairment in either group of patients. We compared cognitive outcome in 46 patients undergoing carotid endarterectomy (CEA = 25) versus carotid artery stenting (CAS = 21) for asymptomatic CS ≥80%. Among them, 35% were women and 54% had right-sided lesions. The 50-min cognitive battery was performed 1–3 days before and 4–6 months after each procedure. The analysis of impact was a normalized change score (change in composite cognitive score vs. baseline). Raw scores from each subtest were transformed into baseline and follow-up Z-scores by using the means and SD of the baseline test scores. The difference between the two was the "change score." A positive change score indicated improved cognition. We found that scores for each test improved after CEA except Working Memory Index which decreased in 20/25 patients. Improvement occurred in all tests after CAS except Processing Speed Index which decreased in 18/21 patients. Both procedures improved overall cognitive function and the scores were not significantly different between the two procedures (0.51 vs. 0.47 SD, p = ns).

6.5.4 Silent Micro-embolization May Result in Cognitive Impairment

In patients with "asymptomatic" carotid stenosis transcranial Doppler (TCD) monitoring frequently identifies silent microembolization to the middle cerebral artery (MCA) [58], and computed tomography scanning identifies silent brain infarctions in 15–19% of such asymptomatic patients [59]. Cerebral microembolization is often seen in patients with vascular dementia and is associated with accelerated cognitive decline [60]. In the Rotterdam scan study, silent cerebral infarcts in elderly people doubled the risk of cognitive impairment [61]. These findings were confirmed by the Atherosclerosis Risk In Communities study and the Cardiovascular Health Study [62, 63]. Furthermore, in animal studies, injection of 50 μm microspheres into rat carotid arteries resulted in cerebral microinfarctions with reduced attentional performance [64]. Therefore, silent microembolization with cerebral microinfarction in patients with otherwise "asymptomatic" CS may result in cognitive impairment.

6.5.5 Cerebral Hypoperfusion May Result in Cognitive Impairment

Chronic cerebral hypoperfusion contributes to the onset of clinical dementia [65]. Verbal, performance, and full-scale IQ are all impaired, as are verbal fluency and Rey figure copy performance, among patients with carotid disease and reduced cerebral blood flow [66]. Carotid cross-clamping also results in EEG waveform flattening and attentional deficit [67]. While chronic or acute cerebral hypoperfusion, and systemic hypotension, are all associated with cognitive dysfunction, it is not certain whether cerebral hypoperfusion influences cognitive outcome in patients with carotid stenosis. As cerebral perfusion pressure falls, cerebral blood flow is maintained by autoregulatory arteriolar vasodilation. When the pressure falls low enough, as in some cases of severe carotid stenosis, the arterioles dilate maximally and vasodilatory challenge with CO_2 inhalation cannot be expected to dilate the arterioles further. Cerebrovascular reactivity (CVR = Δ cerebral blood flow/Δ partial pressure of CO_2) is a standard clinical measure of the ability of cerebral arterioles to respond to changes in $PaCO_2$. Under normal conditions, hypercapnia causes vasodilation and increased cerebral blood flow. A decrease in flow indicates reduced reactivity, indicating an increased risk of hypoperfusive brain injury. These tests can therefore be utilized to assess the role that a fixed carotid stenosis may play in reducing brain perfusion and thereby cognitive function.

6.5.6 Results of the ACCOF Study

The Asymptomatic Carotid Stenosis and Cognitive Function (ACCOF) study is the first attempt to identify the isolated impact of asymptomatic carotid stenosis on cognitive function [68]. Stenosis patients were compared to patients with similar vascular comorbidities but no stenosis. Cerebrovascular hemodynamic characteristics were analyzed to elucidate mechanisms impacting cognition. Sixty-nine patients with ≥50% asymptomatic carotid stenosis and 60 controls with vascular comorbidities without stenosis underwent comprehensive cognitive testing by a trained neuropsychologist. Scores were adjusted for age, sex, education, and race using normative data. An overall index of cognitive function and five domain-specific scores were computed. Breath holding index (BHI), an estimate of cerebrovascular reserve, was measured using transcranial Doppler. Patients were assigned to high versus low BHI groups using a cut-off score of 0.69. The stenosis group performed worse on the overall composite cognitive score ($p \leq .01$) and the domain-specific scores for processing speed ($p \leq .01$) and learning ($p \leq .05$). A trend of reduced performance for executive function and attention emerged ($p = .07$). Within the stenosis group, those with low BHI performed worse on learning ($p < .05$), processing speed ($p < .09$), and overall composite score ($p < .06$). These findings suggest that asymptomatic carotid stenosis is associated with cognitive impairment when compared to patients with similar risk factors but no stenosis. The deficit is driven primarily by reduced processing speed and learning and is mild to moderate in severity. A likely mechanism for this impairment is reduced cerebrovascular reserve.

Additional studies will be required to establish these findings. If substantiated, they have the potential to impact decision-making in the management of patients with asymptomatic carotid stenosis, especially in elderly individuals at higher risk for developing debilitating dementia.

6.6 Conclusions

Chronological age alone should not be utilized as a criterion to exclude patients from consideration for carotid artery revascularization. Current recommendations support optimal medical therapy for symptomatic patients with less than 50% stenosis or in asymptomatic patients with less than 70% stenosis. CEA is preferred over CAS for asymptomatic patients with high grade (≥70% stenosis) when the anticipated perioperative stroke and death rate is less than 3%. In patients that are ≥70 years of age, with a long (>15 mm) lesion, and with preocclusive stenosis, CEA is preferred over CAS. Symptomatic patients with >50% stenosis are generally best treated with CEA. However, in the presence of a prior cervical operation or radiotherapy, a low lesion that extends proximal to the clavicle or a high lesion that extends distal to the C2 vertebral body, prior cranial nerve injury, severe uncorrectable coronary disease, congestive heart failure, or chronic obstructive pulmonary disease, CAS is preferred over CEA (Fig. 6.1).

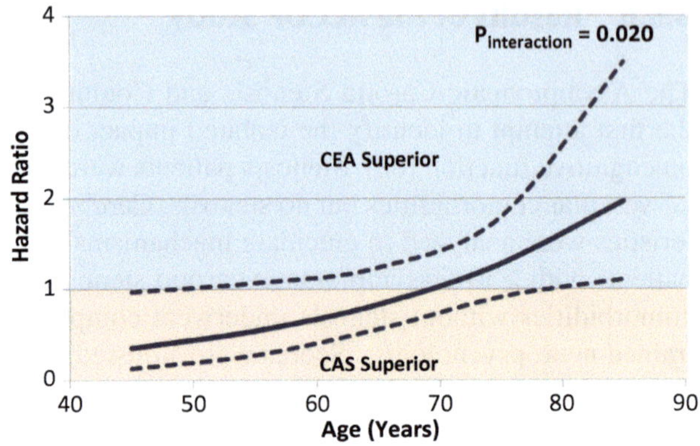

Fig. 6.1 Hazard ratio for stroke and death favors carotid artery stenting in younger patients and carotid endarterectomy in older patients with high grade carotid stenosis

Key Points

- Stroke is an important cause of death and leading cause of disability in the United States
- Risk factors predisposing to stroke are more frequent among elderly
- Stroke is more common among the elderly
- Stroke outcome is worse in the elderly
- Control of risk factors reduces stroke rates regardless of age
- Patients age 75 and older with 50–99% stenosis benefit from carotid endarterectomy more than younger patients with the same degree of stenosis
- Elderly patients with high-grade carotid artery stenosis of 70% or more also benefit from carotid endarterectomy
- Carotid artery stenting in patients aged 70 years or more is associated with an increased risk of stroke and death compared to carotid endarterectomy
- Asymptomatic high-grade carotid artery stenosis may be associated with cognitive impairment, and more information is needed to explore its impact on the functional status of older individuals

References

1. FastStats – Deaths and Mortality. at http://www.cdc.gov/nchs/fastats/deaths.htm.
2. Warlow C, Sudlow C, Dennis M, Wardlaw J, Sandercock P. Stroke. Lancet. 2003;362:1211–24.
3. Centers for Disease Control and Prevention (CDC). Prevalence of stroke – United States, 2005. MMWR Morb Mortal Wkly Rep. 2007;56:469–74.
4. Wolf PA, D'Agostino RB, Belanger AJ, Kannel WB. Probability of stroke: a risk profile from the Framingham Study. Stroke. 1991;22:312–8.
5. Kelly-Hayes M, et al. The influence of gender and age on disability following ischemic stroke: the Framingham Study. J Stroke Cerebrovasc Dis. 2003;12:119–26.
6. Kammersgaard LP, et al. Short- and long-term prognosis for very old stroke patients. The Copenhagen Stroke Study. Age Ageing. 2004;33:149–54.

7. El-Saed A, et al. Geographic variations in stroke incidence and mortality among older populations in four US communities. Stroke. 2006;37:1975–9.
8. Centers for Disease Control and Prevention (CDC). Disparities in deaths from stroke among persons aged <75 years – United States, 2002. MMWR Morb Mortal Wkly Rep. 2005; 54:477–81.
9. Rosamond W, et al. Heart disease and stroke statistics – 2007 update: a report from the American Heart Association Statistics Committee and Stroke Statistics Subcommittee. Circulation. 2007;115:e69–171.
10. Brown DL, et al. Projected costs of ischemic stroke in the United States. Neurology. 2006;67:1390–5.
11. Seshadri S, et al. The lifetime risk of stroke: estimates from the Framingham Study. Stroke. 2006;37:345–50.
12. Heiss G, et al. Carotid atherosclerosis measured by B-mode ultrasound in populations: associations with cardiovascular risk factors in the ARIC study. Am J Epidemiol. 1991;134:250–6.
13. Patel A, et al. Intensive blood glucose control and vascular outcomes in patients with type 2 diabetes. N Engl J Med. 2008;358:2560–72.
14. Laakso M. Benefits of strict glucose and blood pressure control in type 2 diabetes: lessons from the UK Prospective Diabetes Study. Circulation. 1999;99:461–2.
15. Gerstein HC, et al. Effects of intensive glucose lowering in type 2 diabetes. N Engl J Med. 2008;358:2545–59.
16. Wolf PA, D'Agostino RB, Kannel WB, Bonita R, Belanger AJ. Cigarette smoking as a risk factor for stroke. The Framingham Study. JAMA. 1988;259:1025–9.
17. Wolff T, Miller T, Ko S. Aspirin for the primary prevention of cardiovascular events: an update of the evidence for the U.S. Preventive Services Task Force. Ann Intern Med. 2009;150:405–10.
18. Wolf PA, et al. Preventing ischemic stroke in patients with prior stroke and transient ischemic attack: a statement for healthcare professionals from the Stroke Council of the American Heart Association. Stroke. 1999;30:1991–4.
19. Bucher HC, Griffith LE, Guyatt GH. Effect of HMGcoA reductase inhibitors on stroke. A meta-analysis of randomized, controlled trials. Ann Intern Med. 1998;128:89–95.
20. Avellone G, et al. Efficacy and safety of long-term ezetimibe/simvastatin treatment in patients with familial hypercholesterolemia. Int Angiol. 2010;29:514–24.
21. Crouse JR, et al. Measuring Effects on intima media Thickness: an Evaluation Of Rosuvastatin in subclinical atherosclerosis – the rationale and methodology of the METEOR study. Cardiovasc Drugs Ther. 2004;18:231–8.
22. Taylor AJ, et al. ARBITER: Arterial Biology for the Investigation of the Treatment Effects of Reducing Cholesterol: a randomized trial comparing the effects of atorvastatin and pravastatin on carotid intima medial thickness. Circulation. 2002;106:2055–60.
23. Paraskevas KI, Liapis CD, Hamilton G, Mikhailidis DP. Can statins reduce perioperative morbidity and mortality in patients undergoing non-cardiac vascular surgery? Eur J Vasc Endovasc Surg. 2006;32:286–93.
24. Hobson RW, et al. Efficacy of carotid endarterectomy for asymptomatic carotid stenosis. The Veterans Affairs Cooperative Study Group. N Engl J Med. 1993;328:221–7.
25. Endarterectomy for asymptomatic carotid artery stenosis. Executive Committee for the Asymptomatic Carotid Atherosclerosis Study. JAMA. 1995;273:1421–8.
26. Halliday A, et al. Prevention of disabling and fatal strokes by successful carotid endarterectomy in patients without recent neurological symptoms: randomised controlled trial. Lancet. 2004;363:1491–502.
27. Brott TG, Hobson 2nd RW, Howard G, Roubin GS, Clark WM, Brooks W, Mackey A, Hill MD, Leimgruber PP, Sheffet AJ, Howard VJ, Moore WS, Voeks JH, Hopkins LN, Cutlip DE, Cohen DJ, Popma JJ, Ferguson RD, Cohen SN, Blackshear JL, Silver FL, Mohr JP, Lal BK, Meschia JF; CREST Investigators. Stenting versus endarterectomy for treatment of carotid-artery stenosis. N Engl J Med. 2010;363(1):11–23.
28. ACAS Investigators. Beneficial effect of carotid endarterectomy in symptomatic patients with high-grade carotid stenosis. N Engl J Med. 1991;325:445–53.

29. ECST Investigators. Randomised trial of endarterectomy for recently symptomatic carotid stenosis: final results of the MRC European Carotid Surgery Trial (ECST). Lancet. 1998;351:1379–87.
30. Barnett HJ, et al. Benefit of carotid endarterectomy in patients with symptomatic moderate or severe stenosis. North American Symptomatic Carotid Endarterectomy Trial Collaborators. N Engl J Med. 1998;339:1415–25.
31. Alamowitch S, Eliasziw M, Algra A, Meldrum H, Barnett HJ. Risk, causes, and prevention of ischaemic stroke in elderly patients with symptomatic internal-carotid-artery stenosis. Lancet. 2001;357:1154–60.
32. Kim S, et al. Multidimensional frailty score for the prediction of postoperative mortality risk. JAMA Surg. 2014;149:633–40.
33. Audisio RA, et al. Shall we operate? Preoperative assessment in elderly cancer patients (PACE) can help. A SIOG surgical task force prospective study. Crit Rev Oncol Hematol. 2008;65:156–63.
34. Rothwell P, Eliasziw M, Gutnikov S, Warlow C, Barnett H. Endarterectomy for symptomatic carotid stenosis in relation to clinical subgroups and timing of surgery. Lancet. 2004;363:915–24.
35. Mathias K. A new catheter system for percutaneous transluminal angioplasty (PTA) of carotid artery stenoses. Fortschr Med. 1977;95:1007–11.
36. Endovascular versus surgical treatment in patients with carotid stenosis in the Carotid and Vertebral Artery Transluminal Angioplasty Study (CAVATAS): a randomised trial. Lancet. 2001;357:1729–37.
37. Yadav JS, Wholey MH, Kuntz RE, Fayad P, Katzen BT, Mishkel GJ, Bajwa TK, Whitlow P, Strickman NE, Jaff MR, Popma JJ, Snead DB, Cutlip DE, Firth BG, Ouriel K; Stenting and Angioplasty with Protection in Patients at High Risk for Endarterectomy Investigators. Protected carotid-artery stenting versus endarterectomy in high-risk patients. N Engl J Med. 2004;351(15):1493–501.
38. Lal BK, Brott TG. The carotid revascularization endarterectomy vs. stenting trial completes randomization: lessons learned and anticipated results. J Vasc Surg. 2009 Nov;50(5): 1224–31.
39. Voeks JH, et al. Age and outcomes after carotid stenting and endarterectomy: the carotid revascularization endarterectomy versus stenting trial. Stroke. 2011;42:3484–90.
40. Lam RC, et al. The impact of increasing age on anatomic factors affecting carotid angioplasty and stenting. J Vasc Surg. 2007;45:875–80.
41. Ricotta JJ, Aburahma A, Ascher E, Eskandari M, Faries P, Lal BK; Society for Vascular Surgery. Updated Society for Vascular Surgery guidelines for management of extracranial carotid disease: executive summary. J Vasc Surg. 2011;54(3):832–6.
42. Setacci C, et al. Siena carotid artery stenting score: a risk modelling study for individual patients. Stroke. 2010;41:1259–65.
43. Chaytor N, Schmitter-Edgecombe M. The ecological validity of neuropsychological tests: a review of the liter-ature on everyday cognitive skills. Neuropsychol Rev. 2003;13(4):181–97.
44. Rockwood K, Brown M, et al. Societal costs of vascular cognitive impairment in older adults. Stroke. 2002;33(6):1605–9.
45. Gottesman RF, Hillis AE. Predictors and assessment of cognitive dysfunction resulting from ischaemic stroke. Lancet Neurol. 2010;9(9):895–905.
46. Barnett HJ. Carotid disease and cognitive dysfunction. Ann Intern Med. 2004;140(4):303–4.
47. de Weerd M, Greving JP, et al. Prevalence of asymptomatic carotid artery stenosis according to age and sex: systematic review and metaregression analysis. Stroke. 2009;40(4):1105–13.
48. Lal BK. Cognitive function after carotid artery revascularization. Vasc Endovascular Surg. 2007;41(1):5–13.
49. Johnston SC, O'Meara ES, et al. Cognitive impairment and decline are associated with carotid artery disease in patients without clinically evident cerebrovascular disease. Ann Intern Med. 2004;140(4):237–47.
50. Martinic-Popovic I, Lovrencic-Huzjan A, et al. Assessment of subtle cognitive impairment in stroke-free pa-tients with carotid disease. Acta Clin Croat. 2009;48(3):231–40.

51. Benke T, Neussl D, et al. Neuropsychological deficits in asymptomatic carotid artery stenosis. Acta Neurol Scand. 1991;83(6):378–81.
52. Romero JR, Beiser A, et al. Carotid artery atherosclerosis, MRI indices of brain ischemia, aging, and cogni-tive impairment: the Framingham study. Stroke. 2009;40(5):1590–6.
53. Mathiesen EB, Waterloo K, et al. Reduced neuropsychological test performance in asymptomatic carotid ste-nosis: the Tromso Study. Neurology. 2004;62(5):695–701.
54. Murkin JM, Newman SP, et al. Statement of consensus on assessment of neurobehavioral outcomes after cardiac surgery. Ann Thorac Surg. 1995;59(5):1289–95.
55. Ryan CM, Hendrickson R. Evaluating the effects of treatment for medical disorders: has the value of neuro-psychological assessment been fully realized? Appl Neuropsychol. 1998;5(4):209–19.
56. Hachinski V, Iadecola C, et al. National Institute of Neurological Disorders and Stroke-Canadian Stroke Network vascular cognitive impairment harmonization standards. Stroke. 2006;37(9):2220–41.
57. Lal BK, Younes M, Cruz G, Kapadia I, Jamil Z, Pappas PJ. Cognitive changes after surgery vs stenting for carotid artery stenosis. J Vasc Surg. 2011 Sep;54(3):691–8.
58. Spence JD, Tamayo A, et al. Absence of microemboli on transcranial Doppler identifies low-risk patients with asymptomatic carotid stenosis. Stroke. 2005;36(11):2373–8.
59. Brott T, Tomsick T, et al. Baseline silent cerebral infarction in the asymptomatic carotid atherosclerosis study. Stroke. 1994;25(6):1122–9.
60. Purandare N, Voshaar RC, et al. Asymptomatic spontaneous cerebral emboli predict cognitive and functional decline in dementia. Biol Psychiatry. 2007;62(4):339–44.
61. Vermeer SE, Prins ND, et al. Silent brain infarcts and the risk of dementia and cognitive decline. N Engl J Med. 2003;348(13):1215–22.
62. Longstreth Jr WT, Bernick C, et al. Lacunar infarcts defined by magnetic resonance imaging of 3660 El-derly people: the cardiovascular health study. Arch Neurol. 1998;55(9):1217–25.
63. Mosley Jr TH, Knopman DS, et al. Cerebral MRI findings and cognitive functioning: the atherosclerosis risk in communities study. Neurology. 2005;64(12):2056–62.
64. Craft TKS, Mahoney JH, Devries AC, Sarter M. Microsphere embolism-induced cortical cholinergic deafferentation and impairments in attentional performance. Eur J Neurosci. 2005;21(11):3117–32.
65. Ruitenberg A, den Heijer T, van Swieten JC, Koudstaal PJ, Hofman A, Breteler MM. Cerebral hypoperfusion and clinical onset of dementia: the Rotterdam Study. Ann Neurol. 2005;57(6):789–94.
66. Silvestrini M, Paolino I, Pedone C, Baruffaldi R, Gobbi B, Cagnetti C, et al. Cerebral hemodynamics and cognitive performance in patients with asymptomatic carotid stenosis. Neurology. 2009;72(12):1062–8.
67. Marshall RS. The functional relevance of cerebral hemodynamics: why blood flow matters to the injured and recovering brain. Curr Opin Neurol. 2004;17(6):705–9.
68. Lal BK, Dux MC, Sikdar S, Zhao L, AlMuhanna K, Kowalewski G, Hossian M. L1. asymptomatic carotid stenosis impairs cognitive function: preliminary results of the ACCOF study. J Vasc Surg. 2014;59(6):97S.

Aortic Aneurysm Disease in the Elderly

7

Max Wohlauer and Matthew J. Eagleton

7.1 Introduction

Aortic aneurysm disease has remained a challenging clinical pathology for centuries. The primary risk of aortic aneurysmal disease is death from rupture. Currently, there are no medical therapies that effectively prevent rupture, let alone induce regression of the diseased aorta. For decades, surgical repair of the aortic aneurysm has been the mainstay of therapy, at least in patients who were fit enough to tolerate this major operation. In the 1990s, Parodi et al. revolutionized the treatment of abdominal aortic aneurysms (AAA), and ultimately all aneurysm repairs, with the development of endovascular aortic aneurysm repair (EVAR) [1]. The development of this technology has consistently demonstrated decreased short-term mortality when compared to open repair [2]. The decrease in short-term mortality following EVAR, however, is offset by the need for increased rates of reintervention at later time points, which may add to the morbidity and cost of treating aneurysmal disease. With a decrease in perioperative mortality, questions are raised about the futility of treating higher risk patients who may not previously been offered repair – such as the aged population. These questions transcend the endovascular treatment of AAA, and with the evolution of the technology also apply to the endovascular treatment of thoracic aortic aneurysms (TEVAR) and to the use of fenestrated and branched endovascular therapy (F/-B-EVAR) to treat thoracoabdominal aortic aneurysms (TAAA). When considering endovascular or open surgery in the aging population, the untreated

M. Wohlauer
Division of Vascular Surgery, Froedtert & the Medical College of Wisconsin, Milwaukee, WI, USA

M.J. Eagleton (✉)
Department of Vascular Surgery, Cleveland Clinic, Cleveland, OH, USA
e-mail: eagletm@ccf.org

R. Chaer (ed.), *Vascular Disease in Older Adults*,
DOI 10.1007/978-3-319-29285-4_7

aneurysm should be considered the major driving factor in late mortality rather than a patient's other comorbidities [3]. With increasing ability to perform endovascular surgery, perhaps it is prudent to rephrase the question from "Will this patient survive the procedure?" to "Will the procedure prolong the patient's life?"

7.1.1 Definition of "Elderly" Men Versus Women

Elderly is typically defined as age >65 years. This definition is being challenged. For the US population, 65-year-old males have a life expectancy of 18 years and females have a life expectancy >20 years. Overall life expectancy at age 75 is 12 years, at 80 is 9 years, and at 85 years of age it is 6.1 years. For males, life expectancy is slightly lower than females: at age 75 is 11 years, at 80 is 8.2 years, and at 85 is 5.8 years. For females, life expectancy at age 75 is 13.6 years, at 80 is 9.7 years, and at 85 is 6.9 years [4]. As a general principle it has been determined that to garner a "benefit" for repair of aortic aneurysmal disease, patients must have a 2-year survival beyond the time of the repair. Based simply upon age at presentation, all patients would be deemed potential candidates for benefiting from aneurysmal repair.

7.1.2 Who Is at Risk?

It is difficult to define "high risk" with respect to patients with aneurysmal disease. Cigarette smoking is the strongest risk factor for aneurysm development. Other risk factors for the development of aneurysms include advanced age, obesity, atherosclerosis, positive family history, hypertension, and hyperlipidemia. In addition to identifying those at risk for developing aneurysmal disease, surgeons must also determine those who are at risk for repair of aneurysmal disease. Many of the risk factors for aneurysm development also make patient at higher risk for aneurysm repair. A recent review of the Vascular Study Group of New England database showed that advanced age, presence of cardiac disease, COPD (on home oxygen), and renal disease (GFR <30) significantly alter the risk benefit profile away from offering repair. Specifically, the presence of COPD on home oxygen had (hazard ratio of 3, CI 2–4.5, $p < 0.001$), unstable angina or recent MI (hazard ratio [HR] 4.2, CI 1.7–10.3, $p < 0.001$), chronic kidney disease with GFR < 30 (HR 3, CI 1.9–4.7, $p < 0.001$) suggested unsuitability for repair. Age 75–79 had a hazard ratio of 2 (confidence interval [CI] 1.4–2.8, $p < 0.001$), age > 80 (CI 2.7, CI 1.8–3.7, $p < 0.001$) [5]. In this study, the authors found that presence of two or more risk factors was associated with a survival of less than 50% at 5 years despite repair. The authors also found that aspirin and statin use were protective factors, associated with improved survival.

Factoring into the "high risk" equation is determining whether a patient is fit for open surgery. Patients considered unfit for open surgery tend to be offered an endovascular repair. Although it seems intuitive that presence of medical comorbidities and degree of anatomic complexity would determine fitness for open surgery, certain studies challenge this assumption [6].

7.1.3 Basic Indications for AAA, DTAA, and TAAA Repair

An aneurysm is defined as a dilation of an artery greater than 50% beyond its normal diameter. A true aneurysm involves the intima, media, and adventitia of the artery. Fusiform aneurysms are characterized by a symmetric, circumferential dilation, while saccular aneurysms develop as an outpouching of a single portion of the arterial wall. The aorta is considered aneurysmal at 3 cm, or greater than 50% increase in maximum transverse diameter. Several large studies have demonstrated a low risk of rupture in AAA smaller than 5 cm. In the ADAM trial, patients aged 50–79 with aneurysms 4–5.4 cm in size were randomized to surveillance or immediate open repair. Even though operative mortality was low (2.7%), there was no survival benefit for open repair of AAA less than 5.5 cm [7–9]. By convention, aneurysms are typically repaired in asymptomatic patients with fusiform aneurysms when the size is greater than or equal to 5.5 cm. Aneurysm growth more than 1 cm/year is also an indication for repair. Symptomatic, mycotic, and saccular aneurysms are indications for repair due to unpredictable propensity for rupture.

The risk of thoracic aortic aneurysms is not only rupture, but aneurysms in this location also carry with them the risk of dissection. Risks of TAA vary depending upon their anatomic location, varying among ascending, arch, descending, and thoracoabdominal classifications. An understanding of the natural history of the disease in these locations is growing. It is interesting to note that aneurysms in the descending and thoracoabdominal regions have higher growth rates than those in the ascending or aortic arch (0.19 cm/year vs. 0.07 cm/year) [10]. Similar elevated growth rates were identified for those that had dissections compared to those without (0.14 cm/year vs. 0.09 cm/year). Patients with an initial TAA size of 6 cm were associated with nearly a four-fold increase in the rate of rupture. The rate of descending TAA rupture approaches 7% per year and death from rupture 12% per year for those with an aneurysm size of 6 cm [11]. Other univariate predictors of rupture include location of the TAA in the descending or thoracoabdominal aorta and history of AAA, while male gender was protective [10]. Other risk factors for rupture include smoking, chronic obstructive pulmonary disease, age, hypertension, and renal failure [12]. Given these data, it is frequently recommended that repair of descending TAA occur when the aneurysm diameter reaches 6 cm – although other patient-related factors must be taken into account. Thoracoabdominal aortic aneurysms have high risk of perioperative morbidity and mortality with elective operations; however, age alone should not be a contraindication for repair because the complication and mortality rates in the elderly population for emergency surgery become exceedingly high. For example, the 1-year mortality is 35% in patients 70–79 years following elective TAAA repair. This increases to 40% in patients 80–89 years of age. The 1 year mortality increases to 69% when an emergency operation is performed [13].

7.1.4 Preoperative Evaluation

The goal of aneurysm repair is to reduce risk of death from rupture. Patient comorbidities factor into estimating the degree in which someone will benefit from prophylactic repair. Patients with a high risk of rupture and minimal comorbidities should be offered repair. The preoperative work up is discussed more thoroughly in another chapter (See Chap. 2 in this book, *Preoperative optimization of the elderly patient prior to vascular surgery*). Briefly, a thorough history and physical will help target specific problems that need to be addressed before surgery. A complete blood count, basic metabolic panel, and PT/INR are typically performed. An ECG helps to identify those at increased cardiac risk. Dipyridamole-thallium imaging or dipyridamole stress echocardiography may be useful in patients with intermediate to high cardiac risk undergoing vascular surgery. A chest x-ray is useful to evaluate for occult malignancy in patients with a history of cigarette smoking. Pulmonary function tests have shown benefit in patients with COPD undergoing cardiac surgery, although the data for AAA repair are less clear [14].

7.1.5 Discussion of How Age Influences Decision-Making

Although advanced age is one of the risk factors for decreased survival after aortic aneurysm repair, it is often linked to other comorbidities. Increased age alone does not necessarily confer decreased survival. EVAR can be performed with acceptable risk even in patients >85 years [15].

EVAR offers a decrease in short-term mortality compared to open repair at the expense of increased secondary interventions [2]. Surveillance after EVAR usually includes serial CT scans with IV contrast, which is a concern in the elderly population whose renal function may already be impaired. Repeated exposure to IV contrast during secondary interventions and CT scans can threaten renal function to the point of needing dialysis. For this reason, some screening protocols use ultrasound for post-EVAR surveillance to detect aneurysm sac enlargement and presence of endoleaks. CT scans are typically performed at 1, 6, and 12 months and yearly thereafter. Because renal function decreases with increasing age, alternative screening and surveillance protocols using duplex ultrasound may be considered [16].

Open repair of a ruptured aneurysm carries a mortality of 59% and in-hospital mortality of 72% in patients over 80 years of age [17]. Elderly patients are at increased risk for development of delirium. A contemporary study showed decreased delirium following EVAR, compared to open repair [18].

7.1.6 Using Frailty Scores to Risk Stratify and Counsel Patients in Clinic

Because age alone is not a consistent, reliable predictor of outcomes, clinicians have looked at other metrics. In a landmark study, Fried et al. described frailty as a clinical syndrome with three or more of the following criteria: unintentional weight loss (10 pounds in past year), self-reported exhaustion, weakness, slow walking speed, and diminished physical activity. This study, performed in a community setting, showed that presence of frailty was an independent predictor of falls, disability, and death. This study laid the groundwork for future research by showing that presence of comorbidities are risk factors for the development of frailty and that disability is an outcome of frailty, rather than previous notions that frailty, comorbidity, and disability were synonymous [19]. The concept of frailty has moved to the surgical setting, and a recent study found that frailty is an independent risk factor for morbidity and mortality in cardiac surgery patients. The effect of frailty was not dependent on age of the patient [20]. In conclusion, using frailty scores in clinic can help with appropriate patient selection.

7.2 Abdominal Aortic Aneurysm

Abdominal aortic aneurysm is a disease of elderly patients, which begs the question: when is a patient too old for surgery? Although recent publications have stratified according to type of repair and age at time of surgery, the answer remains unclear. What is clear, however, is that 3-year survival in patients with AAA > 5.5 cm turned down for repair is a staggering 17%, with half of all deaths attributable to aneurysm rupture [21]. Current repair strategies continue to offer either open, conventional surgery or endovascular therapy with EVAR. Open surgery requires either a trans-abdominal or retroperitoneal approach with cross-clamping of the aorta in order to halt blood flow thus allowing the aneurysm to be opened and replaced with a graft comprised of artificial material (Fig. 7.1). Alternately, the aneurysm can be repaired in a less-invasive fashion using an endograft (Fig. 7.2). This approach calls for a graft to be inserted through the femoral arteries into the aorta obtaining a seal above the aneurysm in the infrarenal aorta and below the aneurysm, typically in the iliac arteries. This is accomplished either through small incisions over the femoral arteries or in a percutaneous fashion.

Endovascular abdominal aortic aneurysm repair (EVAR) has continued to evolve since it was first described in 1991 [1]. The operative technique and technology has undergone several major advancements, and EVAR is now felt to be a safe and feasible alternative to open repair. Three randomized prospective trials have evaluated EVAR compared to open surgery including EVAR1, the Dutch Randomized Endovascular Aneurysm Management (DREAM) trial, and the Open Versus Endovascular Repair (OVER) Veterans Affairs Cooperative Study Group [22–24]. All three were randomized, prospective trials that enrolled patients who were deemed fit to undergo open surgical repair of an AAA to either EVAR or open repair. All three studies demonstrated lower 30-day mortality rates that were lower in the EVAR group (0.5–1.7%) compared to the open surgical arm (3–5%). By 2 years, however, these differences resolved and survival after EVAR and open surgery were similar. Patients undergoing EVAR, however, had shorter hospital stays, had shorter operative durations, and required fewer blood transfusions. EVAR patients did have increased exposure to fluoroscopy and contrast. Given its promising initial results, it is not surprising that EVAR has become increasingly popular over the past decade.

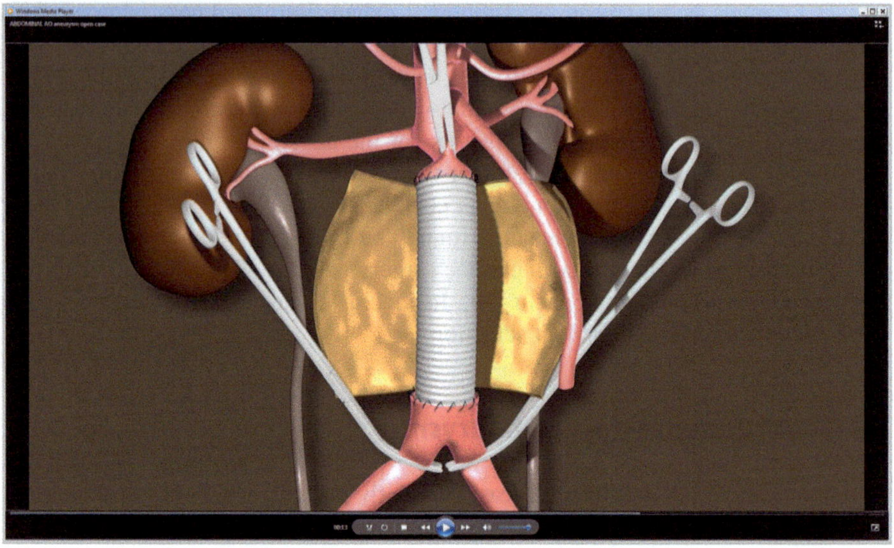

Fig. 7.1 Illustration of an open repair of an abdominal aortic aneurysm. This is accomplished through either a transabdominal or retroperitoneal approach. The aneurysm is exposed and the nonaneurysmal aorta above the aneurysm and iliac arteries below the aneurysm are occluded with vascular clamps. The aneurysm is opened longitudinally and an artificial graft is sutured in place. The aneurysmal segment is not typically resected, but the tissue can be wrapped around the graft material providing an additional layer of biologic material (not pictured)

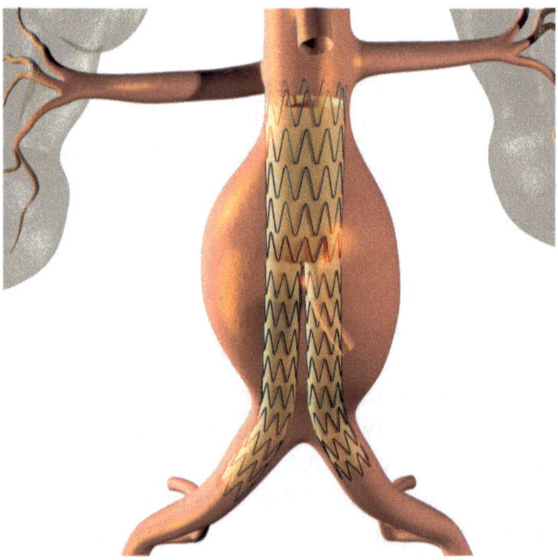

Fig. 7.2 An illustration of an abdominal aortic aneurysm that was repaired with an endograft. The endograft is inserted, in pieces, either through small incisions over the femoral arteries or in a percutaneous fashion. The main body is deployed in the neck of the aorta, below the level of the renal arteries, above the level of the aneurysm. The metal framework of the stent graft provides a radial force that helps it achieve a durable seal and fixation in this location. Extension limbs are then placed that extend into the iliac arteries for a distal seal and fixation

One of the most controversial aspects of AAA repair, however, is when to perform EVAR and when to perform conventional open surgery. Open surgical repair of AAA has long been considered the gold standard, and there is evidence that this option provides good long-term durability [25, 26]. EVAR, however, relative to open surgery, does not have similar time-tested outcomes data. Recently, longer-term outcomes from both EVAR1 and DREAM have been reported [27, 28]. For EVAR1 [27], the median follow-up was 6 years (5–10 year range), and at follow-up the overall aneurysm-related mortality was 1.0 deaths per 100 person-years in the EVAR group and 1.2 deaths per 100 person-years in the open repair group ($p = 0.73$). All-cause mortality was 7.2 deaths per 100 person-years (EVAR) and 7.1 deaths per 100 person-years (open surgery). Graft-related complication rates were higher in the EVAR group (12.6 per 100-person-years) compared to the open surgical arm (2.5 per 100 person-years, $p < 0.001$), and significantly more patients in the EVAR group required re-intervention (5.1 per 100 person-years vs. 1.7 per 100 person-years, $p < 0.001$). In fact, new graft-related complications and re-interventions were reported for as long as 8 years following EVAR. For DREAM [8], at a median follow-up of 6.4 years (5.1–8.2 years), cumulative survival rates were 69.9% for open repair and 68.9% for EVAR. The cumulative rates of freedom from secondary interventions were 81.9% for the open repair group and 70.4% for EVAR ($p = 0.03$). Based on this data, it is clear that EVAR is not without its drawbacks. These factors may change as the technology improves and as we gain a better understanding of the long-term implications of placing an endovascular graft in the aorta. Given this, there is debate over whether repair with endovascular therapy is as durable as conventional repair, and it is not entirely clear when one approach should be used over another. This is especially true for the aged population in which there may be potentially higher risks associated with major surgery.

7.2.1 Open Repair Versus EVAR in Octogenarians

A recent retrospective study from France looked at patients 85–93 years of age undergoing both EVAR and open AAA repair [15]. This population comprised 6% of all AAA repairs at the authors' institution during the study period. Fifty-six percent of patients underwent EVAR, 44% underwent an open repair. Thirty-day mortality was 6.7% (6% with EVAR, 7.6% open repair). Although the mortality was similar, perioperative morbidity in the open repair (OR) group was much higher (42% vs. 15%) than in the EVAR group. Complications in the OR group included MI, respiratory insufficiency, renal failure, stroke, and multiple organ failure. The EVAR group had a higher incidence of midterm complications, which was mostly related to appearance of type II endoleak. Overall survival was 53% at 5 years [15]. Perioperative mortality is higher but considered acceptable in octogenarians when looking at both open and endovascular AAA repair when compared to patients <80 years [29]. EVAR is safe in octogenarians, with a 30-day mortality of 1.5% in a large database. Not surprisingly, octogenarians do experience a significantly longer hospital stay [30]. EVAR can be performed with low perioperative mortality leading some to prefer an endovascular approach [31]. Another study showed no significant difference in operative mortality or long-term survival comparing open repair with EVAR, however, which suggests that either approach may be effective in appropriately selected patients [32].

7.2.2 Open Repair Versus EVAR in Nonagenarians

A review of the Nationwide Inpatient Sample Database evaluated mortality in patients >90 years compared to patients 18–89 undergoing AAA repair. Mortality in patients >90 undergoing open AAA repair was 18.3% compared to 4.6% in patients <90. EVAR in nonagenarians carried a 3.1% mortality compared to 1.2% mortality in patients <90. The authors concluded that EVAR in nonagenarians is preferable to open repair. EVAR in nonagenarians was associated with a higher complication rate compared to younger patients in a recent systematic review [33]. Thirty-day mortality was 4%, considerably higher than the 1.8% mortality in the pivotal EVAR trial and 5-year mortality was 17% [27]. Although complications are higher in the >90 group compared to younger patients, EVAR carries substantially lower mortality compared to open repair and should be offered selectively to appropriate surgical candidates.

7.3 Thoracic Aortic and Thoracoabdominal Aortic Aneurysms

Thoracic aortic aneurysms and their relative the thoracoabdominal aortic aneurysms provide an even greater clinical challenge. Conventional open repair remains a major invasive surgical operation with significant inherent risk. This is frequently related to the requirement of a thoracotomy and the subsequent pulmonary morbidity associated with this in those undergoing TAA repair. TAAA repair has the added morbidity of requiring revascularization of the visceral vessels leading to increased rates of post-operative renal failure and spinal cord ischemia. Similar to AAA, endovascular approaches to these pathologies may significantly alter the short-term outcomes and allow for treatment of those patients at high risk for conventional surgery. Pivotal trials analyzing the outcomes of TEVAR for TAA have demonstrated that endovascular approaches demonstrate a marked reduction in 30-day mortality rates [34–36]. This may translate into reduced long-term aneurysm-related mortality, but not all-cause mortality. Whether these results translate to improved outcomes for the elderly will be discussed in more detail below.

7.3.1 Open Descending TAA and TAAA Repair

Conventional surgery for descending TAA (DTAA) and TAAA has not been limited due to patients' advanced age, but there are limited analyses of outcomes in the markedly aged population. Di Luozzo and colleagues have reported on the outcomes of septuagenarians and octogenarians undergoing repair of DTAA and TAAA [37]. In this series of 93 patients over a 6-year period of time, 22 (24%) had open repair of DTAA, while 71 (76%) underwent TAAA repair. Perioperative mortality was 13.6% for the DTAA group, while those undergoing more extensive repair had a higher rate of 15.5%. Interestingly, the in-hospital mortality was greater in the septuagenarians (16%) compared to the octogenarians (11%). Factors associated with mortality included pneumonia, tracheostomy, and acute respiratory distress syndrome. Long-term survival was equivalent to that of a normal age- and gender-matched population, and male gender provided a survival benefit. Similarly, Huynh and colleagues evaluated the outcomes of patients over the age of 79 years undergoing DTAR and TAAA repair [38]. A total of 56 patients between the ages of 79 and 88 years of age underwent open repair of the descending thoracic aorta ($N = 16$, 29%) or thoracoabdominal aortic aneurysms ($N = 40$, 71%). This represented only 6.6% of the patients undergoing these procedures during that time. Overall 30-day mortality was a striking 25% but was higher in those considered high risk (emergent presentation, diabetes, or congestive heart failure) at 50% compared to those lacking any of these risk factors at 17%. This mortality rate, however, is higher than previously reported for all consecutive patients from this institution (14%) [38]. The mean 5-year actuarial survival rate for this group was 48%. Similar results, however, with a 30-day mortality rate of 21% and a mean survival rate of 61% in patients over 70 years of age, have been reported [39].

7.3.2 Thoracic Endovascular Aneurysm Repair

There are few analyses comparing open repair of DTAA and TEVAR in the markedly aged population. The University of Michigan evaluated outcomes in 93 patients aged 75 years and older undergoing either open ($N = 41$) or endovascular ($N = 52$) descending aortic repair between 1993 and 2008 [40]. Selection criteria for entry into this study were indications for operations were identical in both groups, the extent of pathology was confined to the left chest distal to the left carotid artery, and all patients were initially evaluated for open repair by a thoracic surgeon. The option for TEVAR was offered to patients who were deemed high risk for conventional surgery, who had localized pathology, or who specifically requested endovascular repair. Final suitability for TEVAR was determined by a collaborative multidisciplinary team. While the mean age of the whole group was nearly 79 years, the group undergoing TEVAR were older, had smaller thoracic aortic aneurysms, and had a higher incidence of COPD and prior infrarenal AAA repair. The procedure was observed to be elective in only 63% of patients, and contained rupture was more frequently seen in the TEVAR group (26.9% vs. 4.9%, $p = 0.005$), but a larger proportion of patients undergoing open repaired had an aneurysm involving the distal aortic arch. Technical success was observed in 96% of patients undergoing TEVAR. There was a trend to reduced perioperative mortality in those undergoing TEVAR (5.8% vs. 17.1%, $p = 0.1$), and the incidence of stroke was the same for both groups (14.6% vs. 9.6%, $p = 0.53$). Spinal cord ischemia and renal failure were rare events overall. Crude mortality at last follow-up was 45%, and Kaplan-Meier estimates demonstrate no difference between the open and endovascular cohorts. Endoleaks were observed in 23% of the TEVAR group, and five patients had indications for conversion to open surgery but were considered non-operative candidates. The authors concluded that TEVAR may be a more suitable therapeutic option in this complex elderly group.

7.3.3 F/B-EVAR for Juxtarenal and TAAA

Fenestrated and branched endograft repair began in 1999 in patients with infrarenal aortic necks that were too short for traditional EVAR. The technology has evolved to allow for the treatment of juxtarenal AAA to more complex thoracoabdominal aortic aneurysms. These endovascular surgeries allow for a less-invasive approach to complex AAA and TAAA treatment, but add a complexity of requiring preservation of flow to the renal and/or visceral vessels depending upon the extent of the aneurysm undergoing repair. The preservation of flow is accomplished by incorporating fenestrations or branches on a conventional stent graft (Fig. 7.3). These are connected to their target vessels using a self-expanding or balloon-expandable bridging stent graft. While still fairly early in its development, these procedures have been used to treat patients considered high risk for conventional surgery [3].

A U.S. multicenter trial evaluated fenestrated endograft repair of juxtarenal AAA. Mean age at the time of repair was 74 years and mean aneurysm diameter was 6 cm. Thirty-day mortality was 1.5%. Freedom from all-cause mortality at 5 years was 91%. This multicenter prospective trial showed that fenestrated endograft repair for short-necked AAA can be done with low mortality in experienced hands [41]. Other analyses have analyzed extensive aneurysm repair involving juxtarenal aneurysms as well as TAAA. The French multicenter experience represented a medium-term outcome assessment of prospectively collected data on 134 patients deemed high risk for conventional repair from 16 French academic centers treated between 2004 and 2009 who underwent fenestrated aortic endografting [42]. Unlike the U.S. trial, while the majority of patients were treated for juxtarenal AAA (74%), inclusion of more extensive aneurysms including suprarenal (20%) and type IV TAAA (6%) were included. Median age for this cohort was 73 years (range 48–91 years). Completion angiography confirmed 99% of the target vessels were patent with occlusion of four renal arteries and one celiac artery. Two patients required permanent hemodialysis post-operatively, one related to thrombosis of a renal artery. There was one conversion to open surgery secondary to aortic bifurcation occlusion. The 30-day mortality rate was 2%. Two patients died secondary to multisystem organ failure as a consequence of ruptured iliac artery ($N = 1$) and conversion to open surgery ($N = 1$), while one patient suffered a suspected myocardial infarction after discharge. Twelve- and 24-month survival was 93% and 86%, respectively, with no aneurysm-related mortalities.

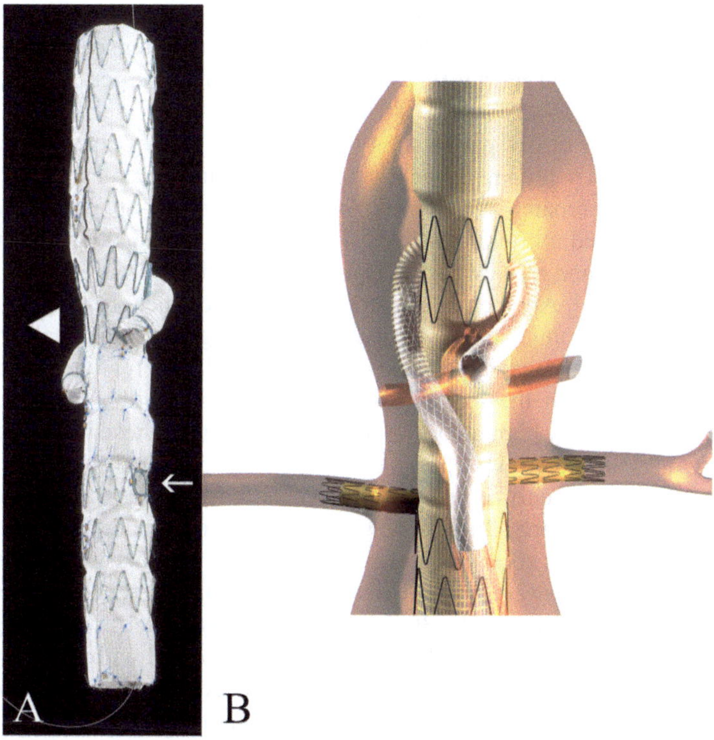

Fig. 7.3 For more complex, extensive abdominal aortic aneurysms, or for thoracoabdominal aortic aneurysms, in which the disease involves the renal or visceral vessels, fenestrated/branched endograft are used. (**a**) Typically these are custom-made grafts that incorporate fenestrations (*arrow*) or directional branches (*triangles*) to allow for preservation of flow to the renal and visceral arteries. (**b**) An illustration of a device with two directional branches and two fenestrations used to treat a thoracoabdominal aortic aneurysm. The branches and fenestrations are mated with their corresponding renal or visceral vessels using balloon-expandable or self-expanding bridging stent grafts

The WINDOWS trial represents the early outcomes of patients treated with fenestrated/branched endografts for complex AAA and TAAA aneurysms in France [43]. This was a multicenter, prospective, single-arm trial of F/B-EVAR for complex aneurysms performed on 268 patients from eight centers between 2009 and 2012. The mean age of those undergoing repair was 72 ± 8.5 years. The population was divided into one of three groups depending on the extent of aneurysm treated: Group 1 ($N = 184$) juxtarenal (51%) and pararenal (18%); Group 2 ($N = 42$) suprarenal (6%) and type IV TAAA (10%); and Group 3 ($N = 42$) type III TAAA (9%), type II TAAA (6%), and type I TAAA (1%). The 30-day mortality rate was 6.7%, and the in-hospital mortality rate was 10.1%. Severe complications occurred in 5.6% of patients and were associated with a 93% mortality rate. Acute renal insufficiency occurred in 18% of patients. Thirty-one (11.6%) patients required aneurysm-related re-intervention due to lower limb ischemia, hemorrhages, infection, and lymphocele. The 30-day combined mortality and severe complications was 22%. The presence of a more extensive aneurysm was predictive of in-hospital mortality, as was the duration of surgery and post-operative events.

In a recent review of 610 patients (349 patients with type IV repair, 258 patients with juxtarenal AAA repair, 3 unclassified) long-term outcomes of fenestrated/branched endograft repair was assessed. At 8 years of follow-up, survival was 20% and aneurysm-related mortality was 2%. The authors concluded that endovascular repair of juxtarenal and type IV TAAA using fenestrated and branched endografts is safe and durable [44]. Another article stressed the importance of selecting patients with appropriate anatomy. Sealing the proximal landing zone in unhealthy aorta or in the juxtarenal aorta was associated with increased risk for type 1a endoleak development. Although the incidence was low, patients with type 1a endoleak (2.8%) had significantly higher aortic-related mortality than those without endoleak (26.9% vs. 6.2%, $p = 0.001$) [45].

There is only one analysis specifically evaluating fenestrated/branched endograft repair in the elderly. In a review of 288 patients undergoing fenestrated branched endovascular aneurysm repair, 11% of the patients were greater than 80 years of age. There were no statistically significant differences in comorbidities between the two groups. The 30-day mortality was higher in the octogenarian group (9% vs. 1.6%, $p = 0.04$). All of the patients who died within 30 days in the octogenarian group had undergone a secondary procedure [46]. The authors conclude that F/B- EVAR is a satisfactory choice of treatment in patients expected to live >2 years. They cautioned that octogenarians with challenging anatomy (who are at higher risk for needing secondary procedures) should be treated with discretion.

7.3.4 Functional Recovery and Quality of Life

The physiologic consequences of open DTAA and TAAA repair are poorly tolerated in the aged population. As the perioperative care of patients improves, in-hospital mortality will continue to decline, and thus more patients will survive in the short-term. The success of these surgeries, however, is not just based on the acute outcomes, but also on the ability to return the elderly patient to the preoperative functional status. Given that, the long-term quality of life improvement is called into question. Quality of life after DTAA and TAAA repair in patients in their 70s and 80s has recently been evaluated by Di Luozzo and colleagues [37]. In a cohort of 48 patients that underwent open repair, 43 patients were living in their homes with family, four were living outside the United States, and one patient was in a nursing home. At a median of 4.1 years from the date of surgery (range 1.1–7.1 years), patients scored slightly lower on quality of life assessment compared to matched United States population, although these did not meet statistical significance. The area of greatest difference was in overall vitality.

7.3.5 Surveillance Protocols

EVAR surveillance typically includes yearly surveillance with CT scans using IV contrast, which can exacerbate underlying renal insufficiency in the aging population. Surveillance using ultrasound has been proposed as a reasonable alternative [15]. The ideal surveillance protocol should be inexpensive, non-invasive, highly sensitive and specific to detect endoleaks, aneurysm growth, and other complications of endovascular repair and should be safe for the patients. Contrast enhanced computed tomography (CTA) is considered the gold standard for surveillance following EVAR. The drawbacks include radiation exposure, contrast nephropathy, and cost. Although Doppler ultrasound (DUS) is less sensitive, it is less expensive and avoids nephrotoxic agents. These qualities make it especially appealing in the elderly population. One institution has modified their protocol using abdominal x-ray and DUS for octogenarians, an approach which has been validated in the general population as well [47, 48]. At our institution, we use color Doppler US + non-contrast CT scan for patients with decreased renal function, which may be an appropriate protocol for elderly patients in general.

Key Points

- Candidacy for aneurysm repair cannot be determined based strictly on age.
- In addition to advanced age, "high risk" factors include cardiac disease, COPD, renal disease, obesity, and unstable angina or recent MI.
- The goal of aneurysm repair is to reduce the risk of death from aneurysm rupture.
- EVAR offers a decrease in short-term mortality, which may be beneficial to patients at "high-risk" for conventional surgery.
- Long-term EVAR is associated with higher rates of re-intervention.
- Open surgical repair of AAA is safe in physically fit elderly patients but is associated with higher perioperative morbidity and mortality.
- While open repair of thoracic aortic aneurysms is possible in the elderly, overall TEVAR appears to be associated with improved perioperative survival.
- Fenestrated and branched aortic endografting is a durable option for patients who present with juxtarenal and thoracoabdominal aortic aneurysms, and it may be particularly beneficial in elderly and high-risk patients.

References

1. Parodi JC, Palmaz JC, Barone HD. Transfemoral intraluminal graft implantation for abdominal aortic aneurysms. Ann Vasc Surg. 1991;5(6):491–9.
2. Becquemin JP, Pillet JC, Lescalie F, Sapoval M, Goueffic Y, Lermusiaux P, et al. A randomized controlled trial of endovascular aneurysm repair versus open surgery for abdominal aortic aneurysms in low- to moderate-risk patients. J Vasc Surg. 2011;53(5):1167–73.e1.

3. Mastracci TM, Greenberg RK, Hernandez AV, Morales C. Defining high risk in endovascular aneurysm repair. J Vasc Surg. 2010;51(5):1088–95.e1.
4. Arias E. United States life tables 2010. Natl Vital Stat Rep. 2010;63(7).
5. De Martino RR, Goodney PP, Nolan BW, Robinson WP, Farber A, Patel VI, et al. Optimal selection of patients for elective abdominal aortic aneurysm repair based on life expectancy. J Vasc Surg. 2013;58:589–95.
6. Greenberg RK, Haulon S, Lyden SP, Srivastava SD, Turc A, Eagleton MJ, et al. Endovascular management of juxtarenal aneurysms with fenestrated endovascular grafting. J Vasc Surg. 2004;39(2):279–87.
7. Lederle FA, Wilson SE, Johnson GR, Reinke DB, Littooy FN, Acher CW, et al. Immediate repair compared with surveillance of small abdominal aortic aneurysms. N Engl J Med. 2002;346(19):1437–44.
8. Lederle F, Freischlag JA, Kyriakides TC, Matsumura JS, et al. Group OVAS. Long-term comparison of endovascular and open repair of abdominal aortic aneurysm. N Engl J Med. 2012;367:1988–97.
9. Ouriel K. Randomized clinical trials of endovascular repair versus surveillance for treatment of small abdominal aortic aneurysms. J Endovasc Ther. 2009;16(Suppl 1):I94–105.
10. Davies RR, Goldstein LJ, Coady MA, Tittle SL, Rizzo JA, Kopf GS, et al. Yearly rupture or dissection rates for thoracic aortic aneurysms: simple prediction based on size. Ann Thorac Surg. 2002;73(1):17–27; discussion -8.
11. Giersson A. Surgical treatment of thoracic aortic disease in the elderly. In: Katlic MR, editor. Cardiothoracic surgery in the elderly: evidenced based practice. New York: Springer; 2011. p. 427–36.
12. Griepp RB, Ergin MA, Galla JD, Lansman SL, McCullough JN, Nguyen KH, et al. Natural history of descending thoracic and thoracoabdominal aneurysms. Ann Thorac Surg. 1999;67:1927–30.
13. Rigberg DA, McGory ML, Zingmond DS, Maggard MA, Agustin M, Lawrence PF, et al. Thirty-day mortality statistics underestimate the risk of repair of thoracoabdominal aortic aneurysms: a statewide experience. J Vasc Surg. 2006;43(2):217–22; discussion 23.
14. Eagleton MJ, Kang J. Preoperative management. In: Cronenwett JL, Johnston KW, editors. Rutherford's Vascular Surgery. 8th ed. Philadelphia: Elsevier/Saunders; 2014. p. 466–79.
15. de Blic R, Alsac JM, Julia P, El Batti S, Mirault T, De Primio M, et al. Elective treatment of abdominal aortic aneurysm is reasonable in patients >85 years of age. Ann Vasc Surg. 2014;28:209–16.
16. Mills Sr JL, Duong ST, Leon Jr LR, Goshima KR, Ihnat DM, Wendel CS, et al. Comparison of the effects of open and endovascular aortic aneurysm repair on long-term renal function using chronic kidney disease staging based on glomerular filtration rate. J Vasc Surg. 2008;47(6):1141–9.
17. Biancari F, Venermo M; Finnish Arterial Disease Investigators. Open repair of ruptured abdominal aortic aneurysm in patients aged 80 years and older. Br J Surg. 2011;98(12):1713–8.
18. Salata K, Katznelson R, Beattie WS, Carroll J, Lindsay TF, Djaiani G. Endovascular versus open approach to aortic aneurysm repair surgery: rates of postoperative delirium. Can J Anaesth. 2012;59(6):556–61.
19. Fried LP, Tangen CM, Walston J, Newman AB, Hirsch C, Gottdiener J, et al. Frailty in older adults: evience for a phenotype. J Gerontol A Biol Sci Med Sci. 2001;56:M146–56.
20. Lee DH, Buth KJ, Martin BJ, Yip AM, Hirsch GM. Frail patients are at increased risk for mortality and prolonged institutional care after cardiac surgery. Circulation. 2010;121:973–8.
21. Conway KP, Byrne J, Townsend M, Lane IF. Prognosis of patients turned down for conventional abdominal aortic aneurysm repair in the endovascular and sonographic era: Szilagyi revisited? J Vasc Surg. 2001;33:752–7.
22. Greenhalgh R, Brown LC, Epstein D, Kwong D, Powell JT, Sculpher MJ, et al. Endovascular aneurysm reapri versus open surgery in patients with abdominal aortic aneurysm (EVAR trial 1): randomised controlled trial. Lancet. 2005;365:2169–86.

23. Prinssen M, Verhoeven EL, Buth J, Cuypers PW, van Sambeek MR, Balm R, et al. A randomized trial comparing conventional and endovascular repair of abdominal aortic aneurysms. N Engl J Med. 2004;351(16):1607–18.
24. Lederle FA. The natural history of abdominal aortic aneurysm. Acta Chir Belg. 2009;109(1):7–12.
25. Conrad MF, Crawford RS, Pedraza JD, Brewster DC, Lamuraglia GM, Corey M, et al. Long-term durability of open abdominal aortic aneurysm repair. J Vasc Surg. 2007;46(4):669–75.
26. Hallett Jr JW, Marshall DM, Petterson TM, Gray DT, Bower TC, Cherry KJJ, et al. Graft-related complications after abdominal aortic aneurysm repair: reassurance from a 36-year population-based experience. J Vasc Surg. 1997;25:277–84.
27. United Kingdom ETI, Greenhalgh RM, Brown LC, Powell JT, Thompson SG, Epstein D, et al. Endovascular versus open repair of abdominal aortic aneurysm. N Engl J Med. 2010;362(20):1863–71.
28. De Bruin JL, Baas AF, Buth J, Prinssen M, Verhoeven EL, Cuypers PW, et al. Long-term outcome of open or endovascular repair of abdominal aortic aneurysm. N Engl J Med. 2010;362(20):1881–9.
29. Henebiens M, Vahl A, Koelemay MJ. Elective surgery of abdominal aortic aneurysms in octogenarians: a systematic review. J Vasc Surg. 2008;47(3):676–81.
30. Pol RA, Zeebregts CJ, van Sterkenburg SM, Reijnen MM, Investigators E. Thirty-day outcome and quality of life after endovascular abdominal aortic aneurysm repair in octogenarians based on the Endurant Stent Graft Natural Selection Global Postmarket Registry (ENGAGE). J Vasc Surg. 2012;56(1):27–35.
31. Prenner SB, Turnbull IC, Malik R, Salloum A, Ellozy SH, Vouyouka AG, et al. Outcome of elective endovascular abdominal aortic aneurysm repair in octogenarians and nonagenarians. J Vasc Surg. 2010;51(6):1354–9.
32. Paolini D, Chahwan S, Wojnarowski D, Pigott JP, LaPorte F, Comerota AJ. Elective endovascular and open repair of abdominal aortic aneurysms in octogenarians. J Vasc Surg. 2008;47(5):924–7.
33. Wigley J, Shantikumar S, Hameed W, Griffin K, Handa A, Scott DJ. Endovascular aneurysm repair in nonagenarians: a systematic review. Ann Vasc Surg. 2015;29:385–91.
34. Fairman RM, Criado F, Farber M, Kwolek C, Mehta M, White R, et al. Pivotal results of the Medtronic Vascular Talent Thoracic Stent Graft System: the VALOR trial. J Vasc Surg. 2008;48(3):546–54.
35. Matsumura JS, Cambria RP, Dake MD, Moore RD, Svensson LG, Snyder S, et al. International controlled clinical trial of thoracic endovascular aneurysm repair with the Zenith TX2 endovascular graft: 1-year results. J Vasc Surg. 2008;47(2):247–57; discussion 57.
36. Makaroun MS, Dillavou ED, Wheatley GH, Cambria RP, Gore TAGI. Five-year results of endovascular treatment with the Gore TAG device compared with open repair of thoracic aortic aneurysms. J Vasc Surg. 2008;47(5):912–8.
37. Di Luozzo G, Shirali AS, Varghese R, Lin HM, Weiss AJ, Bischoff MS, et al. Quality of life and survival of septuagenarians and octogenarians after repair of descending and thoracoabdominal aortic aneurysms. J Thorac Cardiovasc Surg. 2013;145:378–84.
38. Huynh TT, Miller 3rd CC, Estrera AL, Sheinbaum R, Allen SJ, Safi HJ. Determinants of hospital length of stay after thoracoabdominal aortic aneurysm repair. J Vasc Surg. 2002;35(4):648–53.
39. Okita Y, Ando M, Minatoya K, Tagusari O, Kitamura S, Nakajjma N, et al. Early and long-term results of surgery for aneurysms of the thoracic aorta in septuagenarians and octogenarians. Eur J Cardiothorac Surg. 1999;16(3):317–23.
40. Patel HJ, Williams DM, Upchurch Jr GR, Dasika NL, Passow MC, Prager RL, et al. A comparison of open and endovascular descending thoracic aortic repair in patients older than 75 years of age. Ann Thorac Surg. 2008;85(5):1597–603; discussion 603–4.
41. Oderich GS, Greenberg RK, Farber M, Lyden S, Sanchez L, Fairman R, et al. Results of the United States multicenter prospective study evaluating the Zenith fenestrated endovascular graft for treatment of juxtarenal abdominal aortic aneurysms. J Vasc Surg. 2014;60:1420–8.

42. Amiot S, Haulon S, Becquemin JP, Magnan PE, Lermusiaux P, Goueffic Y, et al. Fenestrated endovascular grafting: the French multicentre experience. Eur J Vasc Endovasc Surg. 2010;39:537–44.
43. Marzelle J, Presles E, Becquemin JP. Results and fators affecting early otucome of fenestrated and/or branched stent grafts for aortic aneurysms. Ann Surg. 2015;261:197–206.
44. Mastracci TM, Eagleton MJ, Kuramochi Y, Bathurst S, Wolski K. Twelve-year results of fenestrated endografts for juxtrenal and group IV thoracoabdominal aneurysms. J Vasc Surg. 2015;61:355–64.
45. O'Callaghan A, Greenberg RK, Eagleton MJ, Bena J, Mastracci TM. Type Ia endoleaks after fenestrated and branched endografts may lead to component instability and increased aortic mortality. J Vasc Surg. 2015;61:908–14.
46. Hertault A, Sobocinski J, Kristmundsson T, Maurel B, et al. Results of F-EVAR in octogenarians. J Vasc Surg. 2014;59:1232–40.
47. Visser L, Pol RA, Tielliu IF, van den Dungen JJ, Zeebregts CJ. A limited and customized follow-up seems justified after endovascular abdominal aneurysm repair in octogenarians. J Vasc Surg. 2014;59:1232–40.
48. Verhoeven EL, Oikonomou K, Ventin FC, Lerut P, Fernandes EFR, Mendes Pedro L. Is it time to eliminate CT after EVAR as routine follow-up? J Cardiovasc Surg (Torino). 2011;52(2):193–8.

8 Peripheral Arterial Disease in the Elderly

Jennifer Kaplan, Emily V. Finlayson, and Michael S. Conte

8.1 Introduction

Peripheral arterial disease (PAD), manifesting symptoms from intermittent claudication (IC) to critical limb ischemia (CLI), is predominantly a disease of the elderly and carries a significant healthcare burden. The overall prevalence of PAD in the year 2000 in the United States was 4.3% and 14.5% in those 70 years of age and older, representing at least 4 million individuals [1]. PAD has become a major global health problem in the new millennium, in large part as a result of greater life expectancy. A recent study estimated the global prevalence at more than 200 million individuals, increased by 23.5% from the year 2000 to 2010, spanning all income levels [2]. This study noted that across the world, PAD affects one in ten individuals over age 70, and one in six over age 80. Thus all physicians must be familiar with the disease and its management. These patients have a high comorbidity burden including hypercholesterolemia, hypertension, diabetes, and smoking. In fact, 72% of adults with PAD have at least two comorbidities and 33% had either coronary heart disease, congestive heart failure (CHF), or stroke [1]. The majority of individuals with PAD are asymptomatic, although they are subject to progressive functional decline and are at risk for progression to more advanced manifestations.

Key to a discussion of PAD care in the elderly is the geriatric syndrome frailty, which represents a diminished physiologic reserve and vulnerability to stressors. Among PAD patients in the NHANES dataset, 6.4% were frail, and this subset had the lowest survival probability (48%) at a mean follow up of 58.7 months [3]. In a

J. Kaplan • M.S. Conte (✉)
Department of Surgery, University of California, San Francisco, San Francisco, CA, USA
e-mail: Michael.Conte2@ucsf.edu

E.V. Finlayson
UCSF Center for Surgery in Older Adults, Department of Surgery, University of California, San Francisco, San Francisco, CA, USA

R. Chaer (ed.), *Vascular Disease in Older Adults*,
DOI 10.1007/978-3-319-29285-4_8

study of Medicare beneficiaries with PAD undergoing percutaneous vascular intervention (PVI), the median age was 76 with a sharp increase in outpatient procedures seen in recent years [4]. A recent study reported significant numbers of nursing home patients undergoing revascularization procedures, many of which have cognitive impairment and are nonambulatory at baseline. In this cohort, the majority was nonambulatory or dead within 1 year after surgery [5]. Such reports have increasingly raised questions about the appropriateness of vascular intervention and their clinical benefit, particularly in the frail elderly population. However, other studies have highlighted a relationship between lack of vascular services and amputation rates across disparate hospital referral regions, further demonstrating the importance of defining the optimal level of vascular care [6].

The estimated total cost for PAD care in the United States is $21 billion [7]. At 2 years, the mean cumulative cost per patient with a history of claudication is $7000 and with a history of revascularization is $11,693 [8]. The REACH registry found that average costs for inpatient treatment of PAD exceed those of coronary or cerebrovascular disease. One hospitalization or intervention for PAD is often not definitive and can portend a high rate of additional inpatient and outpatient resource utilization after discharge.

Older patients must balance the desire for symptom relief and functional independence with the risks of intervention and reintervention. The disease itself is associated with high rates of comorbid illness, which more than age alone, put patients at increased risk for complications. In this chapter, we focus on PAD in patients over 70, who represent the majority of subjects in the current vascular literature.

8.2 Evaluation of the Elderly Patient with PAD and Prognosis

8.2.1 Asymptomatic PAD

The American College of Cardiology Foundation/American Heart Association (ACCF/AHA) Task Force on Practice Guidelines outlined the most recent set of recommendations for PAD in 2013 [9]. For those at risk for PAD (which includes patients over age 70), a review of symptoms that includes questions about claudication, rest pain, and nonhealing wounds should be performed as well as a vascular and foot exam. The ankle-brachial index (ABI) test is the accepted standard for making a diagnosis of PAD, and the topic of ABI screening has been controversial. The US Preventive Services Task Force has given ABI screening an "indeterminate" rating [10]. The ACCF/AHA guideline advocates for ABI screening in groups at increased risk. In contrast to ACCF/AHA guidelines, the Society for Vascular Surgery did not recommend ABI screening in asymptomatic patients over age 65 [11]. ABI screening for PAD in the elderly would identify a significant number of asymptomatic individuals, yet it remains unclear if this would lead to direct health benefits.

8.2.2 Intermittent Claudication

If IC symptoms are present, a resting ABI should be performed. If the resting ABI is normal, an exercise ABI should be considered. Segmental Doppler pressures can be useful for preoperative lesion localization. Arterial duplex ultrasound may be used to assess lesion anatomy in patients with known PAD and to consider options for intervention.

The Society for Vascular Surgery (SVS) recently published guidelines for the evaluation of individuals with claudication [11]. These emphasize clinical diagnosis and reiterate the importance of an exercise ABI measurement when resting ABI is normal. This can be done with the patient walking on a treadmill for 5 min, reporting when they are having pain, and encouraging them to finish the test. A PAD diagnosis is made when the exercise ABI is less than or equal to 0.9 or if there is a drop of 30 mmHg with more than 3 min of recovery time.

Exercise testing can be used to quantitate functional limitations in IC and response to therapy. Both pain-free walking distance and maximum walking distance on a treadmill protocol are used, as is a 6-min walk test, which is often more feasible in elderly individuals. A pre- and postexercise ABI can be used to rule out other sources of claudication such as spinal stenosis, also common in the elderly. Exercise testing can also help determine the safety of exercise programs to be used as therapy.

Although many tests for walking impairment exist, the 6-min walk test has been shown to closely correlate to outdoor walking ability ($r = 0.78$, $p < 0.001$) and better reflects quality of life outcomes as compared to other tests ($r = 0.53$, $p < 0.01$) [12]. As discussed by Nordanstig et al., this test is patient regulated and therefore ideal for elderly patients or those with significant comorbidities, which may preclude them from using a treadmill. Other tests include the graded treadmill test, which is highly reproducible and a good test for functional limitations of IC, but should not be used as the sole assessment of walking ability.

8.2.3 Natural History

With new research and follow-up data, we continue to better understand the clinical implications of asymptomatic PAD and IC. PAD is considered a "coronary artery disease equivalent" in terms of long-term risk of mortality and major cardiovascular events. In some individuals it may represent the first manifestation of clinical atherosclerosis. Thus the importance of its diagnosis lies in establishing a framework for guideline-based risk factor and medical management, patient education, and cardiovascular surveillance. A minority of patients with asymptomatic PAD develops severe or limb-threatening disease. However, recent data suggest these individuals are subject to progressive functional decline. The prognosis for many patients with IC is one of symptom stabilization; 25% go on to experience a worsening of symptoms and 1–2% develop CLI [13]. There is also evidence that claudication symptoms do not predict major amputation at 10 years, rather physiologic factors such as decreased ABI and diabetes can better forecast who will progress to limb ischemia [14]. Diabetes is a critical modifier of the prognosis of PAD, portending an increased risk of progression and mandating vascular and podiatric surveillance to reduce amputation risk.

In an observational study of men with a mean age of 69 years and IC, by 18 months of follow-up, pain-free walk distance decreased by 22% ($p < 0.05$), total walk distance by 9% ($p < 0.05$), and resting calf blood flow by 18% ($p < 0.05$). Additionally, 27% of patients reported decreased physical activity ($p < 0.05$), and most importantly, none had a change in their ABI [15]. In a study of over 600 patients with a mean age of 71 with and without PAD, predictors of functional decline included lower starting ABI and worse baseline symptoms of claudication. Even asymptomatic patients with PAD had a greater annual decline in their 6-min walk distance (mean − 76.8 ft, $p = 0.04$) and greater odds of being unable to walk for 6 min (odd ratio [OR] 3.63; $P = 0.002$) as compared to those without PAD [16].

In a study of sedentary elderly individuals (aged 70–89) living in the community, ABIs were measured and correlated with functional walking tests [17]. Only 5.5% of patients with an ABI <0.9 had symptoms; however, even the asymptomatic participants had slower walking times and velocities. The opposite is true for patients who perform self-directed exercise; those with PAD who walk at least three times weekly have less functional decline over the subsequent year [18].

Depression represents another factor contributing to functional decline in elderly patients with PAD [19]. Disability and depressive symptoms go hand in hand, and a Geriatric Depression Score greater than and equal to 6 was present in 21.7% of patients with PAD. After controlling for age and comorbidities, depression was associated with shorter 6-min walk distance and slower walking velocities. In a recent study, depressive symptoms were associated with both prevalent PAD and development of PAD-related events [20]. Some of this association was explained by comorbidities and decreased physical activity, suggesting a potential role for the frailty syndrome in development of PAD in the depressed population.

In summary, despite an apparent stabilization in symptoms, many patients with PAD and IC are undergoing physical decline over time. In older PAD patients, this change may manifest in a shift from independence to partial dependence. It seems intuitive that promotion of a healthy lifestyle by interventions such as smoking cessation, diet, and fitness and walking programs would be of primary import to arrest or slow this decline. Whereas we currently lack evidence to support specific interventions in the large asymptomatic PAD population, there is considerable evidence to support the benefits of exercise therapy in IC [21].

8.3 Noninterventional Management of the Elderly Patient with Claudication

8.3.1 Medical Therapy

Cardiovascular risk reduction is key in the discussion of claudication management as patients are at higher risk for cardiovascular ischemic events than ischemic limb events. Approximately 60–80% of patients with lower extremity PAD have significant coronary artery disease and 12–25% have hemodynamically significant carotid artery stenosis [14].

The main tenets of risk reduction in the PAD population include smoking cessation, lipid-lowering medication, diabetes and hypertension management, and antiplatelet therapy. Current ACCF/AHA guidelines recommend a statin to keep LDL < 100 mg/dL and an antihypertensive to keep systolic blood pressure under 140 mmHg and diastolic under 90 mmHg (unless a diabetic or with chronic kidney disease, in which case blood pressure should be under 130/80) [9]. More recent guidelines suggest that a statin should only be used in asymptomatic patients if the perceived 10-year risk of cardiovascular events is over 7.5% and that in symptomatic patients, statins may improve pain-free walking time [11].

Patients with diabetes should be treated to maintain an HbA1c less than 7% and receive dedicated foot care (podiatric evaluations and early urgent management of any ulcer or lesion). Smoking should be asked about at every visit with cessation counseling and medical therapy if needed. Currently there is no role for homocysteine-lowering medication.

As of 2011, the ACCF/AHA recommend the use of aspirin or clopidogrel for cardiovascular risk reduction in all patients with symptomatic atherosclerotic PAD. Aspirin can be given at doses from 75 to 325 mg, with clopidogrel 75 mg as an alternative. Antiplatelet agents can be given to asymptomatic patients with an ABI <0.9, but benefit has not been shown in those with a borderline ABI between 0.9 and 1. Those at high cardiovascular risk without a concomitant bleeding risk can be given combination therapy of aspirin and clopidogrel. Warfarin dose not play a role in risk reduction for PAD unless needed for a specific indication.

Cilostazol, a phosphodiesterase III inhibitor with antiplatelet and antithrombotic properties, has been recommended specifically for the treatment of claudication. In a systematic review of 15 randomized control trials of cilostazol versus placebo or pentoxyfilline, the Cochrane group found a regimen of 100 mg twice daily to be associated with higher initial claudication distance and absolute claudication distance [22]. As compared to placebo, cilostazol increased resting ABI by 0.06 (95% CI 0.4–0.8). Common side effects included headache, diarrhea, abnormal stools, dizziness, and palpitations all of which were mild and did not require cessation of therapy. Cilostazol is contraindicated in patients with congestive heart failure, renal, or hepatic impairment. Patients in these studies averaged 65–67 years of age; however, the studies included patients up to 85 years of age and can be applied to the elderly population.

Pentoxyfilline given at 400 mg three times is considered second-line therapy, but its effectiveness is less well established [9]. It tends to be well tolerated with mild side effects of nausea, headache, drowsiness, and worsening of hypertension [11]. Medications that have not shown efficacy include prostaglandins, vitamin E, chelation therapy, and levocarnitine. In one randomized trial, ramipril 10 mg given daily for 24 weeks was found to increase pain-free and overall treadmill walking times; however, further work is needed before its use can be recommended to patients with IC (and without evidence of renal artery stenosis) [23].

8.3.2 Exercise Therapy

For many years, the recommendation for patients with mild to moderate claudication has been to "stop smoking and keep walking" [24]. In patients who are able to safely ambulate, supervised exercise therapy is recommended for 30–45 min three times weekly for at least 12 weeks [9]. The presumed mechanism for the benefits of exercise in patients with PAD includes exercise-induced stimulation of collaterals, enhanced bioenergetics of skeletal muscle, and improved nitric-oxide-dependent microcirculatory vasodilatation. Barriers to exercise therapy include compliance, comorbidities, and lack of insurance coverage for supervised programs [11].

A Cochrane review of supervised exercise therapy found significant improvements in maximal walking time, pain-free walking time, and pain-free walking distance [21].

There was only a slight increase in ABI and no significant change to calf blood flow or mortality. A novel finding of this analysis was that maximal improvement in walking distance is seen at 6 months as opposed to three, and therefore this longer period should supplant the 12-week recommendations in current guidelines.

Not every elderly individual is capable of completing supervised walk-based exercise, especially if they have comorbidities such as severe arthritis or COPD. A separate meta-analysis from the Cochrane group examined alternative forms of supervised exercise, which included cycling, strength training, and upper arm ergometry [25]. When these alternatives were compared to supervised walk-based training there was no difference in maximum walking distance or pain-free walking distance (as measured in metabolic equivalents, or METs).

When supervised exercise programs have been compared to nonsupervised or home-based programs, those undergoing supervised exercise had better maximal walking distances and pain-free walking distance [26]. Within the nonsupervised group, those with home-based exercise programs saw more improvement than those who were simply advised to walk on their own. Home-based exercise programs can achieve high adherence rates and similar results to supervised programs [27].

In a study identifying barriers to exercise, Cavalcante et al. found patients over 65, those with low socioeconomic status, diabetes, and baseline low ABI and walking capacity were more likely to experience barriers to activity [28]. These barriers included fear of falling, fatigue/lack of energy, and not having places to sit when experiencing pain. As many of these factors overlap with the frailty syndrome, targeting this group is especially important in preventing further decline. Supervised exercise therapy, whether walking-based or with alternative exercises, should be offered to all patients with claudication, regardless of age, and individualized based on comorbidities.

8.3.3 Open and Endovascular Revascularization for Claudication

The discussion of surgical management for claudication in a patient of any age should begin with three assessments. First, other etiologies of leg pain should be ruled out including arthritis and spinal stenosis. Second, there should be significant disability from claudication that did not resolve with conservative management (e.g. trial of medical therapy and/or exercise). Finally, there should not be another medical condition that would preclude postoperative functional improvement or disability resolution (i.e. severe congestive heart failure). Patients with newly diagnosed intermittent claudication who are considering intervention should complete at least 6 months of risk reduction, medical therapy, and supervised or home-based exercise [11].

Patients should also be counseled that vascular interventions for IC are performed to address their disability and not as prevention against amputation. The risk of ongoing or worsening disability from IC ranges from 20% to 30%, while the risk of critical ischemia is under 5% [11]. Because the affected limb is not threatened, any procedure should have low morbidity and, ideally, good long-term patency. The risk/benefit equation thus also hinges on knowledge of the anatomic pattern of disease in each individual and the likely outcomes of specific interventions. The recent SVS practice guidelines stress the importance of an individualized approach to intervention for IC, stating that the modality offered should provide *a* > 50% likelihood of sustained benefit (patency) for at least 2 years to meet a minimum efficacy threshold [11]. Unfortunately, there are few randomized clinical trials to directly compare effectiveness of various interventions for IC, thus Level 1 evidence is sorely lacking in the field.

The anatomic pattern of disease is an important factor in considering treatment options and likelihood of technical and clinical success. Endovascular therapy is recommended for focal (TASC A, B) femoropopliteal lesions as well as the majority of aortoiliac occlusive lesions [9, 11]. A comparison of bypass surgery to endovascular therapy in 263 patients with femoropoliteal TASC C and D disease (the majority of whom were over 75 years of age) found a higher complication rate in the bypass group (14.4% vs. 3.5%, $p < 0.01$), improved 1- and 5-year primary patency in the bypass group (82.1% and 69.4% vs. 67.8% and 45.2%, $p < 0.01$), but no difference in 1- or 5-year secondary patency rates (93.2% and 79.5% vs. 90.1% and 85.1%, $p = 0.48$) [29]. The authors suggest that endovascular therapy is a preferred option in higher-risk patients.

In a slightly younger retrospective cohort with a full range of TASC disease, bypass grafting as opposed to endovascular therapy demonstrated improved freedom from restenosis at 3 years (73% vs. 42%), but no difference in reintervention at 3 years (77% vs. 66%). In this cohort, use of statins predicted both graft patency and freedom from reintervention. Because the majority of studies comparing bypass to endovascular are retrospective, the patients in each therapy group tend to be quite different, with bypass patients having more complex disease, making a true head-to-head comparison difficult [30].

When risks and benefits are being weighed, age alone should not prohibit patients from undergoing revascularization. When octogenarians with similar risk profiles to patients under 65 underwent endovascular management of intermittent claudication, there was no difference in outcomes (including mortality and reintervention) [31]. Comorbidities and functional impairment as opposed to age likely have more influence on postoperative outcomes for IC.

8.3.4 Open and Endovascular Revascularization for Critical Limb Ischemia

Critical limb ischemia (CLI) is the most advanced clinical syndrome of PAD and portends an increased risk to life and limb. Regardless of chronologic or physiologic age, management of CLI should focus on pain relief, limb salvage, function and quality of life, as well as survival. Patients with CLI suffer greatly from ischemic rest pain, non-healing wounds, and the associated negative impacts on their quality of life. Patients who are chronically nonambulatory, have limited life expectancy, or have very advanced comorbidities may be appropriately treated with palliative care or primary amputation. However, the majority should be considered as candidates for revascularization to relieve symptoms and achieve limb salvage. Whether to choose an open or endovascular approach for revascularization in the setting of CLI depends on the predicted lifespan of the patient, the severity of limb threat, and the pattern of arterial disease. Based on the only level 1 evidence in the field, if the patient is expected to live for more than 2 years, bypass surgery may be considered as first line, versus angioplasty if life span is under 2 years and if there is no suitable vein available for bypass [9, 32]. Vascular disease anatomy obviously plays a critical role in this decision as well. For aortoiliac disease or femoropopliteal type A or B, many prefer to start with endovascular therapy, whereas for more extensive occlusions (e.g. type D anatomy), many would go straight to bypass surgery in an average risk patient [33]. Many if not most patients with CLI have significant below the knee disease, and currently available (limited) data suggest better patency for tibial/pedal bypass but similar midterm limb salvage rates for angioplasty. Table 8.1 provides a summary of open and endovascular outcomes for CLI.

In a recent study of nonagenarians referred for CLI or acute limb ischemia, 83% were living independently prior to surgery, with 72% remaining independent afterwards [34]. Eighty-two percent of the 91% that were ambulatory preoperatively maintained this status postoperatively. Both preoperative living status and ambulatory ability were no different between endovascular and open approaches. Dementia was the single and poor predictor of poor amputation-free survival in this cohort. In a study of septuagenarians and octogenarians with lower extremity CLI undergoing bypass procedures, 5-year survival was 54% and 64%, primary patency 74% and 68%, and limb salvage rate 86% in both age groups [35]. The authors suggest that these age groups stand to benefit from revascularization as a means to relieve symptoms and avoid the morbidity of amputation.

Improved stratification of PAD patients would assist clinical decision-making. To create a prediction score for the composite outcome of amputation and mortality at 1 year, researchers used data from the PREVENT III cohort (Project of Ex-Vivo graft Engineering via Transfection III) [36]. This dataset included 1404 patients with CLI who underwent infrainguinal bypass with autogenous vein. In this model, age greater than or equal to 75 years was an independent predictor of amputation and death in multivariable analysis and given two points in the risk score (HR 1.64, 95% CI 1.21–2.22, $p = 0.001$). Age alone was associated with an amputation-free survival of 89.7%. These results were also confirmed in an observation study of octogenarians with CLI [37]. In this cohort, periprocedural mortality in

Table 8.1 Age and outcome of lower extremity revascularization for critical limb ischemia

Study	*N*	Age range	Procedure/Outcome	Group 1	Group 2	*P* Value
Saarinen (2015) [34]	233	92* (90–100)	*Surgical* vs. *Endovascular*	*Surgical*	*Endovascular*	
			1-year survival	50.9%	48.6%	0.505
			Limb salvage	85.1%	87.9%	0.259
			Amputation-free survival	45.7%	44.4%	0.309
Chang (2001) [35]	383	70–79	*Bypass, Septuagenarian* vs. *Octogenarian*	*Septuagenarians*	*Octogenarians*	
	209	80–89	5-year survival	64%	54%	>0.2
			5-year primary patency	68%	74%	>0.2
			5-year limb salvage	86%	86%	NS
Brosi (2007) [37]	167	85.4** (80–94.9)	*Surgical or endovascular* vs. *medical,*	*Octogenarians*	*Nonoctogenarians*	
	249	69.3** (40.3–79.9)	*Octogenarians* vs. *Nonoctogenarians*			
			Primary clinical success	26.6%	31.2%	NS
			Secondary clinical success	50.6%	55.0%	NS
			Major amputation	22.3%	23.6%	NS
			Repeated revascularization	48.3%	40.4%	NS
Masaki (2014) [33]	131	BY 70* (46–89)	*Bypass* vs. *Endovascular*	*Bypass*	*Endovascular*	
	33	EV 72* (47–89)	3-year primary patency	72%	54%	<0.009
			3-year secondary patency	82%	60%	NR
			3-year limb salvage	86%	82%	NS

(continued)

Table 8.1 (continued)

Study	*N*	Age range	Procedure/Outcome	Group 1	Group 2	*P* Value
Adam (2005) [32]	BY 228	EV 224	*Bypass* vs. *Endovascular*	*Unadjusted*†	*Adjusted*†	
	<70 35%	<70 30%	6-month amputation free survival	1.07 (0.72–1.6)	1.04 (0.69–1.56)	NS
	70–79 39%	70–79 46%	Entire follow-up amputation-free survival	0.89 (0.68–1.17)	0.88 (0.66–1.16)	NS
	≥80 26%	≥80 26%	Entire follow-up all-cause mortality	0.90 (0.66–1.22)	0.95 (0.69–1.29)	NS
Simons (2012) [47]	2110	CLI 69.9* ± 11.4	*Bypass, CLI* vs. *Claudication*	*CLI*	*Claudication*	
	797	IC 64.3* ± 10.4	1-year major amputation	12.2%	1.6%	<0.0001
			1-year primary patency	66.4%	78.9%	<0.0001
			1-year secondary patency	77.4%	89%	<0.0001

Abbreviations: *CLI* critical limb ischemia, *NS* not significant, *NR* not reported
*Median; **Mean; †HR (95% CI) of surgery relative to angioplasty

octogenarians was much higher after surgical bypass as compared to endovascular. Those who did survive had similar outcomes at 1 year as compared to those under 80, suggesting that there may be a cohort of older patients who will benefit from intervention. Other risk scores have identified similar factors from large cohorts, unfortunately none have been prospectively validated on all-comers presenting with CLI [38, 39]. See Table 8.2 for a summary of available prediction scores.

It is often difficult to retrospectively compare outcomes of endovascular and open interventions in the older population, because of the selection bias of older sick patients receiving endovascular therapy. In general, primary patency is superior after bypass surgery; however, limb salvage rate and amputation-free survival are equivalent between endovascular and bypass approaches [33]. Therefore, age alone should not be the determinant for management in these patients with CLI, instead medical comorbidities, life expectancy, degree of limb threat, and severity of the disease should dictate therapy.

8.3.5 Functional Outcomes Following Revascularization for Critical Limb Ischemia

When nursing home residents who were hospitalized for CLI underwent lower extremity endovascular or open revascularization, all saw an initial functional decline after surgery, with patients undergoing open operation having better functional outcomes and faster recovery by 6 months [40]. Factors associated with poor functional outcome included impaired cognitive status, female gender, and worse baseline ADLs. The majority of patients in this study were over age 75.

In a year-long prospective cohort of functional and quality of life (QOL) outcomes after revascularization for chronic CLI in patients with a mean age of 68.1, functional status (as measured by the ALDS score) improved significantly over a year period to a level corresponding to difficult indoor and outdoor activities [41]. In this same cohort QOL (as measured by the VascuQol score) improved in all domains by 12 months of follow-up.

The presence of CLI in any patient mandates therapy, whether palliative or procedural, and therefore the majority of patients appropriately undergo intervention. With a frail elderly patient, goals of care and expectations must be clearly set. In one study, nursing home residents who were nonambulatory at baseline had almost double the risk of being nonambulatory after surgery and over three times the risk of functional decline as compared to those who were ambulatory [5].

8.3.6 Indication for Primary Amputation

Amputation for the primary management of CLI may be appropriate in the setting of refractory rest pain in a high-risk or nonambulatory patient, overwhelming infection, or extensive necrosis [9, 42]. According to the TASC II working group, only 40% of those undergoing below knee amputation will have full mobility at 2 years and 30% will be dead. Primary amputation is often appropriate for the elderly

Table 8.2 Prediction models for patients undergoing revascularization for critical limb ischemia

	Finnvasc [38]	Prevent III [36]	BASIL [39]	CRAB [48]
Variables	One point each for: Diabetes CAD Gangrene Urgent operation	Dialysis = 4 points Tissue loss = 3 points Age ≥ 75 y = 2 points Hematocrit <30 = 2 points Advanced CAD = 1 point	Tissue loss BMI Creatinine Bollinger score Age Smoking History of MI or angina Ankle pressure	Emergent case = 6 points Total functional dependence = 6 points Hemodialysis = 4 points Recent angina/MI = 4 points Age > 75 y = 3 points Prior amputation/revascularization = 3 points Ulceration = 3 points Partial functional dependence = 3 points
Output	0–4 risk points	Low ≤ 3points Medium = 4–7 points High ≥ 8 points	Weibull model predicted survival: http://basiltrial.com/survival_predictor.htm	Low = 0–6 points Medium = 7–12 points High > 12 points
Derivation Cohort	Finnvasc registry	PREVENT III cohort	BASIL trial	ACS-NSQIP 2007–2009
External Validation	Yes	Yes	No	No
Outcome	Major amputation and or death after infrainguinal revascularization for CLI	AFS after infrainguinal vein bypass for CLI	Death at 6, 12, and 24 months after LE bypass or angioplasty for CLI	Perioperative death or major morbidity after LE bypass for CLI

Adapted from Moxey et al. [49]

Abbreviations: *AFS* amputation free survival, *CRAB* comprehensive risk assessment for bypass, *CLI* critical limb ischemia, *LE* lower extremity, *MI* myocardial infarction, *y* years nonambulatory patient with a flexion contracture. Ideally, the amputation is performed at the lowest level possible, allowing for decreased additional energy expenditure and higher likelihood of independent walking.

8.3.6.1 Functional Status and Quality of Life Following Amputation

As with other revascularization procedures, functional status diminishes initially after amputation. However, from 6 to 18 months, walking distance tends to stabilize or improve [43]. Being able to walk then correlates with better QOL metrics including social functioning.

In patients who underwent lower extremity amputation within a year of lower extremity bypass, age was one of the most important predictors of poor functional outcome at hospital discharge (age 70–79 years: OR 0.33 $p = 0.04$, age over 80 years: OR 0.12 $p < 0.001$) [44]. At 1 year follow-up predictors of living at home and ambulating with or without assistance included living at home preoperatively (HR 6.8, 95% CI 0.94–49.2) and taking a statin preoperatively (HR 1.57, 95% CI 1.17–2.11). Comorbidities such as congestive heart failure and dialysis were negative predictors of good functional outcomes and found to have an additive effect.

A meta-analysis of mobility after amputation in patients over age 60 found a dearth of quality data in this field, yet underscored the importance of mobility in this cohort [45]. In general, patients with transtibial amputations performed better than those with transfemoral. A separate meta-analysis of QOL after amputation found a similar lack of quality data and could not conclude whether there is benefit to amputation over revascularization for CLI [46].

Key Points

- Peripheral arterial disease is predominantly a disease of the elderly; therefore, understanding the interplay between functional status, comorbidity burden, overall prognosis and pathology is key in determining management.
- Treating the elderly person with PAD should be a multidisciplinary process with cardiovascular risk mitigation, wound care, skin surveillance, symptom management, and surgical planning.
- Medical management and exercise therapy should start early in patients with claudication, and risk prediction scores should play an important role in honest discussions with patients and their families about more invasive procedures.
- Despite the key caveats noted, chronologic age alone should not be considered a contraindication to vascular intervention in those with severe disability or limb-threatening ischemia.

References

1. Selvin E, Erlinger TP. Prevalence of and risk factors for peripheral arterial disease in the United States: results from the National Health and Nutrition Examination Survey, 1999–2000. Circulation. 2004;110:738–43.

2. Fowkes FG, Rudan D, Rudan I, Aboyans V, Denenberg JO, McDermott MM, et al. Comparison of global estimates of prevalence and risk factors for peripheral artery disease in 2000 and 2010: a systematic review and analysis. Lancet. 2003;382(9901):1329–40.
3. Singh S, Bailey KR, Noheria A, Kullo IJ. Frailty across the spectrum of ankle-brachial index. Angiology. 2012;63(3):229–36.
4. Jones WS, Mi X, Qualls LG, Vemulapalli S, Peterson ED, Patel MR, Curtis LH. Trends in settings for peripheral vascular intervention and the effect of changes in the outpatient prospective payment system. J Am Coll Cardiol. 2015;65:920–7.
5. Oresanya L, Zhao S, Gan S, Fries BE, Goodney PP, Covinsky KE, Conte MS, Finlayson E. Functional outcomes after lower extremity revascularization in nursing home residents: a national cohort study. JAMA Intern Med. 2015;175:951–7.
6. Goodney PP, Holman K, Henke PK, Travis LL, Dimick JB, Stukel TA, Fisher ES, Birkmeyer JD. Regional intensity of vascular care and lower extremity amputation rates. J Vasc Surg. 2013;57(6):1471–9.
7. Norgren L, Hiatt WR, Dormandy JA, Hirsch AT, Jaff MR, Diehm C, Baumgartner I, Belch JJ. The next 10 years in the management of peripheral artery disease: perspectives from the 'PAD 2009' Conference. Eur J Vasc Endovasc Surg. 2010;40(3):375–80.
8. Mahoney EM, Wang K, Keo HH, Duval S, Smolderen KG, Cohen DJ, Steg G, Bhatt DL, Hirsch AT; Reduction of Atherothrombosis for Continued Health (REACH) Registry Investigators. Vascular hospitalization rates and costs in patients with peripheral artery disease in the United States. Circ Cardiovasc Qual Outcomes. 2010;3(6):642–51.
9. Anderson JL, Halperin JL, Albert NM, Bozkurt B, Brindis RG, Curtis LH, et al. Management of patients with peripheral artery disease (compilation of 2005 and 2011 ACCF/AHA guideline recommendations): a report of the American College of Cardiology Foundation/American Heart Association Task Force on Practice Guidelines. Circulation. 2010;127(13):1425–43.
10. Moyer VA; U. S. P. S. T. Force. Screening for peripheral artery disease and cardiovascular disease risk assessment with the ankle-brachial index in adults: U.S. Preventive Services Task Force recommendation statement. Ann Intern Med. 2010;159(5):342–8.
11. Society for Vascular Surgery Lower Extremity Guidelines Writing Group; Conte MS, Pomposelli FB, Clair DG, Geraghty PJ, McKinsey JF, et al. Society for Vascular Surgery practice guidelines for atherosclerotic occlusive disease of the lower extremities: management of asymptomatic disease and claudication. J Vasc Surg. 2015;61(3 Suppl):2S–41S.
12. Nordanstig J, Broeren M, Hensater M, Perlander A, Osterberg K, Jivegard L. Six-minute walk test closely correlates to "real-life" outdoor walking capacity and quality of life in patients with intermittent claudication. J Vasc Surg. 2014;60(2):404–9.
13. Jelnes R, Gaardsting O, Hougaard Jensen K, Baekgaard N, Tonnesen KH, Schroeder T. Fate in intermittent claudication: outcome and risk factors. Br Med J. 1986;293(6555):1137–40.
14. Hirsch AT, Haskal ZJ, Hertzer NR, Bakal CW, Creager MA, Halperin JL, et al. American Association for Vascular, S. Society for Vascular, A. Society for Cardiovascular, Interventions, M. Society for Vascular, Biology, R. Society of Interventional, A. A. T. F. o. P. Guidelines, C. American Association of, R. Pulmonary, L. National Heart, I. Blood, N. Society for Vascular, C. TransAtlantic Inter-Society, F. Vascular Disease. ACC/AHA 2005 guidelines for the management of patients with peripheral arterial disease (lower extremity, renal, mesenteric, and abdominal aortic): executive summary a collaborative report from the American Association for Vascular Surgery/Society for Vascular Surgery, Society for Cardiovascular Angiography and Interventions, Society for Vascular Medicine and Biology, Society of Interventional Radiology, and the ACC/AHA Task Force on Practice Guidelines (Writing Committee to Develop Guidelines for the Management of Patients with Peripheral Arterial Disease) endorsed by the American Association of Cardiovascular and Pulmonary Rehabilitation; National Heart, Lung, and Blood Institute; Society for Vascular Nursing; TransAtlantic Inter-Society Consensus; and Vascular Disease Foundation. J Am Coll Cardiol. 2006;47(6):1239–312.
15. Gardner AW, Montgomery PS, Killewich LA. Natural history of physical function in older men with intermittent claudication. J Vasc Surg. 2004;40(1):73–8. doi:10.1016/j.jvs.2004.02.010.

16. McDermott MM, Liu K, Greenland P, Guralnik JM, Criqui MH, Chan C, Pearce WH, Schneider JR, Ferrucci L, Celic L, Taylor LM, Vonesh E, Martin GJ, Clark E. Functional decline in peripheral arterial disease: associations with the ankle brachial index and leg symptoms. JAMA. 2004;292(4):453–61.
17. McDermott MM, Applegate WB, Bonds DE, Buford TW, Church T, Espeland MA, Gill TM, Guralnik JM, Haskell W, Lovato LC, Pahor M, Pepine CJ, Reid KF, Newman A. Ankle brachial index values, leg symptoms, and functional performance among community-dwelling older men and women in the lifestyle interventions and independence for elders study. J Am Heart Assoc. 2013;2(6):e000257.
18. McDermott MM, Liu K, Ferrucci L, Criqui MH, Greenland P, Guralnik JM, Tian L, Schneider JR, Pearce WH, Tan J, Martin GJ. Physical performance in peripheral arterial disease: a slower rate of decline in patients who walk more. Ann Intern Med. 2006;144(1):10–20.
19. McDermott MM, Greenland P, Guralnik JM, Liu K, Criqui MH, Pearce WH, Chan C, Schneider J, Sharma L, Taylor LM, Arseven A, Quann M, Celic L. Depressive symptoms and lower extremity functioning in men and women with peripheral arterial disease. J Gen Intern Med. 2003;18(6):461–7.
20. Grenon SM, Cohen BE, Smolderen K, Vittinghoff E, Whooley MA, Hiramoto J. Peripheral arterial disease, gender, and depression in the Heart and Soul Study. J Vasc Surg. 2014;60(2):396–403.
21. Lane R, Ellis B, Watson L, Leng GC. Exercise for intermittent claudication. Cochrane Database Syst Rev. 2014;7:CD000990.
22. Bedenis R, Stewart M, Cleanthis M, Robless P, Mikhailidis DP, Stansby G. Cilostazol for intermittent claudication. Cochrane Database Syst Rev. 2014;10:CD003748.
23. Ahimastos AA, Walker PJ, Askew C, Leicht A, Pappas E, Blombery P, Reid CM, Golledge J, Kingwell BA. Effect of ramipril on walking times and quality of life among patients with peripheral artery disease and intermittent claudication: a randomized controlled trial. JAMA. 2013;309(5):453–60.
24. Housley E. Treating claudication in five words. Br Med J. 1988;296(6635):1483–4.
25. Lauret GJ, Fakhry F, Fokkenrood HJ, Hunink MG, Teijink JA, Spronk S. Modes of exercise training for intermittent claudication. Cochrane Database Syst Rev. 2014;7:CD009638.
26. Fokkenrood HJ, Bendermacher BL, Lauret GJ, Willigendael EM, Prins MH, Teijink JA. Supervised exercise therapy versus non-supervised exercise therapy for intermittent claudication. Cochrane Database Syst Rev. 2013;8:CD005263.
27. Gardner AW, Parker DE, Montgomery PS, Scott KJ, Blevins SM. Efficacy of quantified home-based exercise and supervised exercise in patients with intermittent claudication: a randomized controlled trial. Circulation. 2011;123(5):491–8.
28. Cavalcante BR, Farah BQ, Barbosa JP d A, Cucato GG, da Rocha Chehuen M, da Silva Santana F, Wolosker N, de Moraes Forjaz CL, Ritti-Dias RM. Are the barriers for physical activity practice equal for all peripheral artery disease patients? Arch Phys Med Rehabil. 2015;96(2):248–52. doi:10.1016/j.apmr.2014.09.009.
29. Aihara H, Soga Y, Mii S, Okazaki J, Yamaoka T, Kamoi D, Shintani Y, Ishikawa T, Investigators RR. Comparison of long-term outcome after endovascular therapy versus bypass surgery in claudication patients with Trans-Atlantic Inter-Society Consensus-II C and D femoropopliteal disease. Circ J Off J Jpn Circ Soc. 2014;78(2):457–64.
30. Malas MB, Enwerem N, Qazi U, Brown B, Schneider EB, Reifsnyder T, Freischlag JA, Perler BA. Comparison of surgical bypass with angioplasty and stenting of superficial femoral artery disease. J Vasc Surg. 2014;59(1):129–35.
31. Jones DW, Siracuse JJ, Graham A, Connolly PH, Sedrakyan A, Schneider DB, Meltzer AJ. Safety and effectiveness of endovascular therapy for claudication in octogenarians. Ann Vasc Surg. 2015;29(1):34–41.
32. Adam DJ, Beard JD, Cleveland T, Bell J, Bradbury AW, Forbes JF, Fowkes FG, Gillepsie I, Ruckley CV, Raab G, Storkey H; B. t. participants. Bypass versus angioplasty in severe ischaemia of the leg (BASIL): multicentre, randomised controlled trial. Lancet. 2005;366(9501):1925–34.
33. Masaki H, Tabuchi A, Yunoki Y, Watanabe Y, Mimura D, Furukawa H, Yamasawa T, Honda T, Takiuchi H, Tanemoto K. Bypass vs. endovascular therapy of infrapopliteal lesions for critical limb ischemia. Ann Vasc Dis. 2014;7(3):227–31.

34. Saarinen E, Vuorisalo S, Kauhanen P, Alback A, Venermo M. The benefit of revascularization in nonagenarians with lower limb ischemia is limited by high mortality. Eur J Vasc Endovasc Surg Off J Eur Soc Vasc Surg. 2015;49(4):420–5.
35. Chang JB, Stein TA. Infrainguinal revascularizations in octogenarians and septuagenarians. J Vasc Surg. 2001;34(1):133–8.
36. Schanzer A, Mega J, Meadows J, Samson RH, Bandyk DF, Conte MS. Risk stratification in critical limb ischemia: derivation and validation of a model to predict amputation-free survival using multicenter surgical outcomes data. J Vasc Surg. 2008;48(6):1464–71.
37. Brosi P, Dick F, Do DD, Schmidli J, Baumgartner I, Diehm N. Revascularization for chronic critical lower limb ischemia in octogenarians is worthwhile. J Vasc Surg. 2007;46(6):1198–207.
38. Biancari F, Salenius JP, Heikkinen M, Luther M, Ylonen K, Lepantalo M. Risk-scoring method for prediction of 30-day postoperative outcome after infrainguinal surgical revascularization for critical lower-limb ischemia: a Finnvasc registry study. World J Surg. 2007;31(1):217–25; discussion 226–17.
39. Bradbury AW, Adam DJ, Bell J, Forbes JF, Fowkes FG, Gillespie I, Ruckley CV, Raab GM, Participants BT. Bypass versus Angioplasty in Severe Ischaemia of the Leg (BASIL) trial: a survival prediction model to facilitate clinical decision making. J Vasc Surg. 2010;51(5 Suppl):52S–68S.
40. Vogel TR, Petroski GF, Kruse RL. Functional status of elderly adults before and after interventions for critical limb ischemia. J Vasc Surg. 2014;59(2):350–8.
41. Frans FA, Met R, Koelemay MJ, Bipat S, Dijkgraaf MG, Legemate DA, Reekers JA. Changes in functional status after treatment of critical limb ischemia. J Vasc Surg. 2013;58(4):957–65. e951.
42. Norgren L, Hiatt WR, Dormandy JA, Nehler MR, Harris KA, Fowkes FG; T. I. W. Group. Inter-society consensus for the management of peripheral arterial disease (TASC II). J Vasc Surg. 2007;45(Suppl S):S5–67.
43. Fortington LV, Dijkstra PU, Bosmans JC, Post WJ, Geertzen JH. Change in health-related quality of life in the first 18 months after lower limb amputation: a prospective, longitudinal study. J Rehabil Med. 2013;45(6):587–94.
44. Suckow BD, Goodney PP, Cambria RA, Bertges DJ, Eldrup-Jorgensen J, Indes JE, et al.; Vascular Study Group of New England. Predicting functional status following amputation after lower extremity bypass. Ann Vasc Surg. 2012;26(1):67–78.
45. Fortington LV, Rommers GM, Geertzen JH, Postema K, Dijkstra PU. Mobility in elderly people with a lower limb amputation: a systematic review. J Am Med Dir Assoc. 2012;13(4): 319–25.
46. Bosma J, Vahl A, Wisselink W. Systematic review on health-related quality of life after revascularization and primary amputation in patients with critical limb ischemia. Ann Vasc Surg. 2013;27(8):1105–14.
47. Simons JP, A. Schanzer, Nolan BW, Stone DH, Kalish JA, Cronenwett JL, Goodney PP; Vascular Study Group of New England. Outcomes and practice patterns in patients undergoing lower extremity bypass. J Vasc Surg. 2012;55(6):1629–36.
48. Meltzer AJ, Graham A, Connolly PH, Meltzer EC, Karwowski JK, Bush HL, Schneider DB. The Comprehensive Risk Assessment for Bypass (CRAB) facilitates efficient perioperative risk assessment for patients with critical limb ischemia. J Vasc Surg. 2013;57(5):1186–95.
49. Moxey PW, Brownrigg J, Kumar JSS, Crate G, Holt PJ, Thompson MM, Jones KG, Hinchliffe RJ. The BASIL survival prediction model in patients with peripheral arterial disease undergoing revascularization in a university hospital setting and comparison with the FINNVASC and modified PREVENT scores. J Vasc Surg. 2013;57(1):1–7.

Renal Failure in the Elderly

9

Theodore H. Yuo and Mark L. Unruh

9.1 Introduction

Among the elderly, defined as those over 65 years of age, kidney disease is common with between 11% and 30% having chronic kidney disease (CKD) [1]. CKD has been associated with increased risk of death and disability as well as increased surgical risk. A proportion of those with CKD progress to end-stage renal disease (ESRD), at which point kidney replacement therapy is required to sustain life. Among elderly patients with CKD, the cause of kidney disease, severity of albuminuria and glomerular filtration rate (GFR) are associated with the likelihood of progression to acute and chronic kidney failure. Dialysis as a form of kidney replacement therapy for treatment of ESRD is a great triumph of modern medicine, saving lives and providing meaningful improvements in quality of life for many patients. When introduced on a wide scale in the 1970s, ESRD patients treated with dialysis through the Medicare entitlement program were typically young, carefully selected, and did not suffer from multiple other medical comorbidities [2]. Over time, though, the population undergoing kidney replacement has changed, and contemporary reports in the United States suggest that patients over 65 years of age are at least half of incident ESRD patients, with the very elderly, those over 80 years of age, representing a significant and growing fraction of the population [3]. Many elderly patients with ESRD have four or more chronic health conditions when they reach ESRD, and many are not considered candidates for kidney transplantation,

M.L. Unruh
Chair and Professor of Medicine, Department of Internal Medicine, University of New Mexico School of Medicine, Albuquerque, NM, USA

T.H. Yuo, MD MSc (✉)
Assistant Professor of Surgery, Division of Vascular Surgery, Department of Surgery, University of Pittsburgh School of Medicine, Pittsburgh, PA, USA
e-mail: yuoth@upmc.edu

R. Chaer (ed.), *Vascular Disease in Older Adults*,
DOI 10.1007/978-3-319-29285-4_9

suggesting that dialysis will be the patient's kidney replacement therapy for the rest of their lives [4]. ESRD patients in general are fragile, with death rates 8–16 times higher than in the general population [5]. The general challenges of caring for elderly patients, compared to younger patients, have been well documented; these include generalized weakness, increased susceptibility to disease, inability to tolerate adverse environments or minor traumas, loss of agility, and age-related physiological changes in addition to attitudes and beliefs of older adults and their caregivers [6]. Further, within the traditional cohort of elderly patients defined as those over 65 years, there are distinctions between the "young elderly" between 65 and 80 years and the "very elderly" older than 80 years, in terms of comorbidities, frailty, dementia, and institutionalization status [7]. Despite these patient characteristics, dialysis access strategies for the elderly share many features with younger patients. This chapter aims to review the indications and potential modalities for renal replacement therapy (RRT) among the elderly with kidney failure. Further, RRT should be planned in a patient-centered fashion, accounting for patient anatomy, surgical history, medical comorbidities, and patient preferences. We will review the outcomes of vascular interventions in elderly ESRD patients and highlight approaches that may be used to attenuate the risk of contrast. Last, we will focus on individualizing decisions for the elderly with advanced CKD receiving either a dialysis access or other vascular procedures.

9.2 Indications for Renal Replacement Therapy

As in the population as a whole, the most common causes of ESRD in the elderly are diabetes and hypertension. Indications for RRT in the elderly are similar to those in younger patients. Historically, fluid overload and signs or symptoms of uremia, despite the poorly understood nature of the uremic syndrome and its somewhat subjective evaluation, were also considered to be indications for dialysis. As such, it is theoretically appealing to postulate that earlier initiation of RRT can remove these toxins and may be associated with decreased morbidity or mortality, as some observational studies suggested [8]. However, after correcting for lead-time bias, this advantage disappears [9]. The question of timing of initiation of hemodialysis (HD) was also explored in the Initiating Dialysis Early and Late (IDEAL) study, which randomized patients to early or late initiation of dialysis, based on estimated GFR (eGFR) [10]. Patients who started HD early at a target eGFR between 10 and 15 mL/min had similar survival and clinical outcomes as patients who started HD late at a target eGFR between 5 and 7 mL/min, or who started HD due to the development of symptoms associated with kidney failure including fluid overload or uremia. While elderly patients per se were not the target population for this study, the average age of participants in the study was 60 years and the overall findings did not differ between patients who were younger than 60 years and those who were older. Of note, there was substantial cross-over among those randomized to the delayed dialysis initiation so that nearly three-quarters of the group started dialysis at eGFR above 7 mL/min. The degree of cross-over limited the inferences one could draw regarding the impact of delayed start on patient outcomes.

Other authors have noted that assessing kidney function in elderly patients is difficult since the serum creatinine level can be spuriously low due to falling muscle mass, despite steadily declining eGFR as patients age. Further clouding the clinical picture, symptoms associated with uremia are nonspecific, and include anorexia, weight loss, weakness, nausea, and difficulties with sleep and cognition [11].

Given this background, a trial of dialysis in elderly patients may be considered in selected patients who have been well informed of the possible risks and benefits of dialysis, and can cooperate with the treatment and can receive it safely. Recent guidelines published by the Renal Physicians Association (RPA) offer recommendations that incorporate patient preferences and prognostic survival assessments to help guide physicians and patients in the decision-making process [12]. Indications for trials of dialysis include uremia or worsening of congestive heart failure, refractory to maximal medical management. In cases of acute kidney injury, as opposed to chronic kidney disease, when there is a possibility of reversibility of acute kidney failure, dialysis should be offered. Further, patients with atypical presentations of ESRD should be evaluated for treatable causes of kidney failure regardless of patient age. Occasionally, there can be the worry that this attempt at acute treatment may transition inappropriately to a long-term commitment to dialysis. However, while elderly survivors of AKI seem to require more time for total recovery and recover function less completely, they can recover function and generally deserve a trial of dialysis [11]. Ultimately, though, as well described in recent guidelines, "The initiation of dialysis therapy remains a decision informed by clinical art, as well as by science…." [13]

9.2.1 Choice of Dialysis Modality: Hemodialysis (HD) Versus Peritoneal Dialysis (PD)

As in younger patients, the choice of dialysis as kidney replacement therapy in the elderly is influenced by the availability of infrastructure and staff, the burden of comorbidities, specific anatomic contraindications to a particular modality, patient and caregiver ability to adhere to the requirements of the chosen modality, and patient or physician preference. Possible advantages of PD over HD in the elderly include preservation of residual kidney function, avoidance of fluid and electrolyte shifts, more liberal diet, avoidance of vascular access, and decreased transportation time, since this is typically a home modality. On the other hand, HD may be a better choice for patients with hernias, diverticulitis, history of abdominal surgery or other intra-abdominal pathology, morbid obesity, or psychosocial inability to adhere to PD requirements. The requirement for bulky and heavy dialysate consumables is another consideration, which may represent an unanticipated difficulty for elderly patients with limited storage space and physical strength; the employment of home-care assistants may overcome these challenges [14].

Peritoneal dialysis is in general used less frequently than hemodialysis, with approximately 9% of the prevalent US dialysis population using peritoneal dialysis and the balance using hemodialysis. In the elderly, defined as those over 65 years, PD is used even less frequently, with only 7% of the population using PD, though this fraction is growing [15].

There is controversy regarding the possible survival advantage of one modality over the other in elderly patients. In general, there appears to be a benefit to using PD instead of HD initially, but this benefit appears to be lost over time. This has historically been attributed to slower loss of residual kidney function in patients on PD, but more recent analyses have suggested that this effect is overstated and may be due to selection bias [16] or the use of tunneled dialysis catheters (TDCs) in HD patients [17]. In one prospective cohort study of 174 elderly patients older than 70 years in the United Kingdom, the annual mortality and hospitalization rates in PD and HD patients were similar (26.1 vs. 26.4 deaths per 100 person-years and 1.9 vs. 2.0 admissions per person-year, respectively) [18]. Contrary to the reports in younger patients, Windelmayer and colleagues found 16% higher mortality rates for elderly patients that start on PD compared to HD in the first 90 days after dialysis initiation. Mortality rates between 91 and 180 days were equivalent, but were 45% higher after 181 days. This effect was particularly pronounced in those with diabetes [19]. A larger study from Korea with longer follow-up also demonstrated higher mortality in elderly patients started with PD, as compared to patients started with HD, with PD being associated with a 20% higher hazard of mortality. An accompanying meta-analysis again suggested higher mortality with PD, though the magnitude of the increased hazard was only about 10%, but still statistically significant [20]. The possibility of increased mortality rates with PD in elderly patients must be considered and balanced against any possible benefits.

9.3 Selection of Hemodialysis Access: AVF Versus AVG Versus TDC in the Elderly

9.3.1 Kidney Disease Outcome Quality Initiative (KDOQI) Guidelines

The current Kidney Disease Outcome Quality Initiative (KDOQI) guidelines, last updated in 2006, state that patients should have a functional permanent access at the initiation of dialysis therapy. The KDOQI guidelines suggest that a working fistula should have the following characteristics, sometimes called the "Rule of 6s": blood flow adequate to support dialysis (generally greater than 600 mL/min); a diameter greater than 6 mm, with location accessible for cannulation and discernible margins to allow for repetitive cannulation; and a depth of approximately 6 mm [13]. Accordingly, patients should be referred for arteriovenous fistula (AVF) creation at least 6 months before the start of HD. This is in preference to AV grafts (AVG) due to a belief that AVF are superior to AVG due to improved survival, lower costs, better patency, and reduced risk of infection or other complications. This time frame is suggested to allow for both initial access evaluation as well as additional time for revision to ensure that a working fistula is available at initiation of dialysis therapy [13]. Of note, this recommendation is based on expert opinion; a recent meta-analysis was unable to identify any studies that compared early to late referral for access creation [21].

An additional challenge is accurately predicting when dialysis will need to be initiated [22]. A liberal policy of early surgical referral provides more opportunities for successful access creation and can reduce the likelihood of starting HD with a tunneled dialysis catheter (TDC). This is an important consideration in the elderly, who have a lower rate of maturation compared to younger patients [23]. However, this may also be associated with a higher rate of unused AVF due to unexpectedly slow kidney function decline or competing mortality [24]. One study in the United States Department of Veterans Affairs system focused on patients with GFR less than 25 mL/min. In this group, 25% initiated HD over the ensuing year, while a far lower percentage of elderly patients received permanent access. The majority of elderly CKD patients survived without requiring dialysis, and many died before initiating dialysis [25]. A decision analysis model suggests a GFR threshold of 15–20 mL/min; though due to competing mortality risks, later referral at a lower GFR level would be appropriate for elderly patients [26]. Similarly, another resource suggests using a GFR threshold of 20 mL/min at which point a patient should be referred for AV fistula creation [27]. Ongoing work to establish clinically valid prediction rules for the progression to ESRD may help to individualize the approach to access placement.

Compared to AVF creation, AVG placement is considered to be the second best option in patients that have not yet started hemodialysis, but is better than initiating HD through TDC, according to the KDOQI guidelines. This ranking appears to be valid in the elderly, and is supported by data from analysis of data from administrative databases and the US Renal Data system (USRDS) [28, 29]. There is a concern, though, that successful maturation of an AVF may be a marker of overall improved medical status, and not of an effect of the access type [30, 31]. This selection bias may lead to an overestimate of the benefit of AVF over AVG [32]. More recent analyses that account for the influence of selection suggest that AVF and AVG may be equivalent in certain populations, especially the elderly [33–35].

Finally, dialysis through a TDC is considered inferior to both AVF and AVG due to the tendency for patients receiving HD through TDC to suffer increased rates of mortality, infection, and hospitalization compared to patients receiving AVF or AVG [36]. Further, catheters are associated with less efficient dialysis, the development of central venous stenosis, and an increased number of procedures required to maintain a functioning vascular access, leading to increased expense [37, 38]. This dynamic has also been demonstrated in the elderly [34]. The reasons for this increase in adverse outcomes in TDC patients have been postulated to be related to increased risks for catheter-related septicemia and also sterile inflammation even in the absence of infection [39].

The medical rationale for trying to avoid catheters is clear; however, from the patient's perspective, TDC has the distinct advantage of being in many ways the least invasive procedure, as it does not require surgery, a maturation period, or being cannulated thrice weekly with large-gauge needles, as AVF and AVG require [40]. This is especially relevant for elderly patients who may be struggling with multiple other medical challenges [41].

9.3.2 Transitioning Patients from TDC to an Internal Access

Despite KDOQI's goal of 50% AVF as a patient's incident vascular access, in 2010 approximately 80% of patients initiated HD through TDC, with approximately 16% started through AVF, and the balance through AVG. This distribution has remained largely unchanged since 2005, and is also seen among elderly patients [42]. Particularly in the elderly, the challenge of facilitating a transition from catheters to an internal access is complicated by the heavier burden of medical comorbidities that this patient population suffers. Extended TDC dependence after HD initiation is more likely to occur in elderly patients and may be related to longer time to maturation, increased need for secondary procedures, and higher primary failure rates [43].

Because of the known disadvantages of prolonged TDC dependence, AVG placement may be more attractive than AVF creation due to higher maturation rates and shorter time to maturation, leading to earlier TDC removal. However, these advantages need to be balanced against more frequent use of secondary procedures to maintain patency, as demonstrated in one study using administrative data from the USRDS [44]. In the elderly, who have short life expectancy, the longer-term risks of AVG use, including infection, limited primary patency, and potentially higher rates of ischemic steal syndrome, may not be as relevant as for younger patients. Recently, analytic tools to predict mortality rates among ESRD patients on HD have been developed, which may assist clinicians with tailoring vascular access options to particular patient needs [45]. As such, further research is necessary in order to better characterize the role of AVF and AVG, and determine the relative trade-offs, and whether different recommendations should exist based on patient age and preference.

9.3.3 Outcomes of Vascular Interventions in Elderly ESRD Patients

9.3.3.1 General Considerations

Both end-stage kidney disease and increasing age are well-known risk factors after many vascular surgical interventions, including repair of infrarenal abdominal aortic aneurysms (AAAs), carotid artery stenting (CAS) and carotid endarterectomy (CEA), and treatments for lower extremity arterial insufficiency [46–48].

Regardless of the presence of ESRD or advanced age, patients with symptomatic or ruptured aortic aneurysms are nearly always managed with either endovascular or open surgical intervention [49]. In these cases, although the perioperative risks are heightened due to the presence of ESRD and elderly status, the alternative of observation and medical management frequently leads to free rupture and death.

Similarly, symptomatic 50–99% stenosis of the extracranial internal carotid artery is usually treated, with some considerations for medical comorbidities and advanced age. Carotid endarterectomy (CEA) is generally the first option, and is preferred in the elderly, with carotid artery stenting (CAS) being reserved for patients with challenging anatomy or with severe cardiac or pulmonary comorbidities [47].

However, the majority of patients undergoing interventions for abdominal aortic aneurysms and extracranial carotid artery occlusive disease are asymptomatic, and in this population, the increased perioperative risk associated with ESRD and elderly status suggests that observation and medical management can sometimes be appropriate.

9.3.3.2 Asymptomatic, Intact Abdominal Aortic Aneurysms

In general, asymptomatic, intact abdominal aortic aneurysms larger than 5.5 cm should be considered for elective repair. At smaller diameters, the long-term benefit of early repair appears to be outweighed by the perioperative risk. At diameters between 4.0 and 5.4 cm, the UK Small Aneurysm Trial showed that compared to observation, early open surgical repair offered no long-term benefit in survival, while also subjecting patients to approximately 6.8% increased risk of mortality in the first 6 months after randomization [50]. Endovascular abdominal aortic aneurysm repair (EVAR) is associated with lower perioperative risks, leading some to suggest that repair at smaller sizes may be appropriate [51]. On the other hand, more recent publications suggest that patients with overall poor life expectancy and those that cannot safely tolerate a minimally invasive procedure should not undergo AAA repair, though the pre-operative identification of these patients can be difficult [52].

Elderly patients with ESRD over age 65 at HD initiation certainly suffer from abbreviated life expectancy, with a median survival of less than 2 years. Among patients who underwent AAA repair, an analysis of the United States Renal Data System (USRDS) found 1557 patients, 261 who had undergone open surgical repair and 1296 who had undergone EVAR between 2005 and 2008. The 30-day mortality after EVAR was lower than after open aortic repair (OAR) (10.3% vs. 16.1%). This perioperative survival advantage associated with EVAR was quickly lost; survival estimates were similar at 66.5% at 1 year (EVAR, 66.2%; OAR, 68%) and 37.4% at 3 years (EVAR, 36.8%; OAR, 40.0%). Median survival was 25.3 months after EVAR and 27.4 months after OAR [53].

Of note, current European Society for Vascular Surgery clinical practice guidelines state that AAA patients who undergo repair should have life expectancy of at least 3 years, which is longer than the median survival of patients who underwent AAA repair in the USRDS [54]. Meanwhile, American College of Cardiology Foundation/American Heart Association guidelines articulate a life expectancy of 2 years [55]. Ideally, criteria can be developed to assist with selecting patients with the necessary life expectancy, but in the absence of extenuating clinical circumstances, delaying prophylactic repair of asymptomatic AAAs in elderly ESRD patients until the AAAs reach a fairly large size threshold may be an appropriate strategy.

9.3.3.3 Asymptomatic Carotid Artery Occlusive Disease

In asymptomatic patients with 60–99% stenosis of an extracranial carotid artery, the benefit of carotid revascularization in asymptomatic patients can confer durable reduction in the risk of stroke, but this is dependent on excellent surgical technique. Perioperative stroke and death rates need to be less than 3%. However, it is also predicated on the patient's life expectancy, particularly in asymptomatic patients who are only expected to derive the full preventive advantages if they anticipate a life expectancy of at least 3 years [47]. This life expectancy may not be realized in patients with multiple medical comorbidities, particularly elderly patients with ESRD [41]. Although such patients have been shown to have potentially acceptable perioperative outcomes after CEA, long-term survival is poor, leading to calls for a conservative, nonoperative approach to the management of asymptomatic carotid disease for this population [56].

The development of CAS has been presented as an alternative to CEA for certain high-risk patients. Current guidelines define "high risk" as patients with medical risk factors, principally cardiac and pulmonary comorbidities, in addition to challenging anatomy like a high carotid bifurcation, the presence of a tracheal stoma, or extensive scar tissue due to radiation therapy or previous surgery [47]. In the Carotid Revascularization Endarterectomy Versus Stenting Trial, CAS appeared to be associated with lower rates of post-operative cardiac complications, but higher rates of stroke [57]. As such, the use of CAS as opposed to CEA or medical management in asymptomatic patients is still controversial, with specialty guidelines offering varying recommendations [58]. Society for Vascular Surgery guidelines recommend that CAS be reserved for high-risk patients with symptomatic carotid artery stenosis. Asymptomatic patients are best managed with CEA or medical management if they are at high risk for open surgery or if they have limited life expectancy [47].

For a patient with asymptomatic carotid artery stenosis, the relationship between perioperative risk, life expectancy, and the ongoing risk reduction after a successful intervention was recently described mathematically. The investigators of this decision analysis created a generalized model, identifying a critical life expectancy that was a function of perioperative complication rates and the absolute risk reduction that could be expected after successful surgery. As applied to patients with ESRD who have a short life expectancy, in order for either CEA or CAS to be superior to medical management, the intervention would need to be associated with either very low periprocedural complication rates or have very high absolute risk reduction [59].

These challenges were highlighted in a recent analysis of USRDS data, which focused on asymptomatic patients who underwent CEA and CAS. In this study, 2131 asymptomatic patients underwent carotid revascularization (1805 CEA, 326 CAS). Perioperative combined stroke or death rate was similar at 10.1% after CEA and 10.9% after CAS. Median survival after surgery was approximately 2.0 years for CAS and 2.5 years for CEA. Age over 70 years at the time of surgery was predictive of mortality in multivariate Cox proportional hazards modeling. While the rates of stroke with medical therapy alone could not be ascertained in the study, the remarkably short survival after both CEA and CAS is sobering, and is clearly lower than the 3-year guidance offered in contemporary guidelines [60]. As with intact, asymptomatic aortic aneurysm disease, criteria can be developed to assist with selecting asymptomatic, elderly ESRD patients for carotid revascularization. However, in the absence of extenuating clinical circumstances, medical management may be preferable in this population.

9.3.3.4 Lower Extremity Peripheral Arterial Occlusive Disease

Lower extremity peripheral arterial occlusive disease is more prevalent in patients with ESRD, compared to the general population, with rates of approximately 25% in two large prospective studies, in addition to significantly higher rates of cardiovascular morbidity and mortality [61]. Patients with ESRD who undergo lower extremity revascularization are more likely to suffer post-operative morbidity and mortality compared to patients with normal kidney function [62]. An analysis of the Dialysis Mortality and Morbidity Study in the USRDS showed post-operative mortality rates of 12.6% and 7.5% for bypass and angioplasty, respectively [63].

Given these challenging results, some authors have questioned whether lower extremity revascularization is worthwhile in patients with ESRD [64]. The countervailing concern, though, is the fate of the patient in whom limb salvage is unsuccessful. In an analysis of Medicare data from the 1990s, the rate of amputation was 6.2 per 100 person-years. Further, two-thirds died two years post-operatively after an amputation [65]. Clearly, while outcomes after lower extremity revascularization are challenging, amputation is associated with adverse health outcomes, as well.

In general, both endovascular techniques and open surgical revascularization can be used for limb salvage. In the Bypass versus Angioplasty In Severe Ischaemia of the Leg (BASIL) trial, which was a randomized controlled trial (RCT) that compared a balloon-angioplasty-first strategy versus bypass-surgery-first strategy, outcomes in terms of amputation-free survival were broadly similar, though balloon angioplasty was associated with lower costs [66]. However, among patients who survived at least 2 years, bypass surgery was associated with improved survival, leading to the suggestion that bypass surgery should be offered to patients who could be expected to survive at least 2 years [67]. In order to assist with patient selection, a survival model based on BASIL data was created. Elderly status and impaired kidney function were among the most important predictors of mortality [68]. Extending these findings to the elderly ESRD population with symptomatic peripheral arterial disease would suggest that an endovascular-first strategy that spares the patient some perioperative morbidity may be preferable due to the relatively short survival we expect in this patient population.

9.4 Strategies to Prevent Contrast Nephropathy

Contrast-induced acute kidney injury (CI-AKI) has been defined as an acute decrease in kidney function after intravascular administration of an iodinated contrast medium. The change in kidney function manifests as an increase in serum creatinine level of 25% or 50% relative to baseline, or an absolute change in serum creatinine level of 0.5 mg/dL within 2–5 days [69]. Pre-existing renal functional impairment is likely the most important risk factor for developing CI-AKI and the elderly, many with multiple medical comorbidities including diabetes, are certainly at high risk of chronic kidney failure [70].

A single-institution patient series reviewed outcomes after percutaneous coronary interventions. In their analysis of 8357 patients, hypotension, intra-aortic balloon pump, congestive heart failure, chronic kidney disease, diabetes, age greater than 75 years, anemia, and volume of contrast used were identified as risk factors for the development of CI-AKI [71]. While clearly an unmodifiable risk factor, advanced age needs to be recognized as a marker for increased risk of CI-AKI, and appropriate precautions taken to prevent AKI [72].

The mechanism for CI-AKI is not well defined, and is thought to be associated with a combination of renal vasoconstriction, acute tubular necrosis, reactive oxygen species production, and possibly direct toxicity on renal tubular cells. Regardless, the osmolality of the contrast agent appears to be a key modifiable risk factor, and there have been multiple efforts to create nonionic contrast agents, in addition to reducing their osmolality [73]. A recent meta-analysis of 25 trials demonstrated that CI-AKI after intra-arterial injection of contrast was less frequent with use of the iso-osmolar agent iodixanol (Visipaque), as compared to nonionic low-osmolar agents [74]. Iso-osmolar nonionic agents like iodixanol typically have osmolality of 290–320 mOsm, while low-osmolar nonionic agents like iohexol (Omnipaque) and iopamidol (Isovue) have osmolality around 600 mOsm. Finally, the osmolality of older, high osmolar ionic agents like iothalamate (Conray) is around 1600 mOsm; these agents are rarely used in contemporary practice.

The use of pre-exposure volume expansion is widely accepted. Guidelines published by the Kidney Diseases Improving Global Outcomes (KDIGO) initiative recognize the danger of volume depletion in patients who are already at elevated risk of AKI, like the elderly. The use of intravenous volume expansion with isotonic sodium chloride solution or sodium bicarbonate solutions is recommended over using hypotonic sodium chloride solutions, no intravenous volume expansion, or oral hydration alone [75].

N-acetylcysteine (NAC) is related to the amino acid cysteine and acts as a free-radical scavenger, producing antioxidant and vasodilatory effects. It has been studied as a prophylactic agent against CI-AKI in multiple observational and randomized studies with conflicting results [75, 76]. The results of ten randomized controlled trials were recently reviewed in a meta-analysis, which demonstrated that the combination of N-acetylcysteine (NAC) and sodium bicarbonate isotonic solutions reduced the occurrence of CI-AKI overall but not dialysis-dependent kidney failure. While the effect of NAC is not seen consistently across available studies, oral NAC is inexpensive and relatively safe. As such, current specialty guidelines offer cautious endorsement of the use of oral NAC in addition to isotonic intravenous volume expansion in order to prevent CI-AKI [69, 75].

Several investigator teams have studied prophylactic intermittent hemodialysis (IHD) for contrast-media removal. One major RCT demonstrated a benefit from prophylactic hemodialysis in patients with pre-existing chronic kidney disease. This study randomized 82 patients to normal saline intravascular fluid expansion either with or without a 4 h session of hemodialysis immediately after coronary angiography. Baseline creatinine was 4.9 mg/dL in both groups. Patients randomized to HD were noted to have lower peak serum creatinine levels (6.7 mg/dL vs. 5.3 mg/dL), less need for temporary kidney replacement therapy (35% vs. 2%), and lower need for long-term dialysis after discharge (13% vs. 0%) [76, 77]. Multiple authors have challenged the study's conclusions due to the small sample size and the fact that the renal outcome of serum creatinine concentration was directly impacted by the study intervention of prophylactic hemodialysis. Furthermore, the majority of the studies that have been published have not found any benefit from prophylactic kidney replacement therapy. A recent meta-analysis demonstrated that prophylactic HD held no advantages over standard medical therapy in terms of need for permanent kidney replacement therapy or progression to ESRD. In fact, HD appeared to actually increase the risk of CI-AKI [78].

There are other ungraded recommendations from KDIGO that are particularly relevant to the elderly population.

- Clinicians should assess kidney function in order to identify patients with pre-existing, but perhaps underappreciated, chronic kidney disease.
- Alternative imaging methods in patients at increased risk of CI-AKI should be considered.
- The lowest possible dose of contrast medium should be employed in patients at risk of CI-AKI.

The KDIGO recommendations are summarized in Table 9.1.

9.4.1 Considerations for Individualizing Care of Older Patients with ESRD

Dialysis dependence is associated with marked reduction in health-related quality of life (HRQoL) compared to age-matched controls, a finding seen in both North American and international populations [79]. Cross sectional studies have suggested that peritoneal dialysis is associated with improved HRQoL compared to hemodialysis in the general population [80]. While this finding suggests that peritoneal dialysis may be the preferred modality for many patients, it may be related to selection bias, and in any case is difficult to apply to the elderly population, who frequently have difficulty adhering to the self-care requirements. Further, any initial advantage in HRQoL may not be sustained; an observational study focused on

Table 9.1 KDIGO clinical practice guideline for acute kidney injury management associated with radiocontrast administration

Recommendation	Strength of recommendation
Assess the risk of CI-AKI and, in particular, screen for pre-existing impairment of kidney function in all patients who are considered for a procedure that requires intravascular (i.v. or i.a.) administration of iodinated contrast medium	Not graded
Consider alternative imaging methods in patients at increased risk of CI-AKI	Not graded
Use the lowest possible dose of contrast medium in patients at risk of CI-AKI	Not graded
We recommend using either iso-osmolar or low-osmolar iodinated contrast media, rather than high-osmolar iodinated contrast media in patients at increased risk of CI-AKI	1B
We recommend i.v. volume expansion with either isotonic sodium chloride or sodium bicarbonate solutions, rather than no i.v. volume expansion, in patients at increased risk of CI-AKI	1A
We recommend not using oral fluids alone in patients at increased risk of CI-AKI	1C
We suggest using oral NAC, together with i.v. isotonic crystalloids, in patients at increased risk of CI-AKI	2D
We suggest not using theophylline to prevent CI-AKI	2C
We recommend not using fenoldopam to prevent CI-AKI	1B
We suggest not using prophylactic intermittent hemodialysis (IHD) or hemofiltration (HF) for contrast-media removal in patients at increased risk of CI-AKI	2C

Adapted from [75]
Grading scale:
Level 1: "strong"
Level 2: "weak" or discretionary
Quality of supporting evidence: A (high), B (moderate), C (low), or D (very low)

elderly patients found that while initial HRQoL was higher in the PD population, this advantage was not evident at 6 and 12 months after dialysis initiation [18].

For hemodialysis patients, in particular, the causes for reductions in quality of life are likely multifactorial. Pain and depressive symptoms can drive lower mental health scores, and also lead to shortened hemodialysis treatments, increased utilization of emergency services, and hospitalizations [81]. In the recently published Frequent Hemodialysis Network trial, 245 patients were randomized to standard thrice weekly dialysis or a more frequent schedule of dialysis six times per week, with shorter daily sessions. The more frequent schedule was associated with improved self-reported general mental health, although depression scores were not significantly different. Possible mechanisms for this finding include better small molecule clearance, better volume management, reduced inflammation, and more convenient timing of dialysis [82].

Another issue to consider is the impact on caregivers. This is particularly relevant for peritoneal dialysis patients due to the significant home-care that is required.

In one observational study of 201 elderly patients, the caregivers for 84 hemodialysis patients were compared to 40 peritoneal dialysis patients, who were both compared to a control group of caregivers of 77 non-elderly hemodialysis patients. Caregivers of peritoneal dialysis patients scored significantly lower on the mental component of the SF-36 than caregivers of hemodialysis patients. The authors hypothesized that this may be related to the challenges of repetitive dialysis exchanges and other medical responsibilities; these can be onerous and lead to feelings of anxiety, stress, resentment, and guilt [83].

While there have been multiple studies investigating the difference in HRQoL between PD and HD, the HRQoL related to hemodialysis access (i.e., AVF vs. AVG vs. TDC) has not been studied as extensively. The existing measures, including the CHOICE Health Experience Questionnaire (CHEQ) and Kidney Disease Quality of Life (KDQOL), have only a handful of broad questions exploring dialysis access type [84, 85]. More recently, the short-form vascular access questionnaire (SF-VAQ) was developed. This is a validated questionnaire evaluating patient satisfaction in a Canadian setting associated with HD access type. HD through an AVF was associated with the highest overall satisfaction, followed by TDC, with AVG having the lowest scores. Interestingly, the study determined that while AVF scored well in terms of outcomes like concerns around hospitalization and bathing, TDC was preferred when it came to physical complaints like pain, bleeding, swelling, and bruising [86].

Recently, quality of life considerations have been explicitly referenced in contemporary guidelines for the management of patients with ESRD [87]. However, there may still be tension between what might be recommended in guidelines and what an individual patient may find preferable, especially in the elderly [88].

Guidelines for ESRD patients often present a uniform approach to management, prioritizing interventions to reduce mortality and manage disease complications. The overall goal is to provide a simplified pathway to guide management rather than address complex issues that may develop for individual patients. Many ESRD patients have multiple comorbid conditions, which can generate conflicting treatment recommendations [89]. In older patients, an individualized approach that considers competing sources of morbidity and mortality can inform clinical decisions. Clinicians, in conjunction with patients and caregivers, can prioritize patient-centered outcomes, even if these outcomes may not be easily explained by a well-described disease process [90].

Key Points

- With regard to management of vascular surgery issues in the elderly patient with renal failure, most recommendations are similar to those for younger patients. However, current guidelines often present a uniform approach to management, whereas older patients with ESRD may benefit from a more individualized approach due to heavy burden of comorbidities and shortened life expectancy.
- Both hemodialysis (HD) and peritoneal dialysis (PD) are reasonable renal replacement therapies in elderly patients with likely similar long-term outcomes, though PD requires significantly more patient resources and can be difficult for elderly patients and their caregivers to implement.

- In patients receiving HD, both arteriovenous fistulas (AVF) and arteriovenous grafts (AVG) are clearly superior to tunneled dialysis catheters as access modalities. AVF are likely superior to AVG, when they mature, but lengthy AVF maturation time can lead to prolonged TDC dependence. In elderly patients, the long-term benefits of AVF need to be balanced against the effects of prolonged TDC dependence on patients with already shortened life expectancy.
- Repair of asymptomatic, intact abdominal aortic aneurysms in elderly patients with renal failure is associated with poor perioperative and long-term outcomes. Delaying surgical intervention, especially in patients with difficult anatomy requiring open repair, may be reasonable in many cases.
- Medical management is the first choice in asymptomatic elderly patients with carotid artery occlusive disease and dialysis dependence. In well-selected patients with good life expectancy and severe extracranial carotid stenosis, carotid endarterectomy (CEA) is reasonable. The role of carotid artery stenting (CAS) in asymptomatic renal failure patients is unclear, and patients with clinical characteristics that make CEA difficult, and hence favor CAS, are likely best served with medical management alone.

Acknowledgement Dr. Theodore H. Yuo is supported by grants from the NIH, KL2-TR000146 and KL2-TR001856.

References

1. Wiggins J. Why do we need a geriatric nephrology curriculum? Chapter 2. In: American Society of Nephrology Geriatric Nephrology Curriculum. 2009. https://www.asn-online.org/education/distancelearning/curricula/geriatrics/. Accessed 10 Aug 2015.
2. Stevens LA, Weiner DE, Brown WW. The geriatric dialysis patient, chapter 32. In: Henrich W, editor. Principles and practice of dialysis. 4th ed. Philadelphia: Lippincott, Williams & Wilkins; 2009. p. 536–55.
3. O'Hare AM, Bowling CB, Tamura MK. Kidney disease in the elderly. In: Gilbert W, editor. National Kidney Foundation primer on kidney diseases. 6th ed. Philadelphia: Elsevier; 2013. p. 437–45.
4. Singh P, Germain MJ, Cohen L, Unruh M. The elderly patient on dialysis: geriatric considerations. Nephrol Dial Transplant. 2014;29(5):990–6.
5. de Jager DJ, Grootendorst DC, Jager KJ, van Dijk PC, Tomas LM, Ansell D, Collart F, Finne P, Heaf JG, De Meester J, Wetzels JF, Rosendaal FR, Dekker FW. Cardiovascular and noncardiovascular mortality among patients starting dialysis. JAMA. 2009;302(16):1782–9.
6. Kane RL, Ouslander JG, Abrass IB, Resnick B. Chapter 1. Clinical implications of the aging process. In: Kane RL, Ouslander JG, Abrass IB, Resnick B, editors. Essentials of clinical geriatrics. 7th ed. New York: McGraw-Hill; 2013.
7. Kurella M, Covinsky KE, Collins AJ, Chertow GM. Octogenarians and nonagenarians starting dialysis in the United States. Ann Intern Med. 2007;146(3):177–83.
8. Fink JC, Burdick RA, Kurth SJ, Blahut SA, Armistead NC, Turner MS, Shickle LM, Light PD. Significance of serum creatinine values in new end-stage renal disease patients. Am J Kidney Dis. 1999;34(4):694–701.
9. Traynor JP, Simpson K, Geddes CC, Deighan CJ, Fox JG. Early initiation of dialysis fails to prolong survival in patients with end-stage renal failure. J Am Soc Nephrol. 2002;13(8):2125–32.

10. Cooper BA, Branley P, Bulfone L, Collins JF, Craig JC, Fraenkel MB, Harris A, Johnson DW, Kesselhut J, Li JJ, Luxton G, Pilmore A, Tiller DJ, Harris DC, Pollock CA; IDEAL Study. A randomized, controlled trial of early versus late initiation of dialysis. N Engl J Med. 2010;363(7):609–19.
11. Stevens LA, Weiner DE, Brown WW. The geriatric dialysis patient. In: Henrich W, editor. Principles and practice of dialysis. 4th ed. Philadelphia: Lippincott, Williams & Wilkins; 2009. p. 536–55.
12. Guideline recommendations and their rationales for the treatment of adult patients. In: Renal Physicians Association (RPA). Shared decision-making in the appropriate initiation of withdrawal from dialysis. 2nd ed. Rockville: Renal Physicians Association (RPA); 2010. p. 39–92.
13. National Kidney Foundation. KDOQI clinical practice guidelines and clinical practice recommendations for 2006 updates: hemodialysis adequacy, peritoneal dialysis adequacy and vascular access. Am J Kidney Dis. 2006;48(suppl 1):S1–S322.
14. Ho-dac-Pannekeet MM. PD in the elderly – a challenge for the (pre)dialysis team. Nephrol Dial Transplant. 2006;21(Suppl 2):ii60–2.
15. United States Renal Data System, 2014 annual data report: epidemiology of kidney disease in the United States. Bethesda: National Institutes of Health, National Institute of Diabetes and Digestive and Kidney Diseases; 2014.
16. Quinn RR, Hux JE, Oliver MJ, Austin PC, Tonelli M, Laupacis A. Selection bias explains apparent differential mortality between dialysis modalities. J Am Soc Nephrol. 2011;22(8): 1534–42.
17. Perl J, Wald R, McFarlane P, Bargman JM, Vonesh E, Na Y, Jassal SV, Moist L. Hemodialysis vascular access modifies the association between dialysis modality and survival. J Am Soc Nephrol. 2011;22(6):1113–21.
18. Harris SA, Lamping DL, Brown EA, Constantinovici N; North Thames Dialysis Study (NTDS) Group. Clinical outcomes and quality of life in elderly patients on peritoneal dialysis versus hemodialysis. Perit Dial Int. 2002;22(4):463–70.
19. Winkelmayer WC, Glynn RJ, Mittleman MA, Levin R, Pliskin JS, Avorn J. Comparing mortality of elderly patients on hemodialysis versus peritoneal dialysis: a propensity score approach. J Am Soc Nephrol. 2002;13(9):2353–62.
20. Han SS, Park JY, Kang S, Kim KH, Ryu DR, Kim H, Joo KW, Lim CS, Kim YS, Kim DK. Dialysis modality and mortality in the elderly: a meta-analysis. Clin J Am Soc Nephrol. 2015;10(6):983–93.
21. Murad MH, Sidawy AN, Elamin MB, Rizvi AZ, Flynn DN, McCausland FR, McGrath MM, Vo DH, El-Zoghby Z, Casey ET, Duncan AA, Tracz MJ, Erwin PJ, Montori VM. Timing of referral for vascular access placement: a systematic review. J Vasc Surg. 2008;48(5 Suppl):31S–3S.
22. Green D, Ritchie JP, New DI, Kalra PA. How accurately do nephrologists predict the need for dialysis within one year? Nephron Clin Pract. 2012;122(3–4):102–6.
23. Lok CE, Oliver MJ, Su J, Bhola C, Hannigan N, Jassal SV. Arteriovenous fistula outcomes in the era of the elderly dialysis population. Kidney Int. 2005;67(6):2462–9.
24. Tamura MK, Tan JC, O'Hare AM. Optimizing renal replacement therapy in older adults: a framework for making individualized decisions. Kidney Int. 2012;82(3):261–9.
25. O'Hare AM, Bertenthal D, Walter LC, Garg AX, Covinsky K, Kaufman JS, Rodriguez RA, Allon M. When to refer patients with chronic kidney disease for vascular access surgery: should age be a consideration? Kidney Int. 2007;71(6):555–61.
26. Shechter SM, Skandari MR, Zalunardo N. Timing of arteriovenous fistula creation in patients with CKD: a decision analysis. Am J Kidney Dis. 2014;63(1):95–103.
27. Hakim RM. Hemodialysis. In: Gilbert W, editor. National Kidney Foundation primer on kidney diseases. 6th ed. Philadelphia: Elsevier; 2013. p. 437–45.
28. Dhingra RK, Young EW, Hulbert-Shearon TE, Leavey SF, Port FK. Type of vascular access and mortality in U.S. hemodialysis patients. Kidney Int. 2001;60(4):1443–51.
29. Xue JL, Dahl D, Ebben JP, Collins AJ. The association of initial hemodialysis access type with mortality outcomes in elderly Medicare ESRD patients. Am J Kidney Dis. 2003;42(5):1013–9.

30. Murad MH, Elamin MB, Sidawy AN, Malaga G, Rizvi AZ, Flynn DN, Casey ET, McCausland FR, McGrath MM, Vo DH, El-Zoghby Z, Duncan AA, Tracz MJ, Erwin PJ, Montori VM. Autogenous versus prosthetic vascular access for hemodialysis: a systematic review and meta-analysis. J Vasc Surg. 2008;48(5 Suppl):34S–47S.
31. Quinn RR, Ravani P. Fistula-first and catheter-last: fading certainties and growing doubts. Nephrol Dial Transplant. 2014;29(4):727–30.
32. Lee T, Barker J, Allon M. Comparison of survival of upper arm arteriovenous fistulas and grafts after failed forearm fistula. J Am Soc Nephrol. 2007;18(6):1936–41.
33. Chan MR, Sanchez RJ, Young HN, Yevzlin AS. Vascular access outcomes in the elderly hemodialysis population: a USRDS study. Semin Dial. 2007;20(6):606–10.
34. DeSilva RN, Patibandla BK, Vin Y, Narra A, Chawla V, Brown RS, Goldfarb-Rumyantzev AS. Fistula first is not always the best strategy for the elderly. J Am Soc Nephrol. 2013;24(8): 1297–304.
35. Yuo TH, Chaer RA, Dillavou ED, Leers SA, Makaroun MS. Patients started on hemodialysis with tunneled dialysis catheter have similar survival after arteriovenous fistula and arteriovenous graft creation. J Vasc Surg. 2015;62(6):1590–7.e2.
36. Rehman R, Schmidt RJ, Moss AH. Ethical and legal obligation to avoid long-term tunneled catheter access. Clin J Am Soc Nephrol. 2009;4(2):456–60.
37. Lee H, Manns B, Taub K, Ghali WA, Dean S, Johnson D, Donaldson C. Cost analysis of ongoing care of patients with end-stage renal disease: the impact of dialysis modality and dialysis access. Am J Kidney Dis. 2002;40(3):611–22.
38. Eggers P, Milam R. Trends in vascular access procedures and expenditures in Medicare's ESRD program. In: Henry ML, editor. Vascular access for hemodialysis-VII. Chicago: Gore; 2001. p. 133–43.
39. Kaysen GA. Biochemistry and biomarkers of inflamed patients: why look, what to assess. Clin J Am Soc Nephrol. 2009;4(Suppl 1):S56–63.
40. Dinwiddie LC, Ball L, Brouwer D, Doss-McQuitty S, Holland J. What nephrologists need to know about vascular access cannulation. Semin Dial. 2013;26(3):315–22.
41. Wright S, Danziger J. Vascular access for hemodialysis in the elderly. Chapter 21. In: American Society of Nephrology Geriatric Nephrology Curriculum. 2009. https://www.asn-online.org/education/distancelearning/curricula/geriatrics/. Accessed 10 Aug 2015.
42. Lok CE, Foley R. Vascular access morbidity and mortality: trends of the last decade. Clin J Am Soc Nephrol. 2013;8(7):1213–9.
43. Wasse H, Speckman RA, Frankenfield DL, Rocco MV, McClellan WM. Predictors of delayed transition from central venous catheter use to permanent vascular access among ESRD patients. Am J Kidney Dis. 2007;49(2):276–83.
44. Leake AE, Yuo TH, Wu T, Fish L, Dillavou ED, Chaer RA, Leers SA, Makaroun MS. Arteriovenous grafts are associated with earlier catheter removal and fewer catheter days in the United States renal data system population. J Vasc Surg. 2015;62(1):123–7.
45. Floege J, Gillespie IA, Kronenberg F, Anker SD, Gioni I, Richards S, Pisoni RL, Robinson BM, Marcelli D, Froissart M, Eckardt KU. Development and validation of a predictive mortality risk score from a European hemodialysis cohort. Kidney Int. 2015;87(5):996–1008.
46. Patterson BO, Holt PJ, Hinchliffe R, Loftus IM, Thompson MM. Predicting risk in elective abdominal aortic aneurysm repair: a systematic review of current evidence. Eur J Vasc Endovasc Surg. 2008;36(6):637–45.
47. Ricotta JJ, Aburahma A, Ascher E, Eskandari M, Faries P, Lal BK; Society for Vascular Surgery. Updated society for vascular surgery guidelines for management of extracranial carotid disease. J Vasc Surg. 2011;54(3):e1–31.
48. Norgren L, Hiatt WR, Dormandy JA, Nehler MR, Harris KA, Fowkes FG; TASC II Working Group. Inter-society consensus for the management of peripheral arterial disease (TASC II). J Vasc Surg. 2007;45(Suppl S):S5–67.
49. Chaikof EL, Brewster DC, Dalman RL, Makaroun MS, Illig KA, Sicard GA, Timaran CH, Upchurch Jr GR, Veith FJ; Society for Vascular Surgery. The care of patients with an abdomi-

nal aortic aneurysm: the Society for Vascular Surgery practice guidelines. J Vasc Surg. 2009;50(4 Suppl):S2–49.
50. The UK Small Aneurysm Trial Participants. Mortality results for randomised controlled trial of early elective surgery or ultrasonographic surveillance for small abdominal aortic aneurysms. Lancet. 1998;352(9141):1649–55.
51. Finlayson SR, Birkmeyer JD, Fillinger MF, Cronenwett JL. Should endovascular surgery lower the threshold for repair of abdominal aortic aneurysms? J Vasc Surg. 1999;29:973–85.
52. Fillinger MF. Chapter 127 – Abdominal aortic aneurysms: evaluation and decision making. In: Rutherford's Vascular Surgery. 7th ed. Philadelphia: Elsevier; 2010.
53. Yuo TH, Sidaoui J, Marone LK, Avgerinos ED, Makaroun MS, Chaer RA. Limited survival in dialysis patients undergoing intact abdominal aortic aneurysm repair. J Vasc Surg. 2014;60(4):908–13.e1.
54. Moll FL, Powell JT, Fraedrich G, Verzini F, Haulon S, Waltham M, et al. European Society for Vascular Surgery. Management of abdominal aortic aneurysms clinical practice guidelines of the European society for vascular surgery. Eur J Vasc Endovasc Surg. 2011;41(Suppl 1):S1–58.
55. Rooke TW, Hirsch AT, Misra S, Sidawy AN, Beckman JA, Findeiss LK, et al.; Society for Cardiovascular Angiography and Interventions, Society of Interventional Radiology, Society for Vascular Medicine, Society for Vascular Surgery. 2011 ACCF/AHA focused update of the guideline for the management of patients with peripheral artery disease (updating the 2005 guideline): a report of the American College of Cardiology Foundation/American Heart Association Task Force on Practice Guidelines. J Am Coll Cardiol. 2011;58(19):2020–4.
56. Ascher E, Marks NA, Schutzer RW, Hingorani AP. Carotid endarterectomy in patients with chronic renal insufficiency: a recent series of 184 cases. J Vasc Surg. 2005;41(1):24–9.
57. Brott TG, Hobson RW 2nd, Howard G, Roubin GS, Clark WM, Brooks W, Mackey A, Hill MD, Leimgruber PP, Sheffet AJ, Howard VJ, Moore WS, Voeks JH, Hopkins LN, Cutlip DE, Cohen DJ, Popma JJ, Ferguson RD, Cohen SN, Blackshear JL, Silver FL, Mohr JP, Lal BK, Meschia JF; CREST Investigators. Stenting versus endarterectomy for treatment of carotid-artery stenosis. N Engl J Med. 2010;363(1):11–23.
58. Brott TG, Halperin JL, Abbara S, et al. 2011 ASA/ACCF/AHA/AANN/AANS/ACR/ASNR/CNS/SAIP/SCAI/SIR/SNIS/SVM/SVS guideline on the management of patients with extracranial carotid and vertebral artery disease. Circulation. 2011;124(4):e54–e130.
59. Yuo TH, Roberts MS, Braithwaite RS, Chang CC, Kraemer KL. Applying the payoff time framework to carotid artery disease management. Med Decis Mak. 2013;33(8):1039–50.
60. Yuo TH, Sidaoui J, Marone LK, Makaroun MS, Chaer RA. Revascularization of asymptomatic carotid stenosis is not appropriate in patients on dialysis. J Vasc Surg. 2015;61(3):670–4.
61. O'Hare A, Johansen K. Lower-extremity peripheral arterial disease among patients with end-stage renal disease. J Am Soc Nephrol. 2001;12(12):2838–47.
62. O'Hare AM, Feinglass J, Sidawy AN, Bacchetti P, Rodriguez RA, Daley J, Khuri S, Henderson WG, Johansen KL. Impact of renal insufficiency on short-term morbidity and mortality after lower extremity revascularization: data from the Department of Veterans Affairs' National Surgical Quality Improvement Program. J Am Soc Nephrol. 2003;14(5):1287–95.
63. Jaar BG, Astor BC, Berns JS, Powe NR. Predictors of amputation and survival following lower extremity revascularization in hemodialysis patients. Kidney Int. 2004;65(2):613–20.
64. Korn P, Hoenig SJ, Skillman JJ, Kent KC. Is lower extremity revascularization worthwhile in patients with end-stage renal disease? Surgery. 2000;128(3):472–9.
65. Eggers PW, Gohdes D, Pugh J. Nontraumatic lower extremity amputations in the Medicare end-stage renal disease population. Kidney Int. 1999;56(4):1524–33.
66. Adam DJ, Beard JD, Cleveland T, Bell J, Bradbury AW, Forbes JF, Fowkes FG, Gillepsie I, Ruckley CV, Raab G, Storkey H; BASIL Trial Participants. Bypass versus angioplasty in severe ischaemia of the leg (BASIL): multicentre, randomised controlled trial. Lancet. 2005;366(9501):1925–34.
67. Bradbury AW, Adam DJ, Bell J, Forbes JF, Fowkes FG, Gillespie I, Ruckley CV, Raab GM; BASIL Trial Participants. Bypass versus Angioplasty in Severe Ischaemia of the Leg (BASIL) trial: an intention-to-treat analysis of amputation-free and overall survival in patients random-

ized to a bypass surgery-first or a balloon angioplasty-first revascularization strategy. J Vasc Surg. 2010;51(5 Suppl):5S–17S.
68. Bradbury AW, Adam DJ, Bell J, Forbes JF, Fowkes FG, Gillespie I, Ruckley CV, Raab GM; BASIL Trial Participants. Bypass versus Angioplasty in Severe Ischaemia of the Leg (BASIL) trial: a survival prediction model to facilitate clinical decision making. J Vasc Surg. 2010;51(5 Suppl):52S–68S.
69. Palevsky PM, Liu KD, Brophy PD, Chawla LS, Parikh CR, Thakar CV, Tolwani AJ, Waikar SS, Weisbord SD. KDOQI US commentary on the 2012 KDIGO clinical practice guideline for acute kidney injury. Am J Kidney Dis. 2013;61(5):649–72.
70. Mehran R, Nikolsky E. Contrast-induced nephropathy: definition, epidemiology, and patients at risk. Kidney Int Suppl. 2006;69:S11–5.
71. Mehran R, Aymong ED, Nikolsky E, Lasic Z, Iakovou I, Fahy M, Mintz GS, Lansky AJ, Moses JW, Stone GW, Leon MB, Dangas G. A simple risk score for prediction of contrast-induced nephropathy after percutaneous coronary intervention: development and initial validation. J Am Coll Cardiol. 2004;44(7):1393–9.
72. Detrenis S, Meschi M, Bertolini L, Savazzi G. Contrast medium administration in the elderly patient: is advancing age an independent risk factor for contrast nephropathy after angiographic procedures? J Vasc Interv Radiol. 2007;18(2):177–85.
73. Rudnick MR, Goldfarb S, Wexler L, Ludbrook PA, Murphy MJ, Halpern EF, Hill JA, Winniford M, Cohen MB, VanFossen DB. Nephrotoxicity of ionic and nonionic contrast media in 1196 patients: a randomized trial. The iohexol cooperative study. Kidney Int. 1995;47(1):254–61.
74. Heinrich MC, Häberle L, Müller V, Bautz W, Uder M. Nephrotoxicity of iso-osmolar iodixanol compared with nonionic low-osmolar contrast media: meta-analysis of randomized controlled trials. Radiology. 2009;250(1):68–86.
75. Kellum JA, Lameire N, Aspelin P, Barsoum RS, Burdmann EA, Goldstein SL, Herzog CA, Joannidis M, Kribben A, Levey AS, MacLeod AM, Mehta RL, Murray PT, Naicker S. Opal SM, Schaefer F, Schetz M, Uchino S. Kidney disease: Improving global outcomes (KDIGO) acute kidney injury work group. KDIGO clinical practice guideline for acute kidney injury. Kidney Int Suppl (2011). 2012;2(1):6.
76. Fishbane S, Durham JH, Marzo K, Rudnick M. N-acetylcysteine in the prevention of radiocontrast-induced nephropathy. J Am Soc Nephrol. 2004;15(2):251–60.
77. Lee PT, Chou KJ, Liu CP, Mar GY, Chen CL, Hsu CY, Fang HC, Chung HM. Renal protection for coronary angiography in advanced renal failure patients by prophylactic hemodialysis. A randomized controlled trial. J Am Coll Cardiol. 2007;50(11):1015–20.
78. Cruz DN, Goh CY, Marenzi G, Corradi V, Ronco C, Perazella MA. Renal replacement therapies for prevention of radiocontrast-induced nephropathy: a systematic review. Am J Med. 2012;125(1):66–78.e3.
79. Fukuhara S, Lopes AA, Bragg-Gresham JL, Kurokawa K, Mapes DL, Akizawa T, Bommer J, Canaud BJ, Port FK, Held PJ; Worldwide Dialysis Outcomes and Practice Patterns Study. Health-related quality of life among dialysis patients on three continents: the Dialysis Outcomes and Practice Patterns Study. Kidney Int. 2003;64(5):1903–10.
80. Rubin HR, Fink NE, Plantinga LC, Sadler JH, Kliger AS, Powe NR. Patient ratings of dialysis care with peritoneal dialysis vs hemodialysis. JAMA. 2004;291(6):697–703.
81. Weisbord SD, Mor MK, Sevick MA, Shields AM, Rollman BL, Palevsky PM, Arnold RM, Green JA, Fine MJ. Associations of depressive symptoms and pain with dialysis adherence, health resource utilization, and mortality in patients receiving chronic hemodialysis. Clin J Am Soc Nephrol. 2014;9(9):1594–602.
82. Unruh ML, Larive B, Chertow GM, Eggers PW, Garg AX, Gassman J, Tarallo M, Finkelstein FO, Kimmel PL; FHN Trials Group. Effects of 6-times-weekly versus 3-times-weekly hemodialysis on depressive symptoms and self-reported mental health: Frequent Hemodialysis Network (FHN) trials. Am J Kidney Dis. 2013;61(5):748–58.
83. Belasco A, Barbosa D, Bettencourt AR, Diccini S, Sesso R. Quality of life of family caregivers of elderly patients on hemodialysis and peritoneal dialysis. Am J Kidney Dis. 2006;48(6):955–63.

84. Wu AW, Fink NE, Cagney KA, Bass EB, Rubin HR, Meyer KB, Sadler JH, Powe NR. Developing a health-related quality-of-life measure for end-stage renal disease: the CHOICE health experience questionnaire. Am J Kidney Dis. 2001;37(1):11–21.
85. Hays RD, Kallich JD, Mapes DL, et al. Kidney Disease Quality of Life Short Form (KDQOL-SF), version 1.3: a manual for use and scoring. 1997. http://www.rand.org/content/dam/rand/pubs/papers/2006/P7994.pdf. Accessed 16 Aug 2015.
86. Kosa SD, Bhola C, Lok CE. Measuring patient satisfaction with vascular access: vascular access questionnaire development and reliability testing. J Vasc Access. 2015;16(3):200–5.
87. Davison SN, Levin A, Moss AH, Jha V, Brown EA, Brennan F, Murtagh FE, Naicker S, Germain MJ, O'Donoghue DJ, Morton RL, Obrador GT. Executive summary of the KDIGO controversies conference on supportive Care in Chronic Kidney Disease: developing a roadmap to improving quality care. Kidney Int. 2015;88:457–9.
88. Tamura MK, Tan JC, O'Hare AM. Optimizing renal replacement therapy in older adults: a framework for making individualized decisions. Kidney Int. 2012;82(3):261–9.
89. Singh P, Germain MJ, Cohen L, Unruh M. The elderly patient on dialysis: geriatric considerations. Nephrol Dial Transplant. 2014;29(5):990–6.
90. O'Hare AM, Bowling CB, Tamura MK. Chapter 51. Kidney disease in the elderly. In: S. Gilbert, D.E. Weiner (Eds.), National Kidney Foundation primer on kidney diseases. 6th ed. Elsevier; 2014. Saunders

Ethical Considerations 10

Jun Xu and Daniel E. Hall

10.1 Case

An 83-year-old man was transferred to our tertiary care center after reporting to an urgent care center with new onset of back and abdominal pain. A noncontrast CT scan there confirmed a 10-cm juxtarenal abdominal aortic aneurysm with some stranding in the retroperitoneum, indicating a contained rupture. He has significant cardiovascular comorbidities including coronary artery disease that required a 3-vessel coronary artery bypass at age 50. On presentation, the patient is tachycardiac but otherwise stable. He appears to be in mild distress but is otherwise alert and oriented.

10.2 Introduction

This and other situations like it are all too common in vascular surgery. And they are difficult. The right and good course of action is not always clear on the face of facts because what might be good for one patient, might not be good for another patient in similar clinical circumstances. Moreover, such decision making is often caught up in a confusing interface of capacity, consent, and often misguided expectations in and around the end of life. How is a surgeon to navigate this terrain?

Clinical decisions are made through partnerships between physicians and patients. Whether we recognize it or not, each clinical decision includes an

J. Xu
Division of Vascular Surgery, University of Pittsburgh Medical Center, Pittsburgh, PA, USA

D.E. Hall (✉)
Division of General Surgery, University of Pittsburgh, Pittsburgh, PA, USA
e-mail: hallde@upmc.edu

R. Chaer (ed.), *Vascular Disease in Older Adults*,
DOI 10.1007/978-3-319-29285-4_10

ethical choice just to the extent that each decision aims at serving the patient's "good." What is ultimately the right thing to do therefore depends on how each patient and physician understand that "good." The right and good action must not only be informed by the scientific evidence but also take into account the patient's values and the surgeon's own clinical judgment. The following pages lay a foundation for a systemic approach to just this kind of ethically sensitive medical decision making.

10.3 Urgency

Depending on the urgency of the situation, the surgeon and patient may or may not be able to engage each other in every aspect of an ideal decision-making process. In fact, in absolute emergencies, surgeons are empowered to make decisions unilaterally (e.g., the trauma bay). This extraordinary power and responsibility is justified because it is reasonable to assume that most, though not all, patients would prefer to live than to die [1]. Preserving life in these circumstances may also permit patients to make their own choices after the urgency resolves. However, surgeons must exercise this power with extreme care, especially in circumstances where there may be doubt that preserving life is preferable to immanent death. Indeed, a growing literature demonstrates that elderly patients frequently fear invasive treatments and debilitation more than death. For example, one study of seriously ill patients ≥60 years of age found that 99% would agree to a low-burden treatment that was likely to restore current health, but if the treatment was associated with a significant chance of functional or cognitive impairment, 74–94% of patients reported that they would forgo the treatment, even if it meant they would not live as long [2]. The repair of ruptured aortic aneurysms is associated with just these kinds of impairments. Further, the SUPPORT trial demonstrated that many critically ill patients received more invasive treatment than they preferred (e.g., such as surgery) [3], and other research shows that patients often receive treatment that is inconsistent with their values and preferences [4, 5].

The patient in our vignette is hemodynamically stable, but there is a rupture and a decision must be made regarding the next steps. Extensive deliberation is a luxury that neither party can afford. However, there is probably more time to engage in shared decision making (SDM) than is often practiced. For example, the patient could probably wait for an hour or two and weigh his options or wait for the arrival of a trusted family member. But many patients like this will be ready to decide in minutes. Part of the surgeon's responsibility is to discern the time available to make a decision without significant impact on the range of options. If we wait too long, the optimal surgical treatment may no longer be possible. If we act too soon, we may not accurately discern the course of action most suited to the patient's values and goals. Finding the balance between these extremes requires the wisdom of experience.

10.4 Capacity

When time permits, ethical and legal standards require surgeons to involve patients in the decision-making process. To do so, patients need to have decision-making capacity. Capacity is a relatively fluid concept that describes a person's ability to make an informed decision.

In general, four elements are needed to determine capacity, and these are sometimes coupled with the criteria of informed consent: (1) patients must be able to express a choice, (2) understand the surrounding circumstances, (3) appreciate the nature and significance of the decision as well as be able to (4) reason from the understood and appreciated facts to a coherent decision [6–8]. The ability to express a choice is perhaps the least abstract of these criteria: if the patient expresses an opinion, he/she essentially has this capacity. Of course, it is possible to imagine scenarios where patients' understanding and appreciation and reasoning are all intact, yet have no way to express or communicate their informed, reasoned decision, but these instances are rare. Once the patient has expressed a preference for his/her care, the surgeon should then assess the patient's ability to understand the risks and benefits of the clinical options. For capacity to be clearly evident, the patient must go beyond mere comprehension in order to demonstrate an appreciation of what those risks and benefits mean to him/her. That is, patients must recognize that their own lives, values, and futures are at stake, and that the 10% chance of graft infection could *actually happen to them*. Finally, after understanding and appreciating the relevant facts, patients must take those facts and reason with them to choose a course of action that is recognizably coherent. When making a determination about capacity, the focus is not so much on the merits of the decision, but on the integrity of the process by which the decision was reached. Even though the surgeon may disagree with the Jehovah's Witness who chooses to eschew transfusion, that surgeon can recognize that the decision is coherent within the assumptions of the patient's worldview and the relevant facts of the case.

Finally, it is important to recognize that decision-making capacity is always contextual to the decision in question. Patients may be perfectly capacitated to choose clothing or menu items, but incapacitated to choose between open versus endovascular approaches to aortic rupture. Furthermore, during the course of medical treatment, capacity may wax and wane throughout the day or the week with changing orientation and episodic delirium. High-quality shared decision making demands that vascular surgeons attend carefully to patients' capacity to share in the decision making, aware that this capacity may change from patient to patient, and from hour to hour with the same patients.

An example of patient with impaired capacity might look like the following: Mr. Jones understands that his aorta is ruptured and that surgery entails risks of, among other things, renal failure, graft infection, and profound deconditioning requiring long-term rehabilitation in a nursing home, but in justifying his preference for surgery, he repeatedly states he "always beats the odds" and that "these things just won't happen to me." Furthermore, he states his belief that surgery will rapidly restore him to independent living at home. There may be compelling and justifiable reasons to proceed to the operating room, but at this juncture, Mr. Jones does not demonstrate capacity to make that decision by himself, and the surgeon would be wise to contact Mr. Jones' surrogate decision-maker.

10.5 Surrogate Decision-Making

If a patient demonstrates decision-making capacity, then the medical decisions rest with the patient, in consultation with the surgeon. When patients are incapacitated, medical decision falls into the hands of a surrogate. Some patients will formally document their choice for a healthcare power of attorney to serve this purpose. If none is designated, then there are state statutes that rank the applicable hierarchy of surrogates (e.g., spouse, adult child, parent, sibling, family member, and friend). If the statutorily defined surrogate is not available, pragmatic decisions can be made with the patient's family, domestic partner, or close friend. Surgeons should be careful to understand the precise hierarchy established by the state in which they practice. They should also recognize that not all powers of attorney are authorized to make healthcare decisions (e.g., financial powers of attorney). Before accepting the assertion of decision-making authority, careful questioning should clarify that the surrogate is actually the *healthcare* power of attorney.

Living wills and other so-called "advance directives" are another resource for surrogate decision-making, although they are often unavailable during medical emergencies. Generally, a living will is a document that conveys a patient's preferences for healthcare decisions in the event that the patient is incapacitated. It typically includes a list of permitted and/or forbidden technologies and treatments. Although technically precise, the challenge with living wills is interpreting the clinical context in which they should be enforced: Does Mr. Jones' instructions against dialysis apply to the current context of acute renal failure 4 days after cross clamping his aorta at the diaphragm? Living wills generally address only the broad context of end-of-life decisions. They cannot anticipate all the serious medical circumstances the person may face in the future where their preferences for life-sustaining technologies might change.

Further complicating the interpretation of advance directives is the fact that patient preferences can change with the passage of time. Living wills are often created long before serious decisions actually need to be made, so highly specific directions may not have been intended for new and unforeseen circumstances. And even if the living will was recently developed, the psychological phenomenon of "affective forecasting" demonstrates that human beings have only limited abilities to accurately predict future preferences before they actually experience the events that would make those preferences relevant [9]. The preferences recorded in living wills can and should inform clinical decisions, and it is often better to know those preferences than not, but living wills cannot replace good clinical judgment because the details of particular clinical contexts can raise legitimate doubts about the applicability of the living will. Therefore, it is our experience that living wills are most useful when interpreted not in isolation, but in cooperation with a responsible human surrogate who can help clinicians discern if and how the living will should apply.

Surrogates are asked to put their own interests aside and make decisions on behalf of the patient, based on their knowledge of the patient's values, in order to approximate the decision the patient would have made themselves. This emphasis is important to guard against conflicts of interest that lead surrogates to make decisions for personal gain rather than for the patient's interests. However, it is a challenging task to step into somebody else's shoes, and even with a responsible surrogate, substantial obstacles complicate the decision-making process. For example, although surrogates can be trained to predict the healthcare preferences of their loved ones with some accuracy [10], when left to themselves they do so only slightly better than a coin toss [11, 12]. And physicians do even worse than surrogates in predicting their patients' treatment preferences [13]. Thus, although patient preference is always a good place to begin, it is often impossible to know with certainty what patients themselves would choose, and thus surrogates (and physicians) frequently make decisions on their understanding of the patient's best interests. Due diligence is required so that surrogates and physicians do not simply do what is right in their own eyes, and consultation with the patient's primary care physician can often clarify this process. However, in settings such as ours, vascular surgeons are often left to gather the best available information about the patient's values and then discern the course best aligned with their limited understanding of those values.

10.6 Informed Consent

Once the parties sharing in the decision making are determined, the process of informed consent is engaged with either the patient or the surrogate. Informed consent is a relatively new concept for medicine, rising to prominence only in the 1970s. In previous generations, it was generally accepted that the physician's primary task was to inspire the confidence and trust to work in the best interest of the patient. Any disclosure of possible difficulties might erode that trust [14]. However, beginning in the early twentieth century, a series of lawsuits eventually established patients' rights to self-determination regarding medical treatments. One of the earliest precedents in *simple* consent was established in 1914 when a surgeon removed a tumor from the abdomen of a patient who had consented to only a diagnostic procedure. The judge ruled that the physician was liable for battery because he violated an "individual's fundamental right to decide what is being done with his or her body." [15] By the mid-twentieth century, increasing pressure emerged to *inform* patients about the proposed treatment before obtaining their consent. This pressure was partially a reaction against the perceived paternalism of physicians. Surgeons were first required to disclose what other surgeons typically disclosed about the procedure (e.g., the reasonable physician standard). In many jurisdictions, the requirement later shifted to disclosing what the typical patient would want to know (e.g., the reasonable patient standard), including risks, benefits and alternatives of the proposed treatment as well as the risks of not acting or postponing treatment [16].

Regardless of the applicable legal standard, the precise amount of information that needs to be disclosed remains controversial. Some studies suggest [17, 18] (and some courts demand [16]) that physicians disclose risks as rare as 1:14,000.

However, not only would this be impractical, but other studies consistently demonstrate that patients do not remember much of what is disclosed during informed consent [19–22], and that they often overestimate their comprehension [23–25]. Furthermore, there is strong evidence to suggest that patients have varying preferences for information quantity [17, 18, 26–30] and decision-making style [31] (e.g., active vs. deferential). Finally, there is other evidence to suggest that patients' do not always use the information to inform a deliberative decision-making process, opting instead for intuition, instinct [32–35], or a "leap of faith" into the surgeon's care [36, 37]. These and other similar data demonstrate that the ethical and legal ideal of informed consent is rarely, if ever, achieved in practice.

Although the ideal informed consent process is rarely achieved, many surgeons do engage informed consent with substantial effort [38], and those efforts clearly impact patient comprehension and decision making [39–41]. Some surgeons may fear that the legal standards for consent are unattainably high, but it is important to note that deficiencies of informed consent rarely constitute the primary focus of litigation, more often appearing as an adjunct to litigation resulting from bad outcomes. Indeed, legal advice on informed consent is pragmatic, recommending candid communication tailored to each patient's needs rather than to abstract and overly precise risk thresholds [42]. Well-documented, good-faith efforts to involve patients and their families in surgical decision making can satisfy relevant requirements without undue burden to busy clinicians [43].

10.7 Shared Decision Making (SDM)

Although informed consent remains a legal requirement, the concept of "shared decision making" is increasingly influential in both legal and ethical writing [44–46]. Consensus regarding the conceptual model for SDM is still emerging [47], though many elements are shared across the various existing models. For example, Godolfin describes eight elements of shared decision making that describes what the best surgeons have always sought to do (Table 10.1) [48]. The goal is neither to provide a mini-medical education nor to "Mirandize" patients against all possible perioperative risks in an attempt to divest the surgeon from moral responsibility for the decision. Rather, an open discussion describing facts relevant to the decision should be shared so that the patient can participate in the decision-making process. Furthermore, the physician should not shy away from a recommendation, even if it is to do nothing; this also necessitates that the rationale for the recommendation be shared with the patient. If the surgeon thinks that the patient has a significant chance of not surviving the surgery, then the conversation should discuss those risks candidly. The conversation can be framed in a way such that the patient's values are acknowledged in the context of realistic expectations. Such a discussion should empower the patient to take ownership of and share in the responsibility of that decision.

Robust shared decision making is often best achieved in the context of an ongoing relationship of mutual trust and respect. Such a relationship might exist even in the emergent context of our vignette if the surgeon had been managing the patient's

Table 10.1 Eight elements of shared decision making [48]

1. Develop a partnership with the patient.
2. Establish or review the patient's preferences for information.
3. Establish or review the patient's preferences for his or her role in decision-making and the existence and nature of any uncertainty about the course of action to take.
4. Ascertain and respond to the patient's ideas, concerns, and expectations.
5. Identify choices and evaluate the evidence in relation to the individual patient.
6. Present evidence, taking into account points 2 and 3, above, framing effects, and so on; help the patient to reflect upon and assess the impact of alternative decisions with regard to his or her values and lifestyles.
7. Make or negotiate a decision in partnership and resolve conflicts.
8. Agree upon an action plan and complete arrangements for follow up.

peripheral vascular disease while following the seemingly stable aneurysm over time. However, the absence of a long-term relationship does not preclude the possibility of building trust and respect quickly, and engaging an urgent, yet thorough, decision-making process. One technique that has been helpful to improve communication and patient comprehension of the shared decision is to systematically ask patients to "repeat back" their understanding of their prognosis, and what they have understood about the proposed surgical treatment [40, 49–52].

Both the quality and pace of the shared decision will improve when surgeons have a clear view of how decisions are actually shared, including the distinct roles played by both the surgeon and the patient. Surgeons bring to the decision their unique experience treating multiple patients with similar disease. This experience, accumulated through years of practice, endows the surgeon with what Aristotle called "practical wisdom" (Greek: *phronesis*), defined as the capacity to choose the best from among multiple imperfect options [53]. In the same way that a mason, by virtue of his/her long experience mixing mortar and stacking bricks, is uniquely suited to choose the best way to build a wall that stands straight and bears weight, so also, a surgeon, by virtue of his/her long experience caring for vascular disease, is uniquely suited to choose among the available surgical options.

However, practical wisdom does not exist in a vacuum: it can only be exercised toward a specific "goal" (Greek: *telos* from which English gets teleological). The wisdom of the mason's choice is confirmed by the wall standing straight and bearing weight. The wisdom of the surgeon's choice depends on how well it achieves the patient's goals, and thus it is impossible for surgeons to exercise their practical wisdom without first understanding what their patients want to achieve. This requires detailed and rich conversations with the patient: The patient shares his goals, and the surgeon shares his/her practical wisdom. Because they lack experience treating surgical disease, patients cannot have a surgeon's practical wisdom, and forcing them to choose between the multiple imperfect options is a form of moral abandonment against which many patients resist (e.g., "Why are you asking me to decide, doc? You're the one who went to medical school"). On the other hand, presuming to choose a plan of treatment without a rich understanding of the patient's goals is the kind of paternalistic tyranny against which the doctrine of informed consent was erected. Shared decision making requires that surgeons shoulder the moral responsibility of exercising their unique practical wisdom, but doing so also requires clarifying the patient's goals of care in ways that can frequently elude surgeons [54].

10.8 Establishing Goals of Care

For many surgeons, the goals of therapy are most often assumed: restore functional anatomy with minimal morbidity. The surgical literature focuses on survival, complication rates, and quality adjusted life years as the common goals of the profession. Those goals can and do influence surgeons' work. Indeed, they are some of the most important goals that patients hope surgeons can help them achieve. However, the exercise of practical wisdom requires richer, thicker, and deeper discussions that explore what it means for patients to not only live but also flourish. Patients want to keep living, but does flourishing include short (or long) term sustenance on ventilators or dialysis machines? Does flourishing require independence in the patients' own home, or are they open to long-term (or permanent) living in a nursing home? Practical wisdom requires asking patients what makes life worth living. It requires exploring fears, hopes, and dreams, and among the old and seriously ill, it requires asking what patients most want to accomplish with the limited life that remains. In our vignette, if the patient's greatest fear is an extended stay, unconscious in the ICU, the wise choice may direct the patient to hospice rather than the ICU. Likewise, for a frail patient who wants nothing more than to attend his granddaughter's wedding the next day, the wise choice might be to defer his carotid endarterectomy even as he is experiencing crescendo transient ischemic attacks.

Establishing the goals of care is often difficult and uncomfortable, especially among old and frail patients who are approaching the end of their lives. Surgeons have rarely received dedicated training in how to lead these discussions with skill and grace. And in practice environments that do not reward the time and effort spent on setting goals, it is not surprising that the goals of surgical care are frequently underdeveloped. However, the difficulty of establishing goals does not diminish its critical importance.

The skills for clarifying goals can be taught, either through self-directed learning or through interactive simulation [55, 56]. However, given the realities of modern surgical practice, busy surgeons may need help elucidating their patient's hopes, dreams, and goals for surgery. In such circumstances, palliative care consultation may be helpful not only to clarify goals but to ensure that appropriate advance directives are in place, including an identified surrogate. Indeed, there is emerging evidence that early palliative care consultation can improve both quality and quantity of life among those with advanced cancers [57, 58]. In fact, one study has demonstrated significantly increased survival among surgical patients when palliative care consultation is ordered by the surgeon before the operation [59]. All of this suggests that palliative care consultation may be a critical part of the preoperative workup and optimization of high-risk patients, especially when patients are elderly or frail. (See Chap. 2 for further discussion of preoperative workup and optimization of older patients with vascular disease.)

10.9 Intensity of Postoperative Care and Time-Limited Trials

Recovery from a ruptured aortic aneurysm is intense and fraught with complications. Studies repeatedly demonstrate that the risk of complication increases dramatically among the frail elderly [60–64]. As such, older patients considering major vascular surgery need to understand that postoperative complications are not only possible but likely and expected. Therefore, successful recovery from major vascular surgery depends largely on the patient's and surgeon's mutual commitment to treat reversible complications as they arise. Indeed, vascular surgeon Gretchen Schwarze has described how most high-risk surgeons consider the consent process to entail "buy-in" to the index operation *as well as any reasonable rescue therapy* that may be needed in the immediate postoperative period [65–67]. Unfortunately, the data also show that only a minority of surgeons negotiate this buy-in explicitly, and even when they do, patients often fail to understand what the surgeon intends [66]. This failure to communicate can lead to confusion and conflict in the postoperative period, especially when complications render patients temporarily incapacitated.

One helpful way to manage the intensity and duration of postoperative care involves the *explicit negotiation* and *documentation* of a time-limited trial [68]. Time-limited trials are agreements between patients and clinicians to use specific medical therapies over a specific time during which the patient's prognosis can clarify. If the patient is improving, aggressive support continues. If the patient's recovery stalls or deteriorates, support can be withdrawn.

Negotiating time-limited trials requires frank discussions about the expected range of rescue therapies that might be required, including: (1) protracted stays in the intensive care unit (ICU), (2) the need for extended mechanical ventilation and tracheostomy, (3) the chance of acute or chronic renal failure requiring temporary or permanent dialysis, (4) the likelihood of protracted rehabilitation in a nursing facility, (5) the possibility of short-term gastrostomy for nutrition, and (6) the possibility that the best case scenario might include long-term disability and dependence. In much the same way that patients delegate the choice of suture or scissor to surgeons acting as fiduciary agents [69], patients can delegate the choice of rescue therapies to the surgeon and ICU team *for a limited time* to exercise their best practical wisdom in achieving realistic and explicitly described goals for recovery. After the limited time, if the prognosis remains unclear, new decisions can be made to extend, limit, or withdraw support.

Patient's (or their surrogates) are always free to refuse specific therapies as they become necessary, but the principles of distributive justice can impose limited obligations on patients to do what is necessary for an operation to succeed after they have chosen to consume the substantial and limited resources required to complete the index operation. Indeed, part of the surgeon's responsibility is to encourage patients to endure sometimes burdensome therapy that is occasionally necessary to achieve the patient's overarching goals. This discernment requires practical wisdom, and it often requires time for the patient's particular prognosis to emerge.

Ideally, agreements about time-limited trials for postoperative therapy would be reached before the index operation and shared with not only the hospital team but the patient's family and identified surrogate. Early consultation with palliative care specialists can again facilitate this process. Careful planning before the operation can preempt much of the confusion and conflict that attends those patients who experience complication or protracted recovery. Even in instances where a shared decision-making process was inadequately engaged prior to the index operation, instituting a time-limited trial is still useful in negotiating the intensity of treatment postoperatively in circumstances where unanticipated complications put the near and long-term prognosis in doubt. In these cases, negotiating a time-limited trial can afford time for a clearer prognosis to emerge.

10.10 Withdrawal of Support

Not all surgeries go according to plan, and when surgeons operate on elderly patients, some of them will die. Although such deaths are always sobering, they are not necessarily failures because death can be a calculated risk to achieve concrete and mutually agreed benefits. Sometimes the risks are so high that there is no reasonable chance of benefit, and surgeons have always sought to identify these patients preoperatively, steering them to more appropriate, nonoperative management. Unfortunately, traditional strategies for risk stratification systematically underestimate mortality and morbidity in high-risk populations [61, 70–73] and psychological dynamics tend toward a "Lake Wobegon effect" [74, 75] where every patient (and surgeon) is above average. However, an increasing array of powerful risk-prediction models are now available to assist patients and surgeons with patient- and procedure-specific risk profiles that can inform both decisions for or against operative management, as well as strategies for perioperative optimization when surgery is indicated [76, 77].

Although preoperative risk stratification may decrease the frequency of perioperative death among older patients, it will not eliminate it. In these circumstances, withdrawal of care may be indicated. The technical aspects of withdrawal are straight forward and can be managed by the surgeon or ICU team without difficulty, but the decision to act can be challenging. Surgeons develop emotional commitments to patients that sometimes delay recognizing that our best efforts will not help the patient to flourish. Attending to these emotions demands disciplined self-reflection that leads to realistic self-knowledge.

Even when the surgeon recognizes that the time has come to withdraw, it is often difficult to convey the reasons for this decision to the patient, their family, and other members of the healthcare team. Again, skills for communicating bad news can be learned [55, 56], and palliative care specialists can be helpful in this regard. But in the end, the surgeon cannot delegate this critical task because prudent discernment regarding withdrawal depends on the practical wisdom garnered specifically from the experience of practicing vascular surgery. Shouldering this responsibility is one of the greatest privileges and prerogatives of surgical practice, and when done in collaboration with the patient, family, and other medical colleagues, it can also be profoundly rewarding.

10.11 Conclusions

Returning to our case, after evaluating our patient with a ruptured aortic aneurysm, we explained that his condition was likely lethal without an operation, but that the operation itself might very well cause more problems than it solves due to his high risk for postoperative complications. We spent some time asking about the patient's hopes and fears in the twilight of his life.

His initial inclination was to choose surgical therapy, but he first wanted to discuss the matter with his daughter who lived nearby and was currently on her way to the hospital. We waited close to an hour for them to arrive while we completed the ACS NSQIP risk calculator for the proposed procedure in this patient.

By the time the family had arrived, our palliative care colleague had joined us by the patient's bedside where we spent nearly 20 min clarifying the patient's goals, and signing papers making the daughter his official healthcare power of attorney. He had reconciled himself to growing dependence on nursing care, but still found delight in the daily paper, his extensive collection of swing-era jazz, and regular visits from his daughter and grandchildren. His greatest fears were permanent cognitive impairment and dependence on mechanical ventilation. In hopes of restoring him to Duke Ellington and his granddaughters, we negotiated a 21-day time-limited trial beginning with an open repair of his aneurysm. However, we explained that his age and frailty put him at high risk for a number of complications, including death.

Following aortic repair, he seemed to do well initially, but a pulmonary embolus led to protracted ventilation further complicated by pneumonia and sepsis. After 10 days of IV antibiotics, bedside dialysis, and the ICU team's full court press, he started to stabilize and was eventually extubated. However, on postoperative day 15, he suffered a massive stroke that again required intubation to protect his airway. Although still within the negotiated time-limited trial, the stroke eliminated any realistic chance of achieving the patient's overarching goals, so together with the palliative care physician, the patient's surgeon, and daughter decided to withdraw support. The patient died shortly thereafter surrounded by his daughter, grandchildren, and the local parish priest. Although the team was not able to restore the patient to health, the care rendered and the decisions made were nonetheless a model of excellence.

Key Points

- *Ethical Practice Strives for "The Good."* All clinical decisions have ethical content – even if there is no dilemma – because all clinical decisions are directed toward the patient's good. The challenge is to discern the right and good clinical choice in the context of each patient's unique values.

- *Emergencies*: In clinical emergencies when patients cannot speak for themselves, vascular surgeons are empowered to make decisions on behalf of their patient based on the surgeon's good-faith understanding of the patient's good. This power is a heavy responsibility that should be exercised with extreme care, informed by growing data that older patients often receive more invasive and aggressive care than they would have wanted had they been able to speak for themselves.
- *Decision-Making Capacity*: When the patient is able to express an opinion, the vascular surgeon is tasked with assessing the patient's capacity to make the decision at hand. Capacitated patients (1) understand the surrounding circumstances, (2) appreciate that the risks, benefits, and alternatives apply to them, and (3) reason with the information they understand and appreciate to (4) express their preferred course of action.
- *Surrogate Decision-Making*: If a patient does not have capacity, advice from surrogate decision-maker (e.g., healthcare power of attorney) is sought. Surrogates are likely better informed than surgeons about patient values, but they are often inaccurate in predicting what patients would want if they could speak for themselves. It is appropriate to ask surrogates to explain why they think their choices serve the patient's good.
- *Shared Decision Making* combines the surgeon's clinical judgment with patient's values and goals. It recognizes that the surgeon's practical wisdom of experience (*phronesis*) uniquely positions him/her to recommend the option most likely to achieve a specific goal; and that the patient is uniquely positioned to establish the goals for surgical treatment.
- *Goals of Care* guide shared decision making, and they are most effective when they move beyond mere mortality and morbidity to describe in textured ways what it means for patients to flourish and how the proposed surgical treatment can serve that flourishing. Establishing the goals of care starts with the first clinical encounter, and in complex situations, palliative care consultants are often helpful in assessing patient goals. However, ongoing conversations between surgeon, patient, and surrogates are needed to reassess how goals and values change with clinical context. If the right and good choice of action is elusive, time is often best spent elucidating better understanding the goals of care.
- *Time-Limited Trials* are pragmatic tools for discerning the patient's good. In circumstances of diagnostic or therapeutic uncertainty, patients and surgeons can agree to pursue a specific course of action (e.g., initial surgery and 2 weeks of postoperative care) with a plan to reassess the likelihood of achieving the patient's goals at the end of the trial period. If the patient's goals are still achievable, a new trial can be established, but if the stated goals are no longer realistic, the best course of action may require withdrawal of support. Even though such patients do not survive, prudent withdrawal can nonetheless be a model of clinical excellence.

References

1. Mattox K, Engelhardt H. Emergency patients: serious moral choices with limited time, infomraitn and patient participation. In: McCullough LB, Jones JW, Brody BA, editors. Surgical ethics. New York: Oxford University Press; 1998. p. 78–96.
2. Fried TR, Bradley EH, Towle VR, Allore H. Understanding the treatment preferences of seriously ill patients. N Engl J Med. 2002;346(14):1061–6.
3. The SUPPORT Principal Investigators. A controlled trial to improve care for seriously ill hospitalized patients: the study to understand prognoses and preferences for outcomes and risks of treatments (SUPPORT). JAMA. 1995;274:1591–8.
4. Murphy DJ, Burrows D, Santilli S, et al. The influence of the probability of survival on patients' preferences regarding cardiopulmonary resuscitation. N Engl J Med. 1994;330(8):545–9.
5. Weeks JC, Cook EF, O'Day SJ, et al. Relationship between cancer patients' predictions of prognosis and their treatment preferences. JAMA. 1998;279(21):1709–14.
6. Wicclair M. Patient decision-making capacity and risk. Bioethics. 1991;5(2):91–104.
7. Christensen K, Haroun A, Schneiderman LJ, Jeste DV. Decision-making capacity for informed consent in the older population. Bull Am Acad Psychiatr Law. 1995;23(3):353–65.
8. Moye J, Marson DC. Assessment of decision-making capacity in older adults: an emerging area of practice and research. J Gerontol Ser B Psychol Sci Soc Sci. 2007;62(1):P3–11.
9. Gilbert DT, Wilson TD. Miswanting: some problems in the forecasting of future affective states. In: Forgas JP, editor. Feeling and thinking: the role of affect in social cognition. New York: Cambridge University Press; 2000.
10. Kirchhoff KT, Hammes BJ, Kehl KA, Briggs LA, Brown RL. Effect of a disease-specific planning intervention on surrogate understanding of patient goals for future medical treatment. J Am Geriatr Soc. 2010;58(7):1233–40.
11. Shalowitz DI, Garrett-Mayer E, Wendler D. The accuracy of surrogate decision makers: a systematic review. Arch Intern Med. 2006;166(5):493–7.
12. Sulmasy DP, Terry PB, Weisman CS, et al. The accuracy of substituted judgments in patients with terminal diagnoses. Ann Intern Med. 1998;128(8):621–9.
13. Fischer GS, Tulsky JA, Rose MR, Siminoff LA, Arnold RM. Patient knowledge and physician predictions of treatment preferences after discussion of advance directives. J Gen Intern Med. 1998;13(7):447–54.
14. Carter SM, Entwistle VA, Little M. Relational conceptions of paternalism: a way to rebut nanny-state accusations and evaluate public health interventions. Public Health. 2015;129(8):1021–9.
15. Schloendorff v. Society of New York Hospital. Vol 211 N.Y. 125, 105 N.E. 921914.
16. Leclercq WK, Keulers BJ, Scheltinga MR, Spauwen PH, van der Wilt GJ. A review of surgical informed consent: past, present, and future. A quest to help patients make better decisions. World J Surg. 2010;34(7):1406–15.
17. Courtney MJ. Information about surgery: what does the public want to know? ANZ J Surg. 2001;71:24–6.
18. Sulmasy DP, Lehmann LS, Levine DM, Faden RR. Patients' perceptions of the quality of informed consent for common medical procedures. J Clin Ethics. 1994;5(3):189–94.
19. Lloyd A, Hayes P, Bell P, Naylor AR. The role of risk and benefit perception in informed consent for surgery. Med Decis Making. 2001;21(2):141–9.
20. Leeb D, Bowers Jr DG, Lynch JB. Observations on the myth of "informed consent". Plast Reconstr Surg. 1976;58(3):280–2.
21. Lavelle-Jones C, Byrne DJ, Rice P, Cuschieri A. Factors affecting quality of informed consent. BMJ. 1993;306(6882):885–90.
22. Hutson MM, Blaha JD. Patients' recall of preoperative instruction for informed consent for an operation. J Bone Joint Surg Am. 1991;73(2):160–2.
23. Lashley M, Talley W, Lands LC, Keyserlingk EW. Informed proxy consent: communication between pediatric surgeons and surrogates about surgery. Pediatrics. 2000;105(3 Pt 1):591–7.
24. Tait AR, Voepel-Lewis T, Malviya S. Do they understand? (part II): assent of children participating in clinical anesthesia and surgery research. Anesthesiology. 2003;98(3):609–14.

25. Tait AR, Voepel-Lewis T, Malviya S. Do they understand? (part I): parental consent for children participating in clinical anesthesia and surgery research. Anesthesiology. 2003;98(3):603–8.
26. Dawes PJ, O'Keefe L, Adcock S. Informed consent: using a structured interview changes patients' attitudes towards informed consent. J Laryngol Otol. 1993;107(9):775–9.
27. Newton-Howes PAG, Dobbs B, Frizelle F. Informed consent: what do patients want to know? N Z Med J. 1998;111:340–2.
28. Bowden MT, Church CA, Chiu AG, Vaughan WC. Informed consent in functional endoscopic sinus surgery: the patient's perspective. Otolaryngol Head Neck Surg. 2004;131(1):126–32.
29. Chan EC, Sulmasy DP. What should men know about prostate-specific antigen screening before giving informed consent? Am J Med. 1998;105(4):266–74.
30. Wisselo TL, Stuart C, Muris P. Providing parents with information before anaesthesia: what do they really want to know? Paediatr Anaesth. 2004;14(4):299–307.
31. Degner LF, Sloan JA. Decision making during serious illness: what role do patients really want to play? J Clin Epidemiol. 1992;45(9):941–50.
32. Schneider CE. The practice of autonomy: patients, doctors, and medical decisions. New York: Oxford University Press; 1998.
33. Simmons RG, Marine SK, Simmons RL. Gift of life: the effect of organ transplantation on individual, family and societal dynamics. New Brunswick: Transaction Books; 1987.
34. Pierce PF. Deciding on breast cancer treatment: a description of decision behavior. Nurs Res. 1993;42(1):22–8.
35. Nisbett R, Ross L. Human inference: strategies and shortcoming of social judgment. Englewood Cliffs: Prentice-Hall; 1980.
36. McKneally MF, Ignagni E, Martin DK, D'Cruz J. The leap to trust: perspective of cholecystectomy patients on informed decision making and consent. J Am Coll Surg. 2004;199(1):51–7.
37. McKneally MF, Martin DK. An entrustment model of consent for surgical treatment of life-threatening illness: perspective of patients requiring esophagectomy. J Thorac Cardiovasc Surg. 2000;120(2):264–9.
38. Hall DE, Hanusa BH, Fine MJ, Arnold RM. Do surgeons and patients discuss what they document on consent forms? J Surg Res. 2015;197(1):67–77.
39. Fink AS, Prochazka AV, Henderson WG, et al. Predictors of comprehension during surgical informed consent. J Am Coll Surg. 2010;210(6):919–26.
40. Fink AS, Prochazka AV, Henderson WG, et al. Enhancement of surgical informed consent by addition of repeat back: a multicenter, randomized controlled clinical trial. Ann Surg. 2010;252(1):27–36.
41. Hall DE, Hanusa BH, Switzer GE, Fine MJ, Arnold RM. The impact of iMedConsent on patient decision-making regarding cholecystectomy and inguinal herniorrhaphy. J Surg Res. 2011;175(2):227–33.
42. Rozovsky FA. The need for adequate disclosure. In: Rosovsky FA, editor. Consent to treatment: a practical guide. New York: Wolters Kluwer; 2008:§1.02.
43. Hall DE, Prochazka AV, Fink AS. Informed consent for clinical treatment. CMAJ. 2012;184(5):533–40.
44. Gattellari M, Butow PN, Tattersall MH. Sharing decisions in cancer care. Soc Sci Med. 2001;52(12):1865–78.
45. Elwyn G, Edwards A, Gwyn R, Grol R. Towards a feasible model for shared decision making: focus group study with general practice registrars. BMJ. 1999;319(7212):753–6.
46. Towle A, Godolphin W. Framework for teaching and learning informed shared decision making. BMJ. 1999;319(7212):766–71.
47. Makoul G, Clayman ML. An integrative model of shared decision making in medical encounters. Patient Educ Couns. 2006;60(3):301–12.
48. Godolphin W. Shared decision-making. Healthc Q. 2009;12(Spec No Patient):e186–90.
49. Wick JY. Checking for comprehension: mastering teach-back techniques. Consult Pharm. 2013;28(9):550–4.
50. Kripalani S, Bengtzen R, Henderson LE, Jacobson TA. Clinical research in low-literacy populations: using teach-back to assess comprehension of informed consent and privacy information. IRB. 2008;30(2):13–9.

51. Wilson FL, Baker LM, Nordstrom CK, Legwand C. Using the teach-back and Orem's self-care deficit nursing theory to increase childhood immunization communication among low-income mothers. Issues Compr Pediatr Nurs. 2008;31(1):7–22.
52. Flowers L. Teach-back improves informed consent. OR Manager. 2006;22(3):25–6.
53. Aristotle. Nichomachean ethics, Book VI. In: Ackrill J, editor. A new Aristotle reader. Princeton: Princeton University Press; 1987. p. 416–31.
54. Hall DE. The guild of surgeons as a tradition of moral enquiry. J Med Philos. 2011;36(2): 114–32.
55. Back A, Arnold R, Tulsky J. Mastering communication with seriously ill patients: balancing honesty with hope. New York: Cambridge University Press; 2009.
56. Vital Talk. www.vitaltalk.org. http://www.vitaltalk.org. Accessed 11 Aug 2015.
57. Temel JS, Greer JA, Muzikansky A, et al. Early palliative care for patients with metastatic non-small-cell lung cancer. N Engl J Med. 2010;363(8):733–42.
58. Bakitas MA, Tosteson TD, Li Z, et al. Early versus delayed initiation of concurrent palliative oncology care: patient outcomes in the ENABLE III randomized controlled trial. J Clin Oncol. 2015;33(13):1438–45.
59. Ernst KF, Hall DE, Schmid KK, et al. Surgical palliative care consultations over time in relationship to systemwide frailty screening. JAMA Surg. 2014;149(11):1121–6.
60. Adams P, Ghanem T, Stachler R, Hall F, Velanovich V, Rubinfeld I. Frailty as a predictor of morbidity and mortality in inpatient head and neck surgery. JAMA Otolaryngol Head Neck Surg. 2013;139(8):783–9.
61. Makary MA, Segev DL, Pronovost PJ, et al. Frailty as a predictor of surgical outcomes in older patients. J Am Coll Surg. 2010;210(6):901–8.
62. McAdams-DeMarco MA, Law A, Salter ML, et al. Frailty and early hospital readmission after kidney transplantation. Am J Transplant. 2013;13(8):2091–5.
63. Robinson TN, Wu DS, Pointer L, Dunn CL, Cleveland Jr JC, Moss M. Simple frailty score predicts postoperative complications across surgical specialties. Am J Surg. 2013;206(4):544–50.
64. Dwyer JG, Reynoso JF, Seevers GA, et al. Assessing preoperative frailty utilizing validated geriatric mortality calculators and their association with postoperative hip fracture mortality risk. Geriatr Orthop Surg Rehabil. 2014;5(3):109–15.
65. Schwarze ML, Bradley CT, Brasel KJ. Surgical "buy-in": the contractual relationship between surgeons and patients that influences decisions regarding life-supporting therapy. Crit Care Med. 2010;38(3):843–8.
66. Schwarze ML, Redmann AJ, Alexander GC, Brasel KJ. Surgeons expect patients to buy-in to postoperative life support preoperatively: results of a national survey. Crit Care Med. 2013;41(1):1–8.
67. Pecanac KE, Kehler JM, Brasel KJ, et al. It's big surgery: preoperative expressions of risk, responsibility, and commitment to treatment after high-risk operations. Ann Surg. 2014;259(3):458–63.
68. Quill TE, Holloway R. Time-limited trials near the end of life. JAMA. 2011;306(13):1483–4.
69. Joffe S, Truog R. Consent to medical care: the importance of fiduciary context. In: Miller F, Wertheimer A, editors. The ethics of conent: theory and practice. New York: Oxford; 2010. p. 347–73.
70. Anaya DA, Becker NS, Abraham NS. Global graying, colorectal cancer and liver metastasis: new implications for surgical management. Crit Rev Oncol Hematol. 2011;77(2):100–8.
71. Gross CP, McAvay GJ, Krumholz HM, Paltiel AD, Bhasin D, Tinetti ME. The effect of age and chronic illness on life expectancy after a diagnosis of colorectal cancer: implications for screening. Ann Intern Med. 2006;145(9):646–53.
72. Colorectal Cancer Collaborative Group. Surgery for colorectal cancer in elderly patients: a systematic review. Lancet. 2000;356(9234):968–74.
73. Fried LP, Tangen CM, Walston J, et al. Frailty in older adults: evidence for a phenotype. J Gerontol A Biol Sci Med Sci. 2001;56(3):M146–56.
74. Smith TJ. Commentary: "the Lake Wobegon effect, a natural human tendency to overestimate one's capabilities" (Wikipedia). Milbank Q. 2013;91(4):729–37.

75. Wolf JH, Wolf KS. The Lake Wobegon effect: are all cancer patients above average? Milbank Q. 2013;91(4):690–728.
76. Anaya DA, Johanning J, Spector SA, et al. Summary of the panel session at the 38th annual surgical symposium of the association of VA surgeons: what is the big deal about frailty? JAMA Surg. 2014;149(11):1191–7.
77. Bilimoria KY, Liu Y, Paruch JL, et al. Development and evaluation of the universal ACS NSQIP surgical risk calculator: a decision aid and informed consent tool for patients and surgeons. J Am Coll Surg. 2013;217(5):833–42, e831–3.

Index

R. Chaer (ed.), *Vascular Disease in Older Adults*,
DOI 10.1007/978-3-319-29285-4

MIX
Papier aus verantwortungsvollen Quellen
Paper from responsible sources
FSC® C105338

If you have any concerns about our products,
you can contact us on
ProductSafety@springernature.com

In case Publisher is established outside the EU,
the EU authorized representative is:
Springer Nature Customer Service Center GmbH
Europaplatz 3, 69115 Heidelberg, Germany

Printed by Libri Plureos GmbH
in Hamburg, Germany